AM NO' READY FOR THAT

by
Pauline Kennedy

Published by New Generation Publishing in 2023

Copyright © Pauline Kennedy 2023

First Edition

The author asserts the moral right under the Copyright, Designs and Patents Act 1988 to be identified as the author of this work.

All Rights reserved. No part of this publication may be reproduced, stored in a retrieval system or transmitted, in any form or by any means without the prior consent of the author, nor be otherwise circulated in any form of binding or cover other than that which it is published and without a similar condition being imposed on the subsequent purchaser.

ISBN: 978-1-80369-701-7

www.newgeneration-publishing.com
New Generation Publishing

For David.
Simply the best.
Gone but never forgotten.

Introduction

Early August 2017.

I think logically, possess the ability to carve through inane bullshit and problem solve using nothing more than absolute facts. Humour and sarcasm are also thrown in for good measure. I'd like to believe my mother considered these worthy attributes when she asked if I could take her to the hospital, but the fact I had a driving licence, owned a car, and happened to be on annual leave from work, were probably considered more desirable and realistic qualities for this scenario.

To anyone that knows me, it's common knowledge that I have an aversion to hospitals. Never had an overnight stay in one (touch wood) but witnessed a few nightmare-inducing events as a visitor. Sure, I would slip on my 'big girl pants', take one for the team and go along for moral support on this day. Mum fully expected me to bitch and whine about it for the entire duration. I didn't disappoint.

The consultant's words were clipped and sharp. Business-like and why wouldn't they be? I was grateful he was rushing over the details; the busy waiting room we'd just left already had my eyelid twitching. This appointment was merely confirming our suspicions, but the reality check was evident.

My mother (also known as mum, maw, ma and Jan**) never said a word. She didn't have to. Like some unorthodox sign language, a simple glance down at her worsening hand tremor firmly established the diagnosis hadn't gone down well.

"Mrs Kennedy, you have Parkinson's disease."

** For the purposes of the following story, whenever my mother is referred to by her first name, Jan – at that very moment in time, she's being a dick….

Chapter 1 – Harsh Reality

The silence in the consultant's office was deafening, and the awkwardness mildly uncomfortable. Incidentally, I use the term 'office' loosely. If someone had told me it was a janitor's storage cupboard, emptied for today's clinic, I wouldn't have been surprised. The disinfectant smell was overwhelming and suggested the room had been cleaned recently. A thin layer of dust covering the desk told another story.

Armed with my internet-based knowledge, I immediately stormed in with a series of rapid-fire questions. The consultant raised his arms slowly in a makeshift sign of surrender and with the upmost professionalism, spurred himself into verbal action.

"Please understand, Parkinson's disease is not a death sentence and with proper medication it can, and will, be managed," he declared flatly.

"The tremor is apparent in your right hand for the moment, the left appears to be ok. Since Parkinson's disease affects everyone differently, I would advise against internet searches but obviously that's for you to decide."

Too late buddy. That horse had already bolted. When my mum first noticed the hand tremor, and before she underwent a series of neurology tests, I was all over the Google action (other internet search engines are available). My logical brain demanded facts and I felt obliged to feed it, like a decent cocaine dealer would.

It started out as a simple internet search but fast became a rabbit hole from hell, and pretty much every available link featured Parkinson's disease quite heavily.

'Parkinson's disease is a brain disorder that leads to shaking, stiffness and difficulty with walking, balance and co-ordination. Parkinson's symptoms usually begin gradually and get worse over time. As the disease progresses, people may have difficulty walking and talking'.

I'd mentally declared this paragraph 'vague as fuck' and five minutes later, found myself on the Shaky Hand Syndrome page.

I can confirm, it's a thing. Who knew? Perhaps I was searching for a more benign hand tremor explanation or just looking for a light at the end of this grisly web search tunnel but deep down, my gut declared it was Parkinson's disease forty-eight web pages ago.

Mr Consultant and his 'PHD' were finally agreeing with my intuition and link clicking prowess. We were quickly bundled out of the custodian's hideaway – appointment duly over.

* * * * * * *

"You're in some company now mother!" It was a veiled attempt at lifting the sombre mood in the car.

"What do you mean?"

"Well… the only people I know that have Parkinson's disease are famous."

"And what's your point?"

"Woman please! Your dinner party invites are about to get epic!"

A wee smile creased my mum's face and she chuckled. I silently thanked Google and turned the music up. Job done.

Chapter 2 – Now that's a dinner party

Muhammad Ali (boxer), Alan Alda (actor), Neil Diamond (singer/song writer), Ozzy Osbourne (singer), Billy Connolly (comedian/actor/author/legend) and Michael J. Fox (actor) to name but a few. All recognisable people, in their varying fields of excellence, but each of them tethered to Parkinson's disease.

You'll notice the distinct lack of female attendees at this hypothetical dinner party. Recent studies suggest that Parkinson's seems to occur more commonly in men than women. In fact, the risk of developing PD is twice as high in men. It's the second most common, age-related neurodegenerative disorder, affecting about 3% of the population by the age of 65 and up to 5% of people over 85 years. Far higher statistics than I ever imagined them to be. For the enquiring minds among us – Alzheimer's takes the number one slot.

Let's face it, you wouldn't mind any of the aforementioned *turning up at your door wi' a fish supper*, but this story isn't about anyone with celebrity status. If she's famous for anything, it's for being 'the wee wumin wi' the white hair'.

Way back in the 1980s, when Marty McFly was trying to get Back to the Future in a DeLorean, information wasn't readily available and there was no real internet to speak of. Even in the early nineties, and certainly by today's standards, the information superhighway was still worse than useless.

So, if your grandad's left hand started shaking in 1983 and you overheard Parkinson's in a hushed conversation, you were dusting off the library card and making for the infectious disease books, believing your dad's da' wasn't long for this world. The ignorance back then was very much real. It's not infectious, let's just clarify that. Hugs will always be welcomed.

Scottish slang – A person who arrives at your abode, unannounced, with take-away food.

I wholeheartedly admit that, for the best part of this decade, hairspray was considered a life necessity and if you didn't own a ZX Spectrum, Star Wars merch or a pair of roller skates, your street cred was in tatters. Sounds incredibly naïve but we were afforded the luxury of just being kids.

At varying stages throughout this story, I will impart my meagre PD knowledge gradually. Trust me, it's much easier to digest in small batches. Restaurants don't bring all three courses to your table at once and say, "You've twenty minutes to get this lot down you. Go!"

Parkinson's has been kicking around since the early 1800s. Described then as a 'shaking palsy' by English physician James Parkinson. Typically, there's five stages of the disease and I won't question anyone's intelligence but for the record, stage five is… not entirely pleasant.

When PD slowly creeps into your life and touches your world, that's when the awareness kicks in. Prior to that moment, it's not really a go-to genre of reading material when you've unwrapped a lunchtime cheese sandwich and have a half hour to kill, is it? "Oh, I'll just launch a new internet tab and find out what this Parkinson's is all about," said people on a work break. Never.

I did exactly that but only when the hand tremor first became apparent. I remember chowing down on the cheese deliciousness and reading an interview Billy Connolly gave when he was first diagnosed. One line in particular made me laugh, feel empathy and true admiration for the man all at once. "I've got Parkinson's disease. I wish he'd fucking kept it."

My mum, to this day, has never googled the disease and I applaud her for that. Her internet skills are basic at best, and she wouldn't trust her shaky mouse hand with an intrusive pop up either. She did, however, successfully manage to order four air fryers from Amazon because, "The 'buy now' button wouldn't go away." Returning the other three was an absolute pain in the arse.

Our understanding and acceptance of Parkinson's continues daily. It has to, we've little to no choice. We learn something new every day; we accept it, and we deal with it as a family unit.

Humour and laughter have always been our emotional medicine. Some of it politically incorrect. Occasional piss take may be thrown in. It's not considered the 'normal' course of action, and some of the dialogue contained therein may appear harsh but it's our coping mechanism. If you didn't laugh, you'd cry. Personally, I much prefer to see a smile on ma wee maw's face, rather than a tear in her eye.

Chapter 3 – The Crew

Now for some background information. Bear with me please. I'll get you through this section quicker than a good flight attendant working an airplane that's landing in twenty-eight minutes and a trolley load of peanuts to dish out.

In fact, that very thing happened to me on a flight from Manchester to Edinburgh. If I hadn't leaned forward to grab the bag under my seat, I swear those peanuts would've hit me square in the face. She had a good, technical throwing arm. Maybe an Olympian working a day job to supplement her income. The 'benefits' of turning right when you board an airplane. I'm willing to bet there's no business or first-class passenger that has ever been assaulted with a snack bag of any description.

Chapter three is in true recognition of family members and their continuing support.

Roadie JACKIE

Oldest sister. First born and all-round good egg. Like me, she has no filter and I love her dearly for it. There's literally no point in being anything other than yourself throughout life. The alternative is too exhausting. What you see is what you get.

I'm not an avid fan of astrology or concerned about planet alignment. If Jupiter suddenly disappeared down a black hole, I wouldn't be throwing myself forward as a volunteer in the search to find it. Horoscopes, in my opinion, are written by people with too much time on their hands and pent-up angst to get off their chest. Call me cynical.

But I will concede to some mysterious anomalies when it comes to my oldest sister and me. We are separated by exactly five years. Jackie arrived ten days early, whilst I was born the same number of days late. Both times, my mother missed her favourite television series, Crossroads, because there's literally fifteen minutes between my birth time and Jackie's. You think

I'm making this up, right? Either our parents were on some weird exacting sex schedule, or the planets and stars did, indeed, align.

When mother brought me home from the hospital and attempted to pass me off as Jackie's fifth birthday present (the household budget was tight), my loving sister scoffed and flat out announced:

"I want a toy car."

If you're asking Jackie for an opinion, watch out. It will be delivered with the utmost transparency, whether you're ready for it or not. There's no grey area. Diplomacy scale – she's a staunch three. Don't get me wrong. She has diplomacy in her repertoire, she just chooses not to use it.

Roadie LORRAINE

Second in line. The mediator and pragmatist. Sure, she'll draw her sword and enter the fray should you require back-up, but she'll need a minute to consider the available options.

Like a rose between two arseholes (Jackie and I), Lorraine has always been there to steady the ship. Hates confrontation of any sort. Very much prefers the conversational route to actual fisticuffs. Ex-journalist of course, so it's all about the facts and evidence. Could talk her way out of a twenty-five year stretch in jail if the 'opportunity' ever presented itself. Unlikely, now that she works for Police Scotland. She has two sons, Simon and Lewis. Simon has kids of his own now, but Lewis still hovers around granny's purse on the weekend visits.

On the diplomacy scale – our Lorraine is a definite eight but hold on a minute. On the outside she's all sweetness and light but there's an undeniable wicked streak. If you're lucky enough to have a sister, then I'm sure you have some cute anecdotes with reference to your time growing up. Doing each other's hair, borrowing clothes for nights out and having a best friend for life.

Let me tell you, these two have mentally scarred me for life. If you ask them both what it was like growing up together, they'll brandish statements like 'providing essential life skills' or 'toughening her up for the harsh realities of life'.

The following example is just one of many. Please bear in mind, I hate the dark – always have. A hallway light is my eternal friend. My siblings neither understand nor care about any of my fears. Let me tell you why.

I'm halfway up the stairs when the entire hall is plunged into darkness. Unbeknownst to me, my sisters have collected a large pile of soft toys as weaponry. I've instantly balled up into the foetal position, my bottom lip has begun to tremble, and I can feel the sting of tears. Something whistles past my ear. Launched with such purpose, the velocity is undisputable. Another 'missile' bounces off the top of my head. The onslaught is relentless. I can hear scuffles and giggling at the top of the stairs.

"Muuuuuuuuuuuuuuuuuuuuuummmmmmmmmmmmmm!!" It's a shriek of anguish, barely recognisable to my own ears.

Suddenly, the living room door flies opens and a trickle of light filters into the hallway. I am saved.

I can hear mum trying not to laugh as she chastises them both from the open doorway.

"Come on you two! Let your sister get up the stairs, and you better pick those toys up!"

What she failed to do was switch on the hallway light, thereby affording me a half chance at an actual getaway. The living room door closes, the darkness descends once more, and the siege continues. I was ten years old.

So, in conclusion, Lorraine might appear all Switzerland-like but in reality, she'd formulate an attack if she deemed it necessary or found it funny. A younger sister, shit scared of the dark? Well... she'd hit the mother lode.

Roadie BOB

The youngest sibling - living proof that both my father's testicles functioned normally. I'm sure that's how it works. If my brother hadn't arrived when he did, our family could've easily ended up like The Waltons. Clearly my parents were desperate for a son. My sisters and I, relegated to the bench and considered mere practice. The first couple of pancakes you make are always the shabby ones, right?

My brother was born in the back of an ambulance, in the mid-seventies, outside St John's Approved School, Edinburgh Road, Glasgow. Let me explain.

Mum's waters broke in the house and after trailing almost the entire contents of her womb down the tenement stairs, they finally made it to the ambulance. She'd been down this birth giving route three times already and felt it necessary to inform the paramedics 'it was coming'. I'm by no means an expert but perhaps they should've paid attention. She was clearly the most qualified in the 'room'.

I'm also fairly certain that if my brother had entered the world in a somewhat normal fashion (not the shit show that's unfurling here), he'd have been held aloft, high on a Scottish mountain with Elton John chanting in the background about circles and lives. No doubt in my mind, if the Lion King movie was released in 1974, we'd have a brother called Simba. Fact!

Paramedics David and Thomas finally made the decision to pull the speeding ambulance over and, between them both, they extracted the second coming of the Messiah. David and Thomas had their efforts endorsed on Bob's birth certificate (he's the only sibling with middle names). I do often wonder though, if paramedics Morag and Brenda had turned up that day instead of his namesakes, does the same deal apply? He'd have never made it through high school unscathed.

If that's not the purest definition of golden child, then I've no clue what is. Incidentally, that very same GC also stapled his own thumb when he was five and through incoherent sobs, demanded mum call an ambulance. Karma is a bitch.

On the diplomacy scale – Bob is mid table, maybe a five. He's the most laid-back, easy-going person I know, and his sense of humour is legendary. My brother is married to Donna and in 2017 their own ankle biter arrived, Ruby. Mum's middle name. No doubt a lovely tribute but also a silent nod towards the worship he received as a child, the potatoes he never peeled and the dishes he didn't need to wash.

And finally - Roadie ERIC

My partner-in-crime and best friend in life. The carrots to my peas. Has unlimited patience, and the ability to throw in perspective when no one else can see it. In short, he's my polar opposite. One of our many random conversations below explains all.

Me: Do you think it'd be bad if I said that my granny was a bit free with her lady parts – in the book I mean?"
Eric: Ehhh aye. How about... she enjoyed the company of gentlemen?"

Welcome to the support team. Avengers duly assembled.

Chapter 4 – Alice Bond

So, what family doesn't have a few skeletons rattling around in their historical closet? You dig deep enough, you'll find them. A great aunty, blushing January bride and then blessed with a baby in June of the same year? Or a second cousin twice removed, incarcerated for bank robbery?

It's 1946, World War II is firmly in the rear-view mirror and people are, understandably, a bit frazzled. Rationing is still in effect and the second cousin twice removed has obviously ran out of patience. It's also the year my granny (Alice) was 'getting busy' with an American soldier.

Demobilisation of the United States armed forces after WW2 continued through 1946. The US still had a substantial number of armed forces stationed abroad and getting them back home was taking a considerable amount of time. I believe the American public demanded more rapid action, and military personnel were eventually returned to the United States in Operation Magic Carpet. My granny was doing her bit for the war effort and merely keeping one of them entertained, at least.

There's no denying the mystery that surrounded my grandmother. Civil servant apparently, but no one remembers her ever working in an office or stressing about getting there on time. She was partial to a wee drink (functioning alcoholic), smoked four packs of cigarettes a day and even puffed the occasional cigar. She enjoyed the company of gentlemen (see what I did there?) and consistently had a bit of spare cash knocking around. Even by today's standard, she'd be described as fiercely independent.

Taking all this material on board, I've deduced she was British Secret Service. Code name Bond... Alice Bond.

Naturally, I'd like to think my mother was conceived in the throes of true love and unbridled passion. But applying my theory, it's likely that whenever the target (American soldier) was out of the room, Alice was actively rifling through his personal effects and reporting the findings back to HQ. I can see her now, at the bedroom window with her torch in the shape of a lipstick, ripping out morse code to another home-land operative in the building across the street.

Why would British Intelligence be interested in an American soldier? Listen… women were rioting over nylon stockings and men doing the same for pots of hair cream. I don't need to explain why my granny was all over an American like a cheap suit or have knowledge of the highly confidential assignment she had undertaken.

The 'mission' had obviously gone awry at some point, the pregnancy was a curve ball that no one expected. Least of all Alice. Plan B is discarded, not enough manpower. Plan C is dodgy but workable. She'd wait for a sign.

Waiting in line to board a ship bound for America, Alice Bond (now five months pregnant) buys a newspaper at the nearby stand and the vendor suggests that she check out the crossword on page seven. Her service training immediately kicks into action, and she quickly works out the answers to eleven across and nine down. She nods. Her inconspicuous acknowledgement barely visible as she presses her finger to her ear and lifts her sleeve to her lips. Copy that.

American soldier ends up boarding the ship alone. Alice has gone, with all her personal belongings in tow. He would never see her again.

OK, so I fudged the truth a little, call it artistic licence. From the 1930s to 1950s, my gran's living room rug must've been at least two inches thicker than its manufactured spec, such was the amount of bullshit swept underneath it. In those days, facts were side swerved with minimal effort, and indiscretions vanished like cigarette ash in the wind. What we do know was harvested from my great granny and only after my own mother had plied her with a brandy or two.

The American soldier part is genuine and so is my granny leaving him at the dock. Perhaps she had a change of heart, who knows. In my opinion, if you aren't willing to tell the absolute truth when confronted, then expect your granddaughter, some eighty years later, to fill in the blanks with a ludicrous tale. Or is it?

This message will self-destruct in five... four... three... two... Over and out.

Chapter 5 – Mum's the word

It's April 1947 and my mother slides into the world. First half of the covert operation complete. Alice pops open the Cuban cigar case and affords herself a moment of distinction. As the heavy blue-grey smoke fills the room, her carefully cultivated veneer of refinement is solidified once more. Getting the new family addition back home to Greenside Street in Glasgow, without anyone noticing, would be tricky.

When she turns into the cobbled street, it's clear the objective has failed. Batches of crudely positioned neighbours were now all vying for a glimpse of the new arrival. The word was out.

These complex neighbourhood watch counterintelligence measures often go un-noticed and underestimated: Mrs Walker's neighbour has a niece who works in the washhouse, and she was chatting to Jeanie McLaughan. Jeanie's man delivers milk to Doreen who used to date Archie, and his wife was telling Elsie that Alice was pregnant to some American soldier. Left him at the dock, apparently.

Alice could hear them all now,

"Tell ye, I seen the wean wi' ma ain eyes!"

There was never any malice intended. Neighbourhood gossip was a hot commodity and however you came by this precious material, was completely irrelevant. If you weren't fully submerged in someone else's business and using it as a distraction from your own family scandal, then you had no right to wear the apron or hang over a garden fence.

She shrugged her shoulders and rushed inside the house. British Secret Service clearly no match for the proverbial grapevine.

Scottish slang – it's true, I saw the child with my own eyes.

* * * * * * *

Life for Alice continues as normal. The men are still revolving like rotisserie chickens through her front door, and a child in this lifestyle? Undesirable, at best. Like a fly wearing tiny goggles and doing the backstroke in your crystal flute of Dom Perignon champagne.

Margaret (my great granny) found herself babysitting more often and at some point, my mother ended up staying with her permanently. Alice sent money every week to appease the gods of guilt and a couple of months later, parcels containing food and clothes started arriving from the US. For the first couple of months my mum was known, to the gossiping elite, as the best dressed kid on the street. My mother remembers being happy and that's all that mattered.

No judgement please. You may be sucking air through your teeth and shaking your head right about now, but situations like these weren't uncommon. I just happen to be airing the laundry and exorcising demons residing under the living room rug, using humour and a sprinkling of sarcasm.

* * * * * * *

My mother, now sixteen, found herself a job at Timothy Whites pharmacy – a poor man's Boots as she describes it. She'd done well at school, highly intelligent and shrewd by all accounts. The ever-present Margaret was influential in all of it.

However, boys had now become far more interesting and cold hard cash was a major requirement to get out there and mingle. The household biscuit tin also required a cash injection. The Alice payments were sure to dry up soon.

During the last five years, my mum noticed Peter getting robbed to pay Paul more often, and the entire family was considered expert at making a full house appear empty when the Provident man came looking for the weekly instalment. My mother was a full-on accomplice the day she could reach the light switch and throw herself under a windowsill in eight seconds flat.

It wasn't every week but there's no other occasion in her life where she felt more dread cowering under a window or more relief when she could no longer hear footsteps outside. It was an experience that would serve her well in later years.

* * * * * * *

Orange Order Lodge Dance, September 1965

My mum and her two friends were on one side of the dance floor, eyeing their male counterparts on the other.

"I fancy the one on the left," said my eighteen-year-old mother. Sandra declared she'd have the middle one, leaving the one on the right for Lydia, who was none too happy with the leftovers and voiced her disapproval.

"We should've gone to the Dancing Flamingo, whose idea was this?"

Five months later, my mother would discover she was pregnant with our Jackie, to the one in the middle, Robert our dad. Evidence that you could, indeed, get pregnant 'doing it' standing up.

"We'll get married then," said dad. The romance clearly palpable. But in those days, it was considered the right thing to do. Getting to know each other was scribbled down on their to-do lists and the courtship side lined. Welcome to the world of real. We hope you enjoy the trip.

Back home, the news went down like a fart in a spacesuit. Alice, of course, had opinions galore. None of them constructive. Margaret, always known as a gentle sort, was likewise 'slightly peeved' but far less vicious than her own daughter. It was relentless, and all of it completely expected.

Hours later, when the barrage was over and the dust settled, my mother hoped for a little support. It never came and as a result, the defiance within her grew. On that day, in that very moment, our family would never be the same again.

Without any help from her family members, mum cracked on with the wedding arrangements. At the main registry office on Martha Street, Glasgow, she handed over her abbreviated birth certificate and the registrar, 'Frankenstein' (her words not mine), disappeared from the room. A while later he returned with a dishevelled look. Either he'd nipped out for a spot of lunch, and it was windy outside or he'd dragged worried hands, several times, through his now wild mop of hair.

"Do you know the gentleman listed as your father on your birth certificate, is not your actual father?" he announced.

Frank had been gone a while and perhaps he'd entered the wrong room? Who was he directing this matter-of-fact question to? Suddenly, all eyes were focused on mum.

She pointed her thumb to her chest and said, "What? My dad you mean?"

"Indeed," said Mr Stein.

My mother = gobsmacked.

On the bus ride home, amidst swirling thoughts, a revenge plan was formulated. It's a dish best served cold apparently. At an unspecified point in the future, and like a decent gazpacho, she would draw out both barrels.

Two weeks later and Margaret's small kitchen resembled a High Court trial with no judge or gavel. It started with a calmly delivered question from my mother and escalated quickly. Accusations were now flying in all directions and 'you should've told her ages ago' or 'it's all water under the bridge now' were popular rebuttals. As the verbal brawl continued, the room felt thick with self-preservation and deceit. Not one person noticed my mother leaving. She would find out who her father was, just not today or in that kitchen. For a split second she felt alone, like a chick booted from the nest. She quickly reminded herself it was their guilt to carry, and she had no obligation to help with their heavy bags.

Mum and dad married in March 1966. The opinions, of course, still plentiful. 'It wouldn't last. Terrible decision. Utter madness'.

The next eight years were filled with a series of kids arriving and various house moves within Glasgow to accommodate the growing brood. Jackie was born in 1966, Lorraine in 1968, Me in 1971 *extends hand - nice to meet you* and Bob in 1974. For something that wouldn't last – it was going alright, so far.

Chapter 6 – Hawick I: Glasgow Overspill

In 1979, we moved to Hawick, a small town in the Scottish Borders. I often describe our immigration as 'Glasgow overspill' but that actual event took place several years earlier. For those of you not familiar with the term, it was a measure to reduce slum living. Glasgow Corporation's attempt at controlling the overcrowding in the city, thereby improving living conditions.

No, our move was a planned affair. Under the cover of darkness. The moonlight our friend. The neighbours and Glasgow City Council completely unaware we'd even left. My mother will make a mental note when she reads this and be sure to clip me round the ear for writing it. So, for complete transparency. I'm telling fibs. It was all above board with rent paid in full at the time of our departure.

Although, I do find myself wondering why our packed removal van was speeding out of the housing scheme, occasionally on two wheels, with some guy wielding a clipboard pursuing us on foot. Mum had advertised the current venture as a 'nice family day out' but dodging ill-packed furniture in the back of a vehicle that's attempting to break the sound barrier wasn't our idea of fun. I damn near lost an eye to the ironing board and Lorraine wrestled an uncompromising standard lamp for the entire one hundred miles. Sorry! Couldn't help myself. I'll desist immediately. All above board.

My dad is working in the local bakery at the time (the genuine reason for the family upheaval) whilst mum has found herself a job in a clothing store. Jackie slams right into the second year of high school (tough gig), Lorraine is holding her own in the latter years of primary school whereas I'm trying to figure out primary four, bedecked in Lorraine and Jackie's hand-me-downs. Bob has the easy ride in primary one, where the only real challenge is getting through an entire day without soiling your underwear. Much like our weegie accents, Hawick life was very different.

I was young when we moved to Hawick, but I still remember the constant hum of life in Glasgow. People everywhere. Always a minimum of two bus rides if you were going out for the day. Standing under shelters and watching everyone look right for their bus number. Friendly chit chat about the inclement Scottish weather (usually chucking it with rain) or some fellow bus waiter handing you five pence so you could buy a sweetie at the shop. Glasgow was, and still is, the friendliest place I know.

In Hawick, I heard birds chirping in the morning when I woke up and for me, at that point, it felt like the only positive to this move. Fast forward a couple of months and the 'warm welcomes' just kept on coming…

Bob got run over on the main road, just outside the local swing park. He was chasing a stray tennis ball from a game of rounders we were playing. It was horrific. We all ran out of the park on to the road where he lay and I remember traffic still going past, what appeared to be his lifeless body, in both directions. About two hundred yards along the road, I could see the car had stopped. The brake lights were on, and the driver side door opened. A leg appeared, and for a split second, I thought the driver was coming back to help. That same leg quickly disappeared back inside, the vehicle door slammed shut and the car drove off at speed.

We decided to drag him off the road and onto the nearby grass bank. I ran home and when I got there, dad was in the front garden cutting the grass. I could barely speak but between the gasps I managed "Bob been run over. Outside swing park. I think he's dead." Dad dropped the lawnmower and ran down the road. Mum called the ambulance from inside the house.

I remember the two ambulance men running towards the grass bank as I looked down at Bob. I saw a bubble of blood appear from his nostril and in that moment, realised he was still alive. In a flurry of medical activity, bags of fluid, syringes and lots of questions were suddenly important.

"Does anyone know if he went up and over the car? Did his head hit the windscreen?"

We nodded in agreement.

"And the car didn't stop? You didn't see anybody?"

We shook our heads. Someone in the group said the car was a light brown colour. It was all we had.

The medical attention continued, then dad and my little brother were packed into the ambulance. We stood on the pavement in shock and watched it disappear into the distance.

Bob sustained a nasty bleed on the brain and his wrist was shattered. He was in hospital a total of five weeks and for two of those, was unable to communicate. I was too young to appreciate the extent of his injuries or what was going on, but I do remember the day mum came back from the hospital and told us all Bob was sitting up, chatting away. He's now permanently deaf in one ear due to the accident. I had nightmares for two or three months after, where I saw the whole thing over and over in slow motion. The driver was never found. I wonder how they sleep at night.

Move to the countryside they said. Escape the city violence and infinite crime. I'll do the fucking jokes. Welcome to Hawick indeed.

Chapter 7 – Hawick II: Teribus Ye Teri Odin

At some point in this story, I need to explain the Hawick Common Riding. I've decided now is as good a time as any. Good luck me.

When you witness the aforementioned event for the first time, it will have you reeling back and mouthing the words 'what the fuck?' no matter how old you are. I've no doubt Hawick Common Riding historians will scoff at my portrayal of these events but as a disclaimer, this is only my opinion of it. If you want the hard facts, I suggest you buy a book called The Hawick Common Riding and make sure it's written by a local history teacher or a town know-it-all.

I still get confused over the specifics and don't want to antagonise the locals so here's Wikipedia to explain. I'll catch you on the flip side.

The tradition of common riding dates back to the 13th and 14th centuries, during the continual land border wars both with England and against other clans. It was a Border Country custom to plunder and thieve cattle, known as reiving (an historical name for robbing), and commonplace amongst the major Borders families.

In these lawless and battle-strewn times, it became the practice of the day for the local lord to appoint a leading townsperson, who would then ride the clan's boundaries, or "marches," to protect their common lands and prevent encroachment by neighbouring landlords and their peoples.

Long after they ceased to be essential, the ridings continued in commemoration of local legend, history, and are "devoted to pageantry, singing, and unique traditions centered around equestrian events."

In current times, common ridings celebrate each Border town's history and tradition in mid-summer, during a period spanning May through to September. Rideouts now involve hundreds of horses, often ridden in costume to evoke a passion worthy of the reivers of old.

Hawick is traditionally the start of the season of annual common ridings, due to the fact that the community captured a flag from the English army in 1514. Alongside the true common riding towns, other towns which now hold ridings are Currie, Penicuik, West Linton, Peebles, Biggar, Galashiels, Musselburgh, Duns, Kelso, Jedburgh, Melrose, Coldstream, Yetholm, Annan, Dumfries, Lockerbie, Kirkcudbright, Wigtown, Gatehouse of Fleet. One of the most recent common ridings was the Copshaw Riding, formed in 1998.

Each community starts its celebration with the election of that year's principal in the spring, chosen from amongst the community. The leader of the community's celebration once elected and until the end of ceremonies that year in that community, the principal man/woman/ pair is/are an honoured figure(s). The principal is usually an unmarried man of good character. The principals then lead the rideout and celebrate with other towns to show their kinship. Each community often has a different name for their nominated leader/principal. In Hawick, it's the Cornet.

Aaaaaaaaaaannnnnndddddd I'm back!

So... you're nine years old, no internet for material reference, just landed in this strange place and suddenly see two hundred horses fly past you in the High Street? Being honest, I instantly thought invasion.

I saw myself being plucked from the crowd, throat slit and cast away like a used carrier bag. It wasn't until I heard people cheering and saw flags being waved, that I realised the organisation behind it. I joined in. Had no clue what was happening, or the reasoning for it, but the sun was shining and there was nothing else to do.

A year later, I was holding horses and reaping the rewards like a true professional. Each ride out has a destination, so me and a bunch of my mates would hitchhike (or walk) to wherever that was. When the procession arrived, it was time to find your 'horse person rider man'. Then you'd stand for a couple of hours 'holding a horse'. Maybe walk it around some. Said horse rider would return from the social gathering in the local pub and as a thank you for looking after his ride, he'd slip you some cash for your efforts. That money would take you to the Hawick fair (or 'shows' as we called it), where you stuffed your face with too much candy floss, rode the Waltzer, fought nausea and walked home with a goldfish in a bag.

Every Saturday, for the next four weeks or so, that was the order of business. The only difference being the destination of said ride out. Sometime in the final week, the Cornet and the three wise men… no wait… that's wrong, the Cornet, his Right- and Left-Hand men along with the Acting Father would visit your school and ask permission from the headteacher to finish the school day early in preparation for the Friday Mair (I explain this further down, keep reading). Kids were cheering in the main assembly room when the man from Del Monte said yes. Amidst the celebrations, I rattled my lips with a massive sigh.

This early finish was inconvenient. Dad was home but sleeping off a nightshift and mum was busy working. I'd need to go find my little brother and we'd now have to walk the three miles home from school. More lip rattling.

When we arrived home, dad thought someone was breaking into the house and met us at the living room door, wielding a rolled-up newspaper. Naturally, he didn't believe our explanation either.

"The who came to your school?"

I took the offensive 'weapon' from his hands, "The Cornet, dad. He asked our headteacher to let us finish school early."

"Fur wit?"

"The Friday Mair. For the Common Riding."

"The who and the wit now?"

With nothing more to contribute, I shrugged. It was all the answers I'd been given when I asked the kid standing beside me at school. The little shit even had the audacity to throw in some disapproving snorts and I resisted the urge to punch him square in the teeth.

Quick rundown of the Friday Mair. The Mair is a field on the outskirts of Hawick and is common ground belonging to the people of Hawick. It's not the most accessible of places and walking up the hill to get there is lung bursting. On Friday Mair day, beer tents suddenly appear in the field, as do market stalls, and the population of Hawick itself. Packed cars arrive in their droves. Their boots containing essential items like a windbreaker or gazebo and cool boxes stuffed with alcohol. I recently heard that people have started taking port-a-loos now. Wasn't like that in my day. You either relieved yourself behind the dyke wall or took your chance with the makeshift wooden toilet block that some local joiner had thrown together the week before. Perpetual queue at the ladies' end, obviously.

The Cornet and his cavalcade arrive, the horse riders take a circuit of the racetrack in the middle. The Cornet then plants the flag centre stage, and the merriment begins. Bottles of beer are opened; kids are running riot and the Friday Mair is officially underway.

If you were a tourist visiting Hawick on Friday Mair day, you'd arrive in the town centre and think it was a nuclear test site. Not a shop on the High Street is open nor a living soul to be seen. Said tourist would be punching the accelerator and getting the hell out of dodge before they heard a siren, followed by a three-minute warning.

The Saturday Mair is the true culmination of the Hawick Common Riding. Pretty much a re-run of the Friday Mair but with a more poignant feel to it. After the Saturday Mair, the Cornet rides back into Hawick town centre and hands the flag (or standard) back to the people of Hawick at the town hall. I've never actually witnessed the final act but it's a very sad affair by all accounts.

At some point, when you're considered too old to hold horses and alcohol is the new black, your participation in Hawick Common Riding changes. On Friday Mair day, instead of walking up the hill with your cheese spread sandwich for a day of horse holding/money making, you're now arriving with your mates, a two-litre bottle of Scrumpy Jack cider under your armpit and a tartan rug to sit on.

I remember our Lorraine bought a parrot-shaped, helium filled balloon for her son Simon, with the intention of taking it home for him. Someone in the group accidentally burned a hole at the parrot's tail with their cigarette, it started deflating and we all fought over the escaping helium. I grabbed it first, scrunched up the end and sucked a little. Nothing happened. I heard another say, "No, you have to proper suck it, take a lung full."

So, I did, and immediately started singing Abba's Super Trooper. I couldn't hear any difference, but my friends started laughing.

"Is it working?" I asked. Suddenly, mates were pushing me away and holding their sides. Tears of laughter rolling down their faces. We ended up buying another two helium balloons from the market stand and everyone took a lungful. It was hilarious. Lorraine bought another for Simon when we left, and I'm surprised it made it home intact.

Now some thirty odd years later, I wholeheartedly admit, my interest in the Hawick Common Riding was purely for monetary reasons. I wasn't born in Hawick ergo had no real history with the place and because of that, the Common Riding was just something that happened. In the place. Where I lived.

Teribus Ye Teri Odin is popularly believed to have been the war cry of Hawick men at the Battle of Flodden. Yes, the sentiment is undeniable but when you're a young Glaswegian and have no real affiliation with this small town, it's difficult to fully comprehend or immerse yourself therein. Only my opinion, Hawick readers, please, no hate mail.

Chapter 8 – Hawick III: The Midnight Blues

Mum worked in Mackay's on the High Street. A store that, in the early eighties, sold clothing, curtains, bedroom gear and bathroom accessories. The company trades under M & Co. now and only sells clothing I believe. Back in the early eighties, if you needed something for the home or had kids, it was the place to go. We, of course, were like walking adverts for the place. Staff discount.

The store had a shoe shop concession at the back and when the manager left, mum applied for the position. No managerial experience but they were looking for someone to fill the predecessor's shoes quick (no pun intended). Mum was shipped down to Liverpool for three weeks and given the obligatory crash course in management, meaning dad had to step in and look after the pesky kids. We discovered, fairly sharpish, that custard making wasn't his forte. It had the appearance of rice pudding; such were the sizeable lumps in it. I scraped the ginger cake clean, ate that, and left the brain-like matter in the bowl.

Mum returned from Liverpool, she was now the manager of the shoe shop concession and, thereafter, we all had decent footwear. Staff discount.

Between dad doing constant nightshifts and mum's retail hours, we never saw our parents much. We became resilient. Fending for ourselves. Feral, but on a controlled level. My dad was on the committee of the local Liberal Club, so on Saturday nights he and mum socialised.

When they were out, we invited friends over and watched horror films on video. VHS of course. Friday the 13th when the main character was floating down the river in the canoe at the end of the movie everyone in the living room sighed with relief. Then, Jason flies out of the water and grabs her arm… well… you could've picked us all off the ceiling. Sofa cushions were inadvertently launched at the TV and in the panic, a table lamp was knocked over. We all heard the lightbulb pop and that just made it worse. This movie and The Exorcist (shudders) are the reasons I no longer watch films of that genre.

Mum and dad also owned racing greyhounds around this time. More socialising at the local track. Their dog, Midnight Blue, made the final of the big New Year handicap in 1990. The only dog not to win any of its heats, so he was given the outside trap and a sizeable start. Every dog in the race had already earned their owners a minimum of £100 so dad told mum to put the whole hundred on Midnight to win. At the bookie stand, she chickened out and peeled a tenner from her purse instead. He romped home at 5-1. The reduced winnings caused much aggro, but dad eventually got over it and a good night was had by all.

Furthermore, the household earned £250 when yours truly sent a video away to the popular television series 'You've been Framed'. A show where ordinary people would send in home movie clips for the entertainment of others.

At the end of each race, dog owners would stand at the finish and catch the 'unruly' entrants. Midnight, not slowing up this time, ran straight into dad's legs and upended him. It was a full-on, horizontal face plant into the sand. Cirque du Soleil type material. Couldn't even tell you how many times we super-slow-mo'd at the point of impact. I'm surprised the television show was able to extract any useable footage, the tape inside the cassette was worn thin.

When it finally aired on the television show we recorded it, of course. Rewound it and super-slow-mo'd that as well. It still cracks me up to this day. I'd challenge anyone to watch that clip and if you don't leak a bit of pee-pee into your underwear, then you're considered an emotional void to me.

Midnight Blue retired soon after and became the pet dog at home. If he wasn't sleeping, he was up to mischief and that instantly made him the best friend we ever had.

In the mid to late 80s, it was all about roller skates. I was lucky enough to receive a pair from 'Santa Claus', and even though the ground outside was thick with snow and ice, I put those puppies on and out I went. My friend Suzanne also got a pair from the big SC, but she broke her arm on the ice immediately and went home. There was no-one else out playing, so I called it a day and went home. Game over.

A couple of months later and in our roller skates, my friends and I decided to push the roundabout at the local swing park as fast as it would go. You'll notice the local swing park features heavily in our lives. Truth be told, there was nowhere else to go. If you played in your own street, guaranteed some miserable neighbour would open their front door or hang out a window and in no uncertain terms, tell you to 'fuck off' and 'go play somewhere else'. No amount of 'but I live here' claims were ever satisfactory. We'd all leave with heads bowed and a mumbled promise to pick their apple tree clean when it started bearing fruit.

Someone in the group said, "I wonder if we could grab onto one of the rails when it's flying round." I volunteered as tribute. I was the only one to make the leap and successfully managed to hang on. Instantly, I was in the horizontal position and did three full revolutions, thudding my friend's shins on the way round, before my grip failed me. I flew like an Exocet missile through the air. There was no bouncy, marshmallow, child-friendly surface back then, and I felt every inch of the swing park gravel on the crash landing. The seesaw finally halted my forward propulsion. I could've ended up in Dumfries otherwise.

I remember my entire left-hand side being a 'wee bit nippy' for the rest of the day but the streetlights weren't on yet, so I wasn't going home. My mum, armed with a pair of tweezers, spent most of the night picking the swing park ground from my skin. Just so you all know, the gravel extraction from my armpit was excruciating.

Two days later, I was shot in the knee with an air rifle. Sniper unknown. As I looked down at the wound, I instantly saw mum coming at me with the tweezers, so I gouged the pellet out of my kneecap with a 'clean' twig I found on the ground. Feral, but on a controlled level.

* * * * * * *

Both primary and high school alike were a particularly shady time for us all. How Jackie coped going straight into high school, I'll never fully appreciate. She'd left established friendships behind in Glasgow and in this foreign place, had to make new ones. At twelve years old that had to be a monumental task. Lorraine as well, she done a year in primary school before the carnage of secondary education. Bob and I were given half a chance at latching onto an unsuspecting group. You didn't know your arse from your elbow at our age. Best friends came and went, some of them even lasted a couple of hours.

In high school, I wasn't popular material. Wasn't in the far, extreme weirdo section either. Mid table is where I found myself. Average. Un-noticed. The mates I collected along the way remain my best friends to this day.

I had every intention of being a forensic scientist when I left school, but then a careers advisor turned up. I went in for the meeting all gung-ho, this is the job I'll be doing until I retire. I'd watched every episode of Quincy ME on television, knew exactly what I wanted. We discussed the five years of university I'd need to complete and then at the end of it, would still need to find a job. Wait a minute... Say what now?

I ended up leaving school at the end of fifth year and when I announced my decision to maw and paw, needless to say it went down like a lead balloon. Mum jumped right in there with her own career advice,

"You're not sponging off us until you move out, you'll need to find a job."

So... I did. In the payroll department of a local knitwear firm. Wasn't quite the white coat, searching for clues, closing cases, being the hero, I had planned but it kept the parents off my back. I passed my driving test the following year and was duly roped into the chauffeuring-mother-around detail.

I remember a night at home when mum and I inadvertently watched a horror movie called The Fog. Some grisly film about a mist that would roll in from the sea, shroud unsuspecting towns and release the undead who wreaked havoc of epic proportions.

When the creep show ended, mum got up off the sofa to go to bed. If I went to bed now not a wink of sleep would be had that night. We had to watch the end of a crummy sitcom, so I'd retire laughing instead of shitting myself. In a bid to make her stay up, I asked her if she wanted some supper. Toast perhaps?

"That'd be lovely" she said. "Maybe a cup of tea as well if you're making one, and can you bring it up when it's ready?"

Fuck!

She disappeared from the living room, leaving me alone with the fog demons.

Every light within a mile radius of the house got switched on as I made my way to the kitchen. I picked up the kettle, walked over to the sink and turned on the cold water. The sink sat directly under the window; a fine layer of condensation covered the bottom pane. As I began to fill the kettle, I saw what appeared to be two eyeballs and leaned in closer to the window, surely not. I raised a hand to wipe the condensation and was a full inch away from the glass when the finger tapping from outside began.

The involuntary scream came next. I dropped the kettle into the sink and ran to the living room door. The hallway was dark (why did I miss that?), but my over-exaggerating mind declared this fact as the least of my worries. I didn't touch any of the stairs as I flew up the side wall. My ankle knocking against the banister. I'm still screaming at this point. When I burst into mum's bedroom and launched myself onto the end of her bed, she was already asking me what the hell was going on.

In short, sharp bursts I managed,

"Someone...downstairs...kitchen window...they gonny kill us!"

"For God's sake Pauline! Do we really need to do this every time you watch a horror film? You're old enough to know better!"

I was trying to suck air into my deprived lungs and calm the fuck down. Failing miserably. The need to pass out was strong.

When she peeled back the bedcovers and made her way to the bedroom door, I couldn't believe it.

"You're not going down there, are you?"

"What would you have me do? Stick a chair under the bedroom door handle and wait 'til morning?"

It was a sarcastic question, and she was mocking me, but I felt the need to devise a plan. Look for a weapon at least.

Before another thought could enter my head, she was making her way downstairs. I scrambled off the end of the bed, grabbed a huge bottle of Avon perfume from the top of the chest of drawers and followed her. Without fear, courage does not exist.

We crept along the landing, and I found myself wondering if a potato peeler through the undead skull would rid us of this nightmare. If not, we had a tub of supermarket brand margarine in the fridge that could work. Not even bacteria survive on that.

We were halfway down the stairs, me chanting "The power of Christ compels you" over and over behind her, when the front door flew open. Even mum stopped mid step and inhaled sharply. I was hanging onto the back of her bathrobe and wondering if it had lifesaving properties. Fang proof or something. The material felt substantial.

Suddenly, we heard a mixture of laughter and howling wind outside. When we got to the foot of the stairs and turned to look down the hallway at the front door, we saw Jackie doubled over holding a ceramic bowl. Through uncontrollable laughter, Jackie held up the bowl and asked,

"Is there any chance someone could pass me out the rabbit food?"

My sphincter failed me, and I farted a wee bit. Mum reached out a hand and flicked the light switch. It was all too much. Took almost an hour for my heart to beat in a regular fashion. Jackie to this day still can't tell the story without laughing so hard that her ribs and face ache. Bitch.

Lorraine had already left home. She and her pals were sharing a flat in the middle of Hawick High Street. Living the independent life. It was handy if you needed a place to crash when you were out on the town at the weekends and too wasted to go home.

In 1989 she fell pregnant with Simon, and that whole dynamic changed. She moved back home to mum and dads. Not sure if the 'non-sponging off the parents' rule applied to Lorraine but it was nice having her back.

Around the same time, I had a run in with the actual undead. Location: back bedroom (above the kitchen). Creep-o-meter: a firm nine. When Lorraine moved back, I was demoted to the steerage end of the house. The back bedroom was very rarely used and a perfect square in terms of shape, except for the chimney breast that protruded into the room. In front of this sat a chair that I was using to throw clothes on. A makeshift wardrobe if you like.

I'd gone to bed around 10pm and set the alarm for work in the morning. Switched off the bedside lamp and shuffled down the bed, pulling the covers up around my ears. My west highland terrier dog called Hamish was already snoring at the foot of the bed. Just before I dozed off, a small dot of light appeared on the chimney breast wall. I blinked my eyes to dispel the phenomenon, but the dot wouldn't go away. Almost as if in defiance, it started growing bigger. Like…why? How?

Hamish was now awake, witnessing the strange light and couldn't take his eyes off it. I sat upright in the bed. Checked the window for a rogue curtain opening. Nothing. Complete darkness.

Before I knew it, Hamish was whimpering and had taken refuge up on my pillow. When he began clawing at the side of my face and subsequently ripped one of my earrings out of my earlobe, I was mildly aware that something was going on. He was typically a placid dog in nature, but this growing dot of light had freaked him out somewhat.

The two of us stared at the chimney breast wall. A face appeared. Elderly gentleman. Long hair, beard and wearing a ruffled collar. Piece by piece, he showed himself, shoulders suddenly came into view and eventually, the arms. All the while I'm trying to calm down Hamish, but I couldn't take my eyes off the wall. I'm not entirely sure what happened at this point. I heard Midnight Blue running up the stairs, closely followed by mum.

When the bedroom door opened and the hallway light filtered into the room, the elderly gentleman disappeared quickly back into the wall. As if someone had hit the rewind button. Mum said she found me sitting bolt upright and pointing at the wall. Hamish was shaking uncontrollably and apparently, I was screaming. Mum also mentioned the room was absolutely freezing when she first opened the bedroom door, and she could see her own breath. Strange in itself because the back bedroom housed all of the boiler pipes under the floorboards, it was always warm.

Midnight Blue must have witnessed the aftermath and was now barking at the chimney breast wall (he never barked at anything). Mum would tell me later, that it was the first and only time she'd ever seen his hackles raised.

I dragged the covers off the bed. Hamish and I slept in the living room that night. It was a strange occurrence. The back bedroom always had a feel to it. Indescribable.

In the morning, I grabbed my library card and researched the hell out of it. An apparition allegedly. Folks from the other side that are trying to be 're-born' into this world. It was five hours of ghoulish research before I found that out. This elderly person may have been around in the 16th century, but I could still pick him out of a line-up. The image is etched onto my brain. I never slept in the back bedroom again. Nor has anyone else. Validation, perhaps?

My siblings, of course, still rib me to this day over it, but I know what I saw. Soon as the alcohol is flowing, stories of my brush with the afterlife are never too far away. Naturally, their tales are embellished to the point of being ridiculous, meaning no two versions are the same. I believe one interpretation had the old dear wearing tartan slippers and cutting about in a double denim ensemble.

Listen, I know how crazy that story sounds and coming from a logical thinker (says so on the first page of this book) it's just downright weird. Do I believe in ghosts? I didn't until that very moment. I very much believe in what I see but Midnight had decided this invasion wasn't happening on his shift and duly seen the bogeyman off using hackles and greyhound teeth. Me personally, I kinda wanted the apparition to fully appear and listen to his chat, if he had any. Guess we'll never know.

It is what it is. I will continue sucking up the sibling piss takes and wonder if I missed the opportunity of a lifetime. The spooky pensioner wasn't expending that much afterlife energy for nothing. I really do curse my shitebag-ness some days.

Simon was born later that year, and I was in the process of buying my first ever house (also ending my back bedroom heebie jeebies). Since I had two bedrooms, Lorraine and Simon moved in thereafter. We were like a married couple some days. I went out to work, Lorraine stayed home with Simon and when I got back home, dinner was on the table. Family, eh? They'll always be the constant in your life.

* * * * * * *

It was a normal, lazy Sunday in July 2000. Lorraine and Simon were visiting mum and dad for the usual Sunday dinner. The telephone rang in the hallway and dad answered it on his way back to the living room.

"Jan, there's some guy on the phone, says he wants to talk to you." Mum disappeared into the hall and a minute later, she leaned back and closed the open door. It was ages before mum came back into the living room and grabbed the back of the armchair. Lorraine, looking over the top of the Sunday Post newspaper, spoke first, "Are you ok?"

Mum looked around the room, quietly searching for the right words before deciding there was no other way to say it.

"I have a brother."

For her entire life, my mother thought she was an only child. No siblings to confide in or fight with or have your back when you needed it. This telephone call had changed everything. My mother felt happy. She had a brother. It was true and it was real. Alice Bond had tried to sweep an actual human being under the damn rug, but fate had other plans. Karma will always have the last word and on occasion, it even bites back.

Chapter 9 – Uncle Tom (in his own words)

Out of the blue my niece, Pauline, sent me an email with the subject "Hello!" Seemed innocent enough but the content was an eye-opener. She described the situation about her mum's disease and then went on to ask me a pile of questions that were basically about how I found her mum, our first contact and how I felt about it all. I thought "How am I going to answer that?" I decided to ring her.

It was a fairly long telephone call in which she and I discussed the idea behind this book. Then we got around to chatting about how life was for me after my beloved wife, Babs, passed. Pauline raised the point about being a half person and basically, that is it. I am half a person, living a half-life. Luckily, I have the support of my family and friends. Without that support, I probably wouldn't have a life at all.

After the call she sent me her draft of the book. I was gobsmacked – it was brilliant. I replied to her email with my concise answers to her questions and agreed to help as much as I could. I didn't realise what I'd let myself in for.

Away back, when I first started the search for my natural mother, I had to sort out the ever-growing amount of information in a file. A necessary evil, if I was to make any kind of contribution to this story. I was very surprised to see how much correspondence and information I had gathered over the years. Old letters, diaries, and photos. The more I searched, the surprises kept on coming, and coming, and coming. I had forgotten so much, or maybe I had suppressed some of the memories to avoid the emotional reactions I expected when I opened Pandora's box. Most of the contents, moved me to tears. I still cry when I think of Babs. Some of that, I'm sure, has to do with self-pity and maybe I am a wimp after all, but I let it run its course.

As you may gather, I'm an emotional person and this experience has been very affecting. Digging around in my past was not that easy, quite painful sometimes but it needs to be revisited, warts and all.

I think Paul McCartney once remarked that he was surprised how other people had different memories of the same event. Memories are personal and therefore, can easily be 'corrupted' over time. You can research the hell out of something but I'm pretty sure there will still be inaccuracies. Different accounts. I'll stick to what I know. How I remember.

I was born November 1950 in the family house on Greenside Street, Glasgow; with a different name to the one I have now. Then, in 1951, I was put up for adoption and officially adopted by Mr and Mrs C, who lost their second son in 1948 to meningitis. Along with my older brother James, we grew up in the Scotstoun and Yoker areas of Glasgow. George, our dad, was born in Culmore near Derry, a tough Ulsterman and Jane, our mum, was born in Bridgeton, Glasgow. How can I describe my mum? How can I do her justice? Well, she was my mum, a dear sweet person who was always there for us, just as it should be.

When I was two years old, mum fell pregnant with my sister Jeanette and had to go into hospital due to complications. So, I was subsequently shipped off to Dalmarnock Road, Bridgeton to aunty Rita, my dad's sister. Aunty Rita was entirely responsible for discipline in her family. She and her husband, Jim, had a daughter Janet and two sons, John and Jim junior. Whenever aunty Rita took me out anywhere, I was strapped in leather reins which were regularly used to keep me on the straight and narrow. The bare calves got it. Ah, the sting of leather. I would feel it again much later in school.

I daresay my aunty Rita could have driven sheep, cattle or horses. Maybe she did when she was younger in Ireland. She was tough cookie but later on, she spoiled me rotten. Her wonderful husband passed away in 1955, leaving her to raise her young family (with some help from my dad).

My cousin, Janet, often told me I was a blessing to the family. In her opinion, if I hadn't come along, my sister Jeanette might never have been born. Jeanette, like my mother, has always been very special to me.

I still try to keep in touch with family and friends via phone, email, Skype etc. but I get angry with myself when I'm already in bed and remember that I meant to phone or email somebody. Jeanette and I chat regularly. She tells me, quite often, that I talk too much, even more than her best pal Sylvia. Not sure that's an accurate statement. I've experienced Sylvia in full flight, should be subject to debate at least.

Nevertheless, I do tend to ramble on a bit, and I also talk to myself. Trying to be my own psychologist. Been doing that for a long time now; whether it was to help me make decisions or give myself a bollocking for doing something stupid.

At the age of ten, my parents, being honest and decent, told me as much as they knew about my adoption. The identity of my natural parents was protected by law at the time, so the information was sparce. Occasionally over the years, I wondered about my earlier life but never took any serious steps to find out where I came from. It would be several years later before fate forced me to do so.

Lately the thought came to me that when James was five years old, he had lost his younger brother George and I was the replacement. I can't image what sort of effect that would have on him. Understandably, he was spoiled from then on by our doting mum. When I came on the scene, James got the job of looking after me. Couldn't have been a lot of fun running around with a brother eight years his junior. He took me to the 'pictures' a few times. I was thirteen when he took me to Ibrox Stadium for the first time; September 2nd, 1964, to watch the mighty 'Gers beat Red Star Belgrade 3-1. Jim Baxter and the rest, it was impressive.

I think I was around twelve when I got the Saturday job as his assistant driving around the streets of Glasgow on a horse-drawn, flatbed lorry selling coal briquettes. It was hard work running up the tenement stairs with a tray full, but I got a fair number of tips because I was wee and skinny. One Saturday, the lorry had a flat tyre and we had to go to a filling station to have it repaired. That meant uncoupling the horse and I was allowed to ride it around the forecourt. For a full five minutes, I felt like John Wayne or Robert the Bruce!

Sometime later, James left Blythswood Shipyard to join the Merchant Marine. That was good news for me, I finally had the bedroom at Hawick Street to myself. Problems of course when he came home from leave. He'd start ordering me around and complaining about the mess. That was annoying but the situation escalated when he started 'redding up'. James's talent for causing people to lose the rag was rapidly made evident and I lost it… completely: "OK PAL, YOU, OUTSIDE NOW!!!" Mum was really upset but I wasn't in any mood to listen to her.

I charged out the front door, thinking he was right behind me… He was, but only to close the door once I was outside. After kicking the door and swearing loudly for a while, I suddenly thought "Wow, that was cool." I started laughing.

This story, of course, was far too much for his funeral service in May 2021. I didn't really know what to say. He had simply become a grumpy, ungrateful old man because he was sad and lonely, that of course got worse when his beloved wife Lorraine passed away the previous October.

I must admit, I was surprised that our friends remembered him as a kind and gentle person. The fact is, for all his faults, James was not only a decent man, but he was also a kind one. When I was younger, I often judged people harshly. I would end friendships if someone did me wrong. Lately, I have concluded there should only be one criterion for forming an opinion about anyone – are they decent individuals or not? James, Jeanette, and I were brought up by decent people to be decent human beings.

After I left school at seventeen, my dream was to become a navigator and travel the world. That didn't work out, so I decided to apply for a four-year apprenticeship as a draughtsman in one of the local shipyards. At twenty-one, I celebrated my birthday with Terry, my good friend and fellow draughtsman. A lot of parties and copious amounts of alcohol. During this period, in January 1972, my sister Jeanette got married to Billy. As oft times happen at weddings, some people get carried away and make relationship decisions that they may not have done under other circumstances. I was there with my current girlfriend, and I asked her to marry me. She was delighted. I bought the ring and with the help of my dad we found a small flat in Scotstoun and would have set up home there with her toddler daughter, had it not been for the ex-boyfriend still lurking on the side lines, hoping to be brought onto the field as a late substitute. It ended with a broken engagement and a broken hand (mine!).

Jeanette was around to offer sympathy and comfort, but I ended up having Librium prescribed. No medication leaflets. I can't remember whether the doctor told me not to drink alcohol while taking the wee white pills, but the effect was quite relaxing.

In 1973, I was asked whether I would be interested in a student bus trip to Germany. The spot became available because a friend, who was due to go on the trip, had broken his leg playing football. I was only too happy to fill the void, more so when I heard there would be eight guys and thirty-two girl students on the bus!

The coach left St Enoch Square in Glasgow and made its way to Osnabruck where we met up with the German student group to tour the northwest of Germany. We kept in touch with the tour leaders, a really nice couple, who invited us over for Christmas that year. Two of us managed to go and we had a wonderful time.

In the meantime, Terry caught wind of a contract draughting job in a shipyard in Southampton. So, in September 1973, we headed off down south and the lure of the big bucks. More parties and even more alcohol. After six months, I got sacked. It's bad enough going into work with a scorcher of a hangover but infinitely worse when you arrive drunk.

A friend was going to work in London and suggested we flat share until I found another source of employment. I applied for a job at the Ministry of Defence in Bath. The vetting would take some time, so I had to be patient. The money was short and London expensive which meant I had to be careful. The London Underground was an eye-opener. In Glasgow you would frequently find yourself chatting to strangers on a tram, bus or the 'shoogly' subway. On the tube, unlikely you'd ever get that intimate with any of the travellers, but I remember my time in London being quite pleasant.

The acceptance for the MOD finally came through and I was off to Bath. Whilst living and working there, I decided to take a break and go visit my family in Glasgow for the weekend. When I walked into my favourite pub, The Griffin in Bath Street, I was surprised to hear familiar German voices. It was the people from the group I'd been on the tour with the year before. I was invited to join their tour of Scotland which included trips to Largs and Hamilton. The trip to Hamilton was a disco night at Hamilton Accies Football Club on July 31st, 1974. It was then and there that I first encountered the girl from Nuremberg. Barbara (Babs) was drinking a scotch on the rocks, smoking a cigarette and chewing gum. I asked her for a dance, she accepted.

The German students were staying at the Baird Hall of Residence in Sauchiehall Street, Glasgow, and it's where Babs and I spent the night together. She suggested that I could travel with her in the group's bus to London, which I did. We parted there with the promise to write, which we both did. During Easter of the following year, I took the train to visit her in Nuremberg where I met her boyfriend who would then become her ex.

In 1975 I moved to The Netherlands and a new job in The Hague. I quickly learned that Holland was just a region of The Netherlands and not a country. A few months later, Babs gave up her further education studies to join me. She found a good job for a Dutch/Austrian company, and we got to know each other a lot better. There was a whole bunch of other British contract draughtsmen working there and most of them thought Babs was Scottish. I hadn't noticed she had taken on a Scottish accent.

When Babs arrived, we shared a rented house with a pal and his girlfriend. Later we found a lovely little flat in Scheveningen on the coast. One day Babs and I were walking along the beach, and it took us no time at all to notice that everyone around us was naked. It was a nudist beach. The Netherlands was pretty liberal. At parties we noticed hash and then rows of powder on tables also. We occasionally dabbled with the weed on offer but stayed well clear of other recreational drugs.

After the job contract ended and we had spent a summer at the coast, Babs talked me into moving to her hometown of Nuremberg. We agreed it would only be for a year or so. In 1978, we packed a minivan; Babs and our good friend Charlie from Yorkshire took turns in driving us to Franconia. Initially we stayed in a basement room of Babs' parents then found a rented flat, got married in July and after that, found jobs. Slightly unconventional but that was us. I had learnt a few expressions in German from Babs, but we knew that wouldn't be enough to live and work in Germany. So, I went back to school to learn the lingo. If I remember correctly, the course was once a week and most of us usually ended up in the local pub with Detlef our teacher. I had the advantage that Babs helped me with the crazy German grammar. We got to know the couple who ran the pub, Olga and Bernd, really well. A lot of the students, Detlef, Olga and Bernd became our friends. Over the years most of the students moved on or back to their native countries. One of the Americans, a lovely lady from Philadelphia who was married to a German doctor, and Olga sadly passed away. To this day, the Hungarian couple, Laci and Martha, are two of our best friends.

In 1975, the law had changed allowing people to find their natural parents but living in Germany complicated the process. To become a resident in Nuremberg, I requested and received copies of my birth/adoption certificates in March of 1978. When I found out about the new law, I contacted Strathclyde Council for more information.

It would be 1984 when I received letters from the council with regards to my adoption and my natural mother. After my birth in 1950, I lived with my mother for almost six months before I was placed with my adoptive parents in October 1951. The council informed me they could be of no further help, and I was referred to the Salvation Army, local press etc. I did place a personal ad in the Scottish Daily Record newspaper but without success.

In the same year, I was over in Scotland for a funeral when I found out from the general registrar that I had a half-sister, Janice Chapman who was married and had four children! Their last known address was in Errogie Street, Glasgow from 1974. Unlikely they would still be living there so I went back to Strathclyde Council – they were unable to confirm the address. I had to go back to Germany and couldn't research it any further, so I hired a research student in Edinburgh. Gave her all the information I had and requested that she also ran a search for my punitive father, Joseph Wynne; there was no trace. She found, amongst other things, the death of Margaret Cumming McInnes with a last known address in Armadale Court. Glasgow Housing Department couldn't confirm it. A year later, I requested a copy Alice Chapman's birth certificate – my natural mother.

I received a letter from Strathclyde Council social work department in July of 1985. Mrs Chapman had visited the council offices. She was nervous but had told them she would like to hear from me. The social worker went on to describe my mother's appearance: "she seems a pleasant lady, small, around 5ft tall, quite plump, well dressed and groomed." She went on to say that my mother worked for many years in the teachers' salaries department in Bath Street. She lives alone and has done for a long time. The overall impression was that she's not very close to her immediate family and for that reason, hasn't been able to talk to anyone about what happened or the circumstances behind the decisions made.

The social worker agreed with Alice that I should write to her via their council department. In effect, I wasn't allowed to communicate with my mother directly. I duly wrote a letter to my mother and the council worker handed it over to Alice in August 1985. I can't find any reply and I don't remember receiving one. I had suggested a telephone call, maybe via the council offices but Alice didn't respond to that either. It seems my mother was reluctant to have any direct contact with me.

A relative who was working for the Post Office found a telephone number for William McInnes, my mother's brother. I called but he wasn't too pleased to hear from me. He eventually reneged and gave me my mother's address at Langside Road. I wasn't sure what to do with this information.

When I was back over in Scotland for a visit, I met up with the research student in Edinburgh again. It was finally my cousin John, who talked me into knocking on my mother's door. "If you don't, you may never get a chance later," he said.

At first nobody answered the door and I said "Well, we tried!" John wasn't giving up that easily, knocked on the neighbour's door and she opened it right away. Alice must be home she said. The neighbour knocked on Alice's door and said, "It's me Alice."

The front door opened, and Alice appeared with obvious suspicion. I tried to explain who I was, she murmured something like "no…" and then simply closed the door. It wasn't quite the first meeting I had been hoping for. I was disappointed but had to accept the fact, she didn't want to know me. We left. I would never see her again.

After the disappointing meeting with my mother, the family search stagnated for a few years. I knew of them, but I didn't know where they were. In July 2000, I found an address and telephone number for "Kennedy, R F" at Heronhill Crescent in Hawick. It was my sister Jeanette who found out the residents of the address in September; all the names I was looking for. So, I telephoned and subsequently, followed the call up with a letter.

I received a letter from my sister Jan soon after, thanking me for the telephone call. In it, she told me she was delighted to hear from me. She also said that the last time she was in Glasgow was to arrange her mother's funeral. Alice had passed away in April 1994 and is buried in Riddrie Cemetery beside her gran and grandpa. The letter included family photos and a list of relatives. I was over the moon.

We arranged a meeting in Galashiels – August 11th, 2008. For moral support (and transport) I asked my sister Jeanette and my cousin John to accompany Babs and I to the Scottish Borders where we met up with Jan and Pauline (Jan's moral support and transport perhaps?).

It was just great to finally meet my sister, Janice, in the living flesh and I had an immediate feeling that we were soul mates, bonded, on the same wavelength, close siblings. We were going to get along very well indeed.

I have always been a people watcher and, nervous as I was, I got the (first) impression that Pauline was pretty wary about it all. I might have been wrong, could be that she was as nervous as I was, but I thought to myself, "If I didn't behave myself here, I would maybe have to break her jaw to get her fangs out of my neck." Turns out, she was just as nice as her mum, harder, but nice. We had a lovely meal at Jan's favourite restaurant, Macari's. What a wonderful day, I was so happy.

All of that wouldn't have happened without the help and everlasting support of my sister Jeanette, my cousin John and my beloved better half, Babs. Yes, despite her depression, she was better, more compassionate, and stronger that I will ever be. Women are in any case, stronger, and more resilient than men. If you can imagine how women deal with labour pains and compare that with how men whimper and whine squeezing out a hard shite, you get my drift.

I was privileged and honoured that Babs and I were invited to Bob and Donna's wedding in September 2012. A crowd of lovely (and interesting) people in a wonderful setting. It was great to see my new part of the family, whether it was in Edinburgh or Galashiels.

At some point, I do need to wind this part of the book up. I've rambled on as per usual. When I started writing this chapter and sent initial drafts to family and friends, a couple of them said, "You should write your own book." Nope, this is where the story belongs. I somehow feel it's our story. The story of, as Jeanette put it, our 'blended' family. How we found each other, how we got to know and love each other, the history that formed us and ultimately made us who we are.

My good friend Armin is blind from birth. He studied, amongst other things, music at the Institute for the Blind in Nuremberg. The first time I met him was at a friend's birthday party. He was playing guitar and singing Scottish/Irish folk songs, some of which I'd never heard before. Armin and I often go for walks and Indian lunches. He would often start singing a Sottish song when we were out, and I of course had to join in. I am in no way a good singer but the effect that had on people around us was amazing. Smiles, lots of smiles. I encounter people who smile at me, and I always make a point of smiling back. Costs nothing and makes my day, sometimes even leads to friendly chit chat. Armin's perspective of things is something else, a different slant on life. Never fails to surprise me. Through Armin, I've got to know quite a few sight impaired people and have always been impressed by their positive outlook. Lately, due to Corona virus restrictions, I have been spending more time in his company than anyone else. He listens patiently to me ranting on and then usually comes back with something that I hadn't considered. It's a pleasure being Armin's friend.

As part of their English language course my good friends Ernst and Fiona, Jenny and Gerhard organised a ceilidh every year from 2007 until 2020 to commemorate Robert Burns' birthday. Fiona and Jenny gave English language courses for the further education department of the Oberasbach Local Council. Music was performed by my good friends Thomas and Susy (highland pipes, dance), Armin (guitar, vocals) with his band Cauldron or solo.

In the earlier years, Babs drove me, Armin and his band to the venue. It wasn't a lot of fun for Babs. Later, she didn't feel safe driving at night as her vision had deteriorated, so we arranged alternative transport. At some point, I was asked to read a Burns poem, 'Tae A Moose'. Latterly it was 'A Red, Red Rose' (dedicated to Babs). At the ceilidh in 2019, I managed to bungle it and missed a line. I told Ernst that I wasn't sure whether I would be able to read any poems again. As always, he and Fiona were very understanding about it.

Nevertheless, when it was nearing the time for the 2020 ceilidh, I didn't want to let them down. Ernst and Fiona suggested a less emotional (for me) Burns poem, 'Up in the Mornin' Early' maybe? I had been thinking of trying to write my own poem about Babs and I was surprised that it came so easily to me. I showed 'Tae Babs' to Ernst and read it out to Armin. Ernst got a bit emotional. At the ceilidh, Ernst gave me all the poem sheets. I had free choice. Determined to get it right this time, I read out all three. It went down well.

Afterwards, I was approached by a woman who said she was collecting stories about people who had lost their loved ones. She asked me to explain the poem and my thoughts about Babs. I agreed when she asked if she could use the story (anonymously) for her magazine article.

Around the year 2000, Babs was diagnosed with depression. She required therapy. That meant she had to find a therapist. She did but unfortunately that therapist had, to put it mildly, marital problems and Babs being Babs, ended up trying to help her! As in most cases, that led to psychotropic drugs. A lot of people mistakenly believe that depression is somehow a figment of the imagination or maybe just a bad mood. "Buck up!" is what you usually hear when the black dog turns up.

After a major ten-hour operation, a month in intensive care and without fully regaining consciousness, my beloved wife passed away in July 2017, ten days after her sixty-seventh birthday and twelve days after our thirty ninth wedding anniversary. It was a terrible experience for our kids and I, but we struggled through it together and are still doing so. I can only imagine how it would have been without the support of my (double) family and the best friends you could ever hope for in this world. God bless them all.

'Tae Babs', read out by her loving husband on Friday 24th of January 2020 at the Scottish ceilidh in the primary school in Oberasbach-Altenberg.

Tae Babs – A poem wi a bit ae prose *In the spirit o' Rabbie Burns*

Fae fair Nuremberg she came tae Glesca
 – an' tae me
She stole ma hert an' tak ma breath aw a'
Wis ma safe haven an ma anchor an' aw

Mither ae ma weans an' healer ae ma pains
Builder ae oor hoose an' hame, never looked fur fame

A wis a helper in need, wis a taxi fur aw
 (especially me)
Drove me everywhere, drove me crazy an' aw

Aye, she pit up wi' aw ma failings;
 Suffered hardship an' pain withoot complaint
She told me she loved me, every day
Ah tell her ah love her, every night.
Aye, my love is like a red, red rose

 So my dear friends —
 If you love someone, hug them,
 kiss them, tell them you love them,
  every day

Chapter 10 – Alice Chapman

In 1993, Alice was diagnosed with Alzheimer's Disease and moved to a private nursing home. Mum visited her as much as she could. On one occasion, my granny handed Bob fifty pence and a tangerine, telling him to share it with his sisters. In 1994, and after a couple of chest infection battles, she passed away peacefully in her sleep. Seventy-eight years young. RIP Alice Chapman. When we meet again, you and I will have a chat.

Chapter 11 – William Harold Schaeppi (American soldier)

After my granny's funeral, mum went to the nursing home and collected her personal items. The nursing staff couldn't have been more helpful. People dealing with Alzheimer's disease in any capacity will always have my true admiration. It's a tough grind.

My granny would often recall stories from yesteryear with pinpoint accuracy. She'd know what colour the handkerchief square was in her brother's suit pocket when she first got married and even how it'd been folded. She'd tell us who delivered her milk, on what days and when she paid for it. But… if my mother broached the subject of her real father, the Alice guard would instantly go up. You'd see true sadness in her weary eyes and recognition of a past she didn't want to revisit.

In the small box that contained my granny's life, we found a name. William Harold Schaeppi from Ramsay, St Paul, Minnesota. The name Schaeppi was also important enough to make its way onto my mother's birth certificate. Sherlock Holmes could sit this one out. Written on a piece of paper, inside a box, belonging to my gran – my mum had found her father.

Perhaps the gods of guilt appeared to my granny while she, with great fondness, was remembering a time where she almost sailed across the Atlantic Ocean to be with the man she adored. In my mind, I can see Alice smiling as she grabbed that very piece of paper and asked a passing nurse for a loan of her pen. Maybe my granny had finally found some peace as she scribbled down his name. Whatever the reason, I thank her for it.

Mum and I had started the family tree history some two years previous, but the search had stalled on her dad's side for obvious reasons. Back in the mid-nineties, every couple of months, we paid £10 at the Registry House in Edinburgh and sat there from dawn 'til dusk, researching our family history on their computers. It's sad to say but the most 'valuable' information we ever found was on death certificates.

The person who registered that death would take you on another course and you'd find yourself immersed in their life; if they were married, if they had kids etc. What their relationship was to mum and would they find themselves a branch on our family tree. Then, five hours later, you'd have to disconnect from that person and remember who you were looking for in the first place. The staff at the Registry House would quite often have to throw mum and I out. Me, running to the printer and grabbing our search efforts from the tray before we were manhandled onto the pavement outside.

We'd go home and start filling in names on a makeshift family tree constructed out of old wallpaper rolls (the blank side), a pencil and sticky tape. The length of the wallpaper strip afforded us the luxury of adding in family members that appeared during our subsequent searches and meant we didn't have to disturb any of the information we'd found the month before. Much like everything in life, we discovered width matters. Wallpaper provided just that.

The further back you go in your family history, (mid 1800s to, say, the 1940s) you'd find that a married couple having one kid was just plain weird. So, we'd cut another piece of wallpaper from the roll and add it on to the end of the existing chart to accommodate the multitude of humans brought into the world around that entire period of time. I genuinely got sick of re-writing the whole tree every time we found someone new with twenty kids. Incidentally, I had to rub out/erase an aunty Betty from the ancestral line because she wasn't really our aunty. My siblings and I promoted a neighbour to that rank without realising she wasn't even a blood relative. It was a cut-throat/enlightening kind of day.

Whenever the wallpaper chart slid off the wall and you'd catch a glimpse of the 70's throwback pattern adorning the other side, I'd always say, "God, mother did you really have this on your walls?" That memory still makes me smile to this day. Given the current fashion trend and if she still had rolls of it in the cellophane, she'd make a fortune. We upgraded to normal lining paper a few years later. It was lighter in weight and adhered to the wall for longer periods of time.

I've gone off track now... Where was I? If you ever research your family history – you'll say that very line A LOT.

Yes... William Harold Schaeppi. Armed with this new information, we visited the Registry House again with renewed hope. We had his name and a hometown, albeit in the United States of America but surely, we'd find something to go on.

We quickly cursed our naivety and optimism. Everything we searched; telephone directories, census details, marriage registers, death certificates, birth certificates and even our neighbour's crystal ball the night before, turned up a series of depressing nothingness. Finding anyone not belonging to nor living in the UK was going to be a challenge. The registry staff kicked us out, again. Mum and I went home.

We wrote to a company called TRACE in America – even getting an address for them was frustrating but we managed. I believe they occasionally teamed up with the American consulate and rooted around in war service records in a bid to supply details. Everything done by letter and post on a dot matrix printer. I refuse to explain that technological masterpiece. The postage costs were also of the eye-watering variety. I once asked the post office clerk if she had her foot on the weigh scale when she was calculating the charge. I laughed. She didn't.

It was months later when we finally received a reply. A two-sided letter with very little content. Informing us, the name Schaeppi was fairly common in Minnesota and that without an address, there wasn't any significant information they could provide. They did, however, suggest we contact The London Library as they housed all the telephone directories for overseas as well as the UK.

I can truly hear every millennial saying, "Like actual?" Right about now. Enough already with the eye rolling. It's called doing all you can, with what you had available in the early to mid-nineties. *Get o'er yersels.*

Mum called The London Library not expecting very much but a couple of days later, she was given a list of possible suspects. No William Schaeppi mentioned, so we selected the first candidate (as you do), a Mary F Schaeppi from St Paul, Minnesota and cranked up the dot matrix once again.

The first letter was important, so it took us an age to compose. We had to include details of relevance, be vague, yet supply enough information that would pique the interest of any relative in the know and reading it. Three weeks later and with the printer ink ribbon in shreds – we dropped our literary genius in the post-box.

Early December 1994 we were contemplating candidate number two on the list, when a letter bearing the familiar blue 'By Air Mail - Par Avion' sticker arrived. Several months had passed, so mum and I stared at the letter for a while. We each took a turn feeling up the contents before mum finally opened it.

In the letter, Mary told us she had been married to one of William's brothers (twelve siblings in total) and that her husband had died two years prior to our letter arriving. She had been talking to other members of the Schaeppi family and trying to find out some information for us. Mary asked mum to supply a couple of things, the age of Alice in 1946 and the area where my granny lived at that time. We replied with the answers and thanked Mary for her response.

Almost a year later, another letter from Minnesota arrived. This time different handwriting and the sender's details on the back of the envelope said Maryjo Schaeppi. When my mother opened this correspondence and we finally read the contents – words failed us both. You dig deep enough, right?

Scottish Slang – One should get over the shock and be sympathetic to ancient processes.

Maryjo was doing her own family history and she called Mary to help fill in some blanks. Mary had dropped into the conversation that she'd received a letter from Scotland, and this intrigued Maryjo. After much research, she found out that my mum's dad was her uncle William! Furthermore, William had three children Lyle, Gordon and Barbara and they all knew about their half-sister – my mother. Maryjo supplied addresses for all three of them and suggested to mum that she should get in touch with them directly. She also said that William had sadly died in 1969 – he was fifty-one years old. My mother had been duly added to Maryjo's family tree and she would endeavour to send a copy when she'd taken it as far as she could. If mum needed any further information, Maryjo would help in any way she could. She asked mum to keep in touch and said welcome to the family! We both read the letter multiple times and with a touch of bewilderment, it was my mother who spoke first.

"Can you believe this?"

"It's... outrageous! The mid 1900s were wild!" I replied.

With letter in hand and arms thrown outwards in despair my mother remarked, "I'm forty-eight years old Pauline, just finding brothers and sisters now?"

My wild 1900s chat probably wasn't the best reply. Likewise, it certainly wasn't the time to tell her that someone had left the back door open, and Midnight was now in the garden, running around with a flower bush in his mouth. Mum had planted that very same bush the week before and I could see the gaping hole in the soil where it once resided.

"They all knew about me, and I find out in a letter that my father is dead?" Her voice wavering.

I didn't need to say anything else. She knew we'd accomplished everything we set out to do when she found her father's name. All events prior to this moment in time, were a product of years gone by. Decisions made by the people who brought her up. The reasons for which unknown but had to be respected. Sort of.

We had pursued this information for a couple of years using all the grit and determination we possessed. Yes, it wasn't easy but against all the odds, we had uncovered a multitude of truths.

The best she could do, was draw a line in the sand of historical shitness and embrace the start of this new chapter. Amidst my mother's hurt and frustration, we'd found two more half-brothers and a half-sister. Getting to know them was the new objective.

Midnight tossed the newly evicted shrub high in the air and trapped it between his two front paws. At least his day was a happy one. For now.

Chapter 12 – Hawick, the latter years

Between 1996 and early 2005, mum got to know her half siblings through various letters and Christmas cards exchanged over the years. The dot matrix printer was finally retired and replaced with a laser jet. Printing in colour was now an option but very rarely utilised because 'it cost an absolute fortune'. Progress never comes at affordable prices.

In 1999, Jackie came back to Hawick after her stint in the NAAFI. For us civilians, this is The Navy, Army and Air Force Institutes. An organisation created by the government in 1921 to run recreational establishments required by the British Armed Forces, and to sell goods to servicemen and their families. In short, supplying alcohol, cigs and food to our serving heroes.

She'd been 'deployed' in various places throughout the UK and even got a wee stretch in Bielefeld, Germany. I went over for a visit while she was there and couldn't believe my ears when she started talking fluent German! I figured some old-time war veteran had possessed her body and instantly began searching for a divine intervention to eject the old soul. "It's just easier to learn the language when you actually live here," she said.

I eyed her suspiciously and made the decision. It was time for Flight Lieutenant Schmidt to go find someone else to inhabit. He'd freaked me out long enough.

Lorraine is busy reporting for the local rag, The Southern Reporter, and a single parent to Simon at this time. If we were ever out in the car together and saw an ambulance or police car speeding past, I'd always shout, "get your note pad out!" and pretend to do a handbrake turn in the road. It was probably funny the first couple of times and flat out irritating thereafter but she would always humour me. "You do know my jobs isn't like that?" she'd ask.

Sure. I knew. In later years I would even roll down the window and pretend I was sticking a flashing light on the roof of the car just to add more flair. No doubt in my mind, that action pissed her off as well, but I didn't care. I was, and still am, proudly annoying.

September 2001 – Lorraine had just bought her first flat and wanted to sand the wooden floors. She called me on a Friday night asking if I would collect the floor sander from the hire company in the morning. She didn't sound very well on the phone and when I asked her if everything was alright, she told me the doctor had just been to her house. A touch of food poisoning the doctor had said and he'd given her an injection to stop her being sick.

"Fuck's sake Lorraine. You still want me to pick this sander up?"

"Yeah, I'll be fine tomorrow. Just feel out of sorts right now," she said. I hung up but wasn't entirely convinced.

When I called her in the morning, it was Steven the paramedic who answered. I could hear Lorraine moaning in the background.

"We're just taking Lorraine to the hospital," he'd declared. "Going to the Borders General, if you're following behind, go straight to the accident & emergency department." The phone line went dead.

I called mum. She asked me to pick her up and we'd go over together. My mother hates travelling at speed in the car but on this occasion, she never said a word. I could see her hanging onto the car door handle whilst I drove like an absolute lunatic for the eighteen miles or so to the hospital.

The A&E department was busy when we finally arrived. I could hear Lorraine in one of the curtained booths, her pain obvious to all who were sitting in the waiting area. The receptionist wasn't much help, but she'd find out what was going on. Mum and I sat down. We got chatting to this young lad who was sitting in a hospital wheelchair. He'd broken his leg playing rugby with his mates. When he lifted the blanket to let us see (we didn't ask but there was no stopping him) I saw his leg in what can only be described as an 'S' shape. Mum was horrified and I gave him my best 'ouch' face. He was oddly proud of his misshapen limb.

Mum and I were ushered into a side room about ten minutes later with the promise that a doctor would come see us soon.

Mum in her infinite state of optimism asked, "Is this not the room they use when people have died?"

"You went right there huh?" I decided nonchalance was the route of choice. I could see my mother getting worked up, so I was attempting to level it out. I started reading posters on the hospital room wall.

"Did you hear our Lorraine screaming in that booth?"

"I think the entire A&E department waiting room heard it mother."

The tension was marginally relieved when a student doctor appeared at the door. He looked like a twelve-year-old playing doctor in a white coat and wearing his stethoscope as a fashion accessory.

"We believe Lorraine has suffered a ruptured appendix and that's not good. She's been rushed to emergency surgery, we'll have more information when that's over," Mr Twelve-year-old said.

"Can you explain why 'that's not good' as you so vaguely describe it?" I was annoyed but diplomatic. Mum had burst into tears.

"It depends on whether the appendix has ruptured or not. If it's still intact, they will remove it and she'll be good to go home in a couple of days. If not, then she may suffer blood poisoning and that's a downright nasty affair."

"Please regale the group on your definition of nasty affair," more annoyance from me.

"It could be several weeks before she makes a full recovery and the road back to health will be tricky for sure," he said flatly. I could tell from his demeanour he wanted to be somewhere else.

"So, what do we do now?"

"Go home is probably the best idea. We'll let you know how everything goes." He scurried out of the room. Mum was trying to compose herself and I (ever sympathetic) rolled my eyes.

"You need me to get my slapping hand out, mother?"

"No. I'm fine!" She said through incoherent sobs.

On the way out, I told 'S' leg that I hoped his operation went well and he was back playing rugby soon. He smiled and sealed the deal with a thumbs up.

It would be a couple of days before we could visit Lorraine. Her appendix had, indeed, ruptured and she did have blood poisoning. Simon (aged eleven) insisted on going to visit her and who was I to stand in the way.

We'd just walked down a long corridor and turned into the hospital ward when Simon asked,

"Is my mum going to be alright aunty Pauline?"

I put my arm around his shoulder as we entered Lorraine's room,

"She'll be fine pal and out of here in no time!"

That's when Lorraine opened her eyes and instantly vomited what can only be described as dark material, all down her front, onto the bedsheets and subsequently, the floor. Classic timing. There's no choreographing that shit. Simon and I shuffled to the foot of the bed and stared at the gruesomeness while my mum took off out the room, shouting for a nurse.

By the fifth visiting day we were getting the hang of it. Even managed to get some of the cardboard sick bowls under her chin before the offensive matter hit the floor. Mum was no longer sprinting to the nurse's station for help whenever we heard the familiar gurgling noises emanating from my sister. Progress. Simon was an absolute trooper throughout the entire ordeal, despite my fraudulent 'she'll be fine' declaration.

She was in hospital for twelve days in total and most of it was, indeed, a 'downright nasty affair'. In hindsight, the first student doctor we met at the A&E had described it perfectly. Thankfully, Lorraine made a full recovery. I dislike hospitals – quite intensely.

Chapter 13 – Unlucky for some

Early 2005 – mum and dad felt like they were rattling around in the house we grew up in, so the decision was made to downsize. The three gardens were a lot of work and more so now that they were both approaching sixty. It was no doubt a difficult choice for them, but it made perfect sense. Thirty odd years of memories all packed away in cupboards, and the attic was full to bursting. A sentimental exorcism if you like. The effort was monumental. It's only when you move house do you realise the garbage you hang onto for various reasons. 'That might come in handy one day' or 'can't throw that out - your sister made that in her woodwork class at school'. My mother did surrender some items, but I could tell most of it she desperately wanted to keep.

Once it was cleared of the family clutter, the house went on the market and sold very quickly. They bought another property in Hawick, literally three hundred yards away from where I lived. It was nice. Like having a convenience store down the road whenever I ran out of milk or bread. I would occasionally saunter down in my slippers, say hello on entry, collect milk from their fridge, and bid them both a wonderful evening on the way back out with the 'purchases' tucked under my arm. Mum got into the habit of buying extra in her own weekly food shop because she knew that I'd appear at some point.

Around this time, Mum and I are both working in the town of Galashiels – eighteen miles north of Hawick. I'm employed with a small business travel agency and mum is working at a chartered accountants' firm.

In the winter months, the daily commute was a complete ball-ache. I'm not a huge fan of driving in the snow and mum, as previously explained, isn't the best of passengers either. At night, when we were navigating the road home, in the heavy snowfall and wind, it felt like I was driving Miss Daisy in the

Millenium Falcon. I'm refusing point blank to explain any of those references.

It's a journey that would normally take twenty minutes, but some nights were close to an hour in the heavy snow. Mum would be grabbing my arm and saying incredibly supportive things like 'can you not slow down a bit' or 'god this will take us ages to get home'. We'd argue of course. I'd occasionally ask her if she wanted to drive the fucking car, or I'd suggest pulling the vehicle over mid trip so she could find her own way home. She'd always decline said offers and then follow it up with 'we should've taken the bus'. The dispute would rumble on.

Lorraine worked in Selkirk, a small town in between Hawick and Galashiels, so she'd quite often get roped into the commuting detail. We'd then trade 'passenger mum' horror stories and laugh about it. I'm not entirely sure why my mother is the epitome of the anti-Christ when travelling by car. I've certainly never given her reason to push the invisible brake pedal or hang onto the internal door handle like her life depended on it. Those are life choices only she can rationalise.

Not long after my parents moved into their new home, my mum was signed off her work with pleurisy for five weeks. I travelled to and from work alone. The music was up to full volume and the Millenium Falcon occasionally jumped to lightspeed. Weather permitting, naturally.

* * * * * * *

June 2005 – Saturday morning and mum appeared at my front door. Sounds like a perfectly natural occurrence, right? Let me give you a couple of reasons why this situation was odd.

I can count the number of times my mother has visited my house on one hand. She's never in her own home very often, let alone mine. Number two reason, she accepted a cup of tea when I awkwardly offered (caught off guard by the surprise visit). This meant she was intending to stay a while and for someone constantly on the go and busy, this whole setting meant only one thing. Bad news. Maybe a family member had died, or she required a kidney, and I would need to go for compatibility tests immediately.

I was in the kitchen stirring the teas when, from the living room, I heard my mother say very calmly,

"I'm thinking about divorcing your father."

The teaspoon ground to a halt inside the cup. See. Told you. News, of the bad kind.

Chapter 14 – Tech Wiz?

In April 2006, after forty-one years of marriage, my parents called it a day and divorced. As The Rolling Stones affirmed, 'It's All Over Now'. Mum relocated to Galashiels, meaning no more daily commute or quarrels over how fast I was or wasn't going in the car.

She was now living on her own. Strangely, the fact she had full management of the TV remote and no longer had to endure televised football games gave her the most joy. I'm sure there's a whole host of other factors that led up to this life-changing split but I, personally, didn't want to know. There was no family meeting where we all sat around the dining room table, and everyone got a chance to air grievances (if any) over their decision. I know. Some of you will be shocked by that revelation but in my opinion, it was my parents' business, not anyone else's. There was no collateral damage or custody battles over furniture that once belonged to someone's great aunt. They split everything down the middle and went their separate ways. If Carlsberg did divorces.

Mum's new house came with a list of requirements. She had to be sixty or over to qualify for one of the properties and only just made that age when she'd applied. When she moved in, the average age of those already living in the development surely would have plummeted. She was the youngest resident by a country mile. It wasn't long before helping elderly neighbours back to their feet also became part of the requisite.

She bought wallpaper and paint for the new digs with no intention of decorating it herself – after all, what are children for? She changed your diapers so that, one day, you would change her décor. We visited one Saturday morning, mum literally handed us paint brushes and a bag of wallpaper paste, while she put the kettle on. Lorraine (pregnant with her second child) and I traded 'fucking knew it' glances and ten minutes later, the decoration works commenced. In all fairness, it didn't take us long. I went home with clumps of wallpaper paste in my hair and a new t-shirt design I wasn't too keen on.

Mum is still working full time at the chartered accountants' firm, but the role is becoming increasingly more difficult for her. So, a full year later, she bows out and retires gracefully. At sixty-one years of age and having worked her entire life, it was well deserved.

She joins the committee of the housing development's curricular activities, and it wasn't long before she was running up member lists for the weekly bingo and printing menu choices for the day trips away.

With her basic computer skills in the current environment, she instantly becomes the 'tech wiz' which is akin to calling the only university student in the dorm who can make edible scrambled eggs, a Michelin star chef. Previously handwritten coffee morning tickets are soon replaced with printed versions. Obligatory pic of the steaming coffee cup now included. In later years, a cake slice appeared, sometimes a cookie and then a 'fancy' border that framed the important coffee morning details. When the tickets were printed on different-coloured card it was an instant hit. Perhaps even increased sales.

Life is good. Mum is happy in her retirement and with single life in general. She's meeting new friends and feeling useful. She couldn't ask for more.

Chapter 15 – English, but not as we know it

Late July 2006 and Lorraine is rushed into hospital. Again.

Pre-Eclampsia. The reason why I'm driving to the city of Newcastle like Vin Diesel in Fast & Furious 75 (or whatever the current sequel number is). Lorraine is thirty weeks pregnant, and the Borders General Hospital in Melrose have waved the white flag due to a lack of neo-natal intensive care beds, so she's dispatched to The Royal Victoria Infirmary in Newcastle, almost a hundred miles south of Melrose.

It was the dead of night; I was driving this nightmare of a road without any sleep. Most of it is classified as an 'A' road by the Standards for Highways, but I can assure you, whoever graded this particular horror show misplaced their spectacles that day. There are parts of the road that are single track. Straight sections are as rare as hen's teeth and throwing stray sheep over the car bonnet, a complete possibility. If you owned a factory producing ready-made shepherd's pies, this road is your larder. I raced over a cattle grid; it woke me up at least.

I can't even begin to imagine how Lorraine felt doing the same trip in the back of that ambulance, not knowing if her child was going to live. Her due date was early October and I'd previously joked about my sister hanging onto her offspring for a couple more days and then 'setting it free' on Jackie and I's birthday. Stars and planets aligning once more. In retrospect, this entire scenario was a gigantic head fuck.

When we finally arrived, Lorraine was already in theatre having a caesarean section. Jackie, mum and I were directed to the waiting area. Mum was doing her usual verbal worrying and every door that opened had her head swivelling like an R2D2 unit. Jackie and I chatted about a whole host of uninteresting stuff in a bid to pass the time. We checked out the posters on the wall. Reading all about the invariable pitfalls of pre-mature births. I appreciate the medical awareness implications but good grief, really? I made some comment about how good the wall space was for advertising and the NHS were missing a trick with regards to hospital revenue. Jackie laughed. Mum tutted.

We went on to debate whether nurses, doctors, surgeons, and even consultants should get personal sponsorship deals with Nike or Adidas for their uniforms and scrubs. They were professionals after all. Not in the sports sense but did that matter?

I braved a coffee from the vending machine and was midway through it when someone approached us. Lorraine had given birth to a baby boy, and both were doing as well as could be expected. Baby was going to the neo-natal intensive care and Lorraine was currently still in recovery. Mum, right on cue, started crying. Jackie and I cheered 'Ya beauty!' simultaneously, then we all hugged. A mix of pure relief and happiness.

It was almost four in the morning, and as we weren't permitted to see Lorraine or the new arrival, we went home. Jackie and I travelled back to Newcastle a couple of days later and managed to check in on them both.

I remember someone handing me a hospital gown and paper elastic hat to put on. We were then directed to a small sink in the corner of the dark intensive care unit to wash our hands. The intensive care unit itself, looked like the bridge of the Starship Enterprise. Lights of varying colours, monitors, bleeping noises everywhere. I fully expected Captain Kirk to appear from the darkness, yelling "Shields up!"

Right next to the sink was an incubator containing a small, new-born baby with transparent skin. Pointing at the occupant inside and turning to Lorraine, I whispered,

"God look at that. Looks like a wee skinned rabbit."

"That's Lewis," she replied in a hushed tone. "Your nephew."

"Really? That's him?"

I smiled at Jackie, and everyone shuffled around the incubator. He was tiny but perfectly formed. Every now and then his little hand would move, maybe a leg. All sorts of machinery surrounded us. Cables and wires everywhere. Us three numpties, in our paper hats, just staring inside. It was well worth the five hours round trip in the car. Even with my hatred of hospitals, I wouldn't have missed that visit for the world.

On the journey home, Jackie slipped a CD into the car stereo (yes, there's still no Bluetooth or downloaded music yet in my ageing vehicle), and we sang 'If I Could Dream' so loudly that poor Elvis, for the entire three minutes, was demoted to a mere backing singer. That song is still on my playlist today and every time it plays from the random shuffle, I smile. A simple tune that will always evoke a lovely memory in all our lives.

Lewis was in the neo-natal intensive care in Newcastle for two weeks and when he was finally stable enough to travel, he went back to the Borders General. He did some more sprouting in the incubator, amid a series of complications, but seven weeks later my sister took him home.

History dictates the Scots, and the English are considered 'The Auld Enemies'. Nah, not in my opinion. On his birth certificate, my nephew is considered English *shrugs*. If he ever gets to play a sport on an international level, he knows where his roots are *winks*.

Chapter 16 – The odds & sods

For the decade that spanned the years from 2007 to my mums Parkinson's diagnosis in 2017, there was plenty going on.

I relocated to Edinburgh in 2007 and employed at a chartered surveyors' firm. Eric came along in 2008 and he was undergoing a series of corneal transplants around this time. He's been seriously sight impaired from an early age, so these surgeries were necessary. More hospital drop offs and collections for me though. The irony. I should start 'hating' St Lucia or the Maldives. Or disliking big lottery wins. Might start reaping some rewards.

Lorraine and Lewis became regular visitors to the Scottish capital and a year later, they decided to move here and stay. We'd travel to visit mum in Galashiels at the weekends. Occasionally for more decorating works. Mother would define it as 'freshening up'. Lorraine and I describing it (more accurately) as 'taking the pure piss'.

Bob is doing the whole 'single bloke' thing. If he wasn't out around the Hawick pubs at the weekends, he was away on lads' holidays doing the exact same. You're not truly loving life until some Spanish bar owner is attempting to move you out of their pub doorway at 6am using a broom and words of encouragement like 'time to go home'.

My brother would return from these trips, face sunburnt to hell and start entertaining us with horrifying stories of 'great nights out' through bursts of laughter. We'd be sitting there, mouths hanging open and wondering how he'd survived these ordeals.

He met Donna in early 2011 and some semblance of order was finally restored. They got married in 2012 at the Mansfield House Hotel in Hawick. It was a brilliant day.

Jackie is living her independent life. She had a couple of trips away to Australia, visiting friends and family. Never too far away from a glass of wine or gin and tonic though.

My nephew Simon, still living in Hawick, was bringing new life into our worlds. Carly was born in 2014 and Kayla arrived in 2017. Suddenly we're all promoted to the level of 'greatness'. 'Cept Lorraine. She just had to make do and get to grips with being a granny.

July 2014 and absolutely nothing to do with the pressure of being a great aunty, it all went a bit pear shaped.

Eric, Lorraine, Lewis and I arrived at mums for our weekend visit. We were literally five minutes in (the kettle was still boiling) and Jan was poking for an argument. I obliged, as always. My mantra in life, if you're going to do a job, might as well do it properly.

Looking back on it now, the whole outburst was over nothing. Just one of those days where she needed to vent, and I should've recognised it. Hindsight.

Anyway, it kicked off and instead of defusing the situation as I normally would, I threw in a gallon of petrol and struck a match. In the metaphorical sense, of course. When a gap in the verbal blitz arrived, I stormed out of her house mumbling a host of expletives as I went. Since I'd driven them all down, Lorraine, Eric and Lewis had no choice but to follow me out. I sat in the car and watched them all file out of Jan's house. Eric was fighting to get his coat back on and Lorraine looked like a deer in the headlights. On the drive home, conversation was minimal, a nerve pulsed at the side of my forehead for the entire trip. Patience is a virtue. Some people have it. Some people don't. Me? I continually hover around the lower end of the patience scale, if a scale of this nature exists.

Jan and I wouldn't speak to or see each other for a year and a half. During this time, she got her leg caught in the bedcovers and fell, headfirst, into a bookcase shelf in her bedroom. Jackie took her to the hospital for an x-ray, nothing broken but her face was badly bruised, and her eyes were swollen. I'd quite often ask Lorraine or Jackie how she was doing, and they'd always update me without judgement.

Christmas 2014 – Eric and I spent it together. The rest of the family went to Bob's house for dinner. Given that it was the first Christmas without the family, I didn't know what to expect. On

Christmas Eve, Eric and I went to Newmains, North Lanarkshire (about thirty miles west of Edinburgh) to his mum's house and dropped off the presents. Heavy snowfall in the two days previous had made the night-time return journey on the M8 precarious. More so when I discovered the windscreen wash reservoir was empty. Chris Rea was busy singing about 'Driving Home for Christmas' on the car stereo and making it sound like a truly pleasurable experience.

Back in the here and now though, I have a hole the size of a thumb print by way of visibility and even that's reducing rapidly with every car that flew past us. It's quarter past eleven at night on Christmas Eve so there's no hope of a petrol station being open for business. When I found myself sitting at a weird, forty-five-degree angle and my nose almost touching the windscreen, we agreed drastic measures were required. Eric searched the car for a rogue bottle of water. Nothing. On the back seat was a twelve pack of tonic water for our Christmas day gins. He cracked open a tin, rolled the window down and hung out. Naturally, most of the contents went down his arm but just above the howling wind noise, I heard him shout,

"Did any of it reach the windscreen at least? It's freezing out here!"

Unbelievably, a couple of tonic droplets had made it, so I hastily turned on the wipers. A single clear streak appeared right before the wiper blades stuck to the windscreen, in the upright position. We burst out laughing. Eric rolled the window back up and I hit the accelerator. Go on Chris Rea, I dare you to write a ballad about this cluster-fuck.

We made it home in time for Christmas, with five minutes to spare, eleven tins of tonic and a partridge in a pear tree. Eric didn't know it yet, but he was having five G&Ts to my six.

As it happens, our Christmas turned out to be one of the best days ever. We spent the entire day in our pyjamas, watched a selection of feel-good movies and ate a fillet steak dinner from our laps. Even took turns at 'going to the bar'. It was a completely relaxed affair.

Late September of the following year, I swallowed my pride and went down to mums. She had no idea we were coming for a visit and I'd mentally prepared for a variety of outcomes. For example, if she was in the middle of preparing vegetables using a large knife, I'd walk out backwards, real slow and try again some other time.

Lorraine, Eric, Lewis and I sauntered into her living room and when she saw me, her bottom lip crumpled. I gave her a huge cuddle, told her that I missed her large and then ruffled her hair. It's never been mentioned again. Well... until now. Does that even count?

Mid-February 2016 and Bob steps into the 'limelight' again. He and Donna came up to Edinburgh for a weekend visit. Eric's nephew, Kerr (aged ten, same as Lewis) was also staying at our house. Saturday night, so it wasn't long before the chilled beers were out, and the Xbox was fired up. Usual footballing trash talk during games of Fifa and the inevitable family bickering when everyone had an opinion on working through the puzzles in the Tomb Raider game.

Sunday morning, and Bob offered to take us all out for breakfast at Toby Carvery – all you can eat buffet style. We piled in the front doors like the Clampetts and were quickly shown to a table. Kerr sprung up from his chair and encouraged everyone towards the food counter. Bob gently pulled him aside and offered up some advice,

"Little and often is the way to go with these buffets," he said. "There's no sense in grabbing what you can on the first visit. Space it out lad, there's no rush." Eric laughed and winked at Kerr. We carefully selected a few items, under the solid Bob advisement, and made our way back to the table. The conversation, between mouthfuls of sausage and bacon, was pretty much what we were picking on the second visit to the hotplates of wonder. It wasn't long before our plates were clear, and cups drained. We were unsure of the plate etiquette; do we leave them on the table or take them with us? Kerr didn't care, he was already making for the counter.

Bob was walking in front of me when he stopped abruptly and placed the palm of his hand on the side wall. I pointed at the buffet in the opposite direction and said something like, food is this way, Bob. That's the exact point where it all got a bit… messy.

I walked around to face Bob and saw him grab the top of his left arm. Beads of sweat were visible on his forehead and top lip. I grabbed a chair, from the nearby table, and made him sit down. Two off-duty firemen, enjoying their breakfast, came over to help. Bob managed to tell them that he had a pain in his arm, he felt lightheaded and that his view momentarily flipped upside down. It was so disorientating that he'd scrunched his eyelids shut. Someone called an ambulance and when it arrived, Bob and Donna were ushered inside.

The paramedics went through a series of tests (FAST) in the back of the ambulance. They asked Bob to smile at Donna and she confirmed his face had drooped. Eric, Kerr and I were standing in the carpark, staring at the ambulance back doors, when the blue lights and siren started up. One of the paramedics appeared from the side door and said they were going to Edinburgh Royal Infirmary. The three of us watched the ambulance disappear out the carpark. I made a crummy joke to disguise the obvious shock,

"That was a bit extreme," I said. "He could've just asked us to pay the bill, eh?" I turned to face Eric and noticed Kerr's mouth was hanging open. "Guess we're off to the hospital then!" We made our way to the car. Just a typical Sunday morning.

The waiting area of the A&E department was busy. We managed to find three empty chairs and sat down. A man, sitting at the end of our row, was holding a heavily bandaged arm in the air and a woman sitting opposite us, had an obvious swollen foot. Kerr was sitting in between Eric and I, trying not to stare at the wounded around us. The conversation was minimal. Not entirely sure how long we'd been sitting there, when Donna appeared,

"They are still doing tests on Bob," she said. "They don't think it's a stroke or heart attack, the doctor said his heart is strong."

"Where is he now?" I asked. "Still in resus?"

She nodded, "I think they are moving him to A&E soon," she replied. "You guys should be able to see him then. I'll come back when he's been moved."

Thirty minutes later we made our way in to see him. Bob was sitting up; a cardboard sick bowl was lodged between his legs. He was hooked up to a monitor, various numbers on the screen and flashing lights. Several balls of cotton wool were taped to the inside of both his arms. Apart from the lack of colour in his face, he looked alright, considering.

"The manager at Toby Carvery was running after customers fleeing down the drive when you left," I said. "Took him ages to convince them all that it wasn't the food." Bob laughed a little, but I could tell he was worried. We all heard a strange gurgling noise and that's when the shit truly hit the fan. In these current times, we refer to this particular moment as mild vomiting, because the actual volume expelled has traumatised Kerr for life. He pretty much hid behind the cubicle curtain for most of the ordeal.

Donna stood at Bob's bedside and disposed of the full sick bowls in the small sink on the side wall, while passing empty ones over. It was an impressive production line. In between waste disposal dumps, she wiped his mouth and nose. I've never actually witnessed vomit coming out of someone's nose before or considered the lack of oxygen implications because of said act.

Bob would sit upright on the hospital bed and quickly suck in gulps of air on the momentary phases where nothing was being ejected. Donna would use these infrequent times to complain about the leaning tower of full sick bowls in the small sink and insist that someone clears them away before the next deluge. A nurse walked quickly past, pointed in Bob's direction and shouted that, "More anti-sickness drugs were required here!" It was a hive of activity. Eric and I did nothing but stand at the end of the bed and wonder if the cubicle curtain was big enough for the three of us to hide behind.

It would be three different types of anti-sickness medication before the vomiting subsided and Bob fell asleep. We figured he'd be kept in for the night, so the three of us went home. Donna stayed on behind.

At around three in the afternoon, Donna called us to say that Bob had been given all clear and with that, permission to go home, back to Hawick. I was surprised but picked them both up at the Royal Infirmary and Bob (unbelievably) drove the fifty-odd miles back to Hawick.

Monday morning and Bob went to work as he normally would. By lunchtime he'd developed pain across his forehead and at the base of his skull. He gave up an hour later and went home. Tuesday, the symptoms had gradually got worse, so he made a doctor's appointment for the next day and stayed at home. Wednesday, he visited the doctor who advised that Bob had a viral infection and prescribed painkiller medication until the symptoms had passed.

It would be the Thursday evening when he eventually called NHS 24. An ambulance arrived and Bob was carted off to the Borders General Hospital. He doesn't remember a great deal of what happened when he arrived, but he does have a vivid memory of being surround by doctors. He heard labyrinthitis (inflammation of the inner ear) being mentioned but one of the doctors advised doing an MRI scan as he'd noticed that Bob's eyes were flickering.

They carried out an MRI, discovered a swelling on his brain and because the situation may have required a drain, Bob was rushed to Edinburgh's Western General Hospital. More detailed scans were carried out and they confirmed a blood clot on his brain which later turned into a bleed on the lower cerebellum. For us mere mortals without PHDs, and in simple terms, my brother had suffered a big, fat, fuck-you, stroke.

He doesn't recall much of his time at the Western General, but we all do. I remember the first visit where we all filed into a 'quiet' room for the obligatory sit down. There are parts of that conversation where I watched the doctor's lips move but didn't hear any words. Mum was doing her level best to appear strong but as per usual, she was failing miserably. I'd read every poster on the wall behind the doctor's head before I re-joined the conversation and heard about the loss of sensation in his left-hand side. Thereafter, it was all about Bob's young age (forty-two) and intensive physiotherapy being huge factors in his recovery. Of course, I done my own Google research at home and once I had digested the facts, we tackled it head-on, in the typical Kennedy style. We downplayed the seriousness and made jokes at every opportunity.

Three days later and on an evening hospital visit, Bob was in a small ward containing four patients. His bed was the one closest to the ward door. Only two people were allowed in to see him, so the rest of us stood outside in the corridor and peered in the small window. It must have been quite a sight from inside the ward, there was five of us on the other side, all vying for position and noses pressed against the glass. We saw Donna and mum sitting on either side of Bob's bed inside.

Bob lifted his head from the pillow and gently coaxed mum closer so she could hear what he had to say. Someone from our small window gathering outside in the corridor, wiped the condensation from the glass and everyone fell silent. You could've heard a mouse fart when Bob said, "Mum, if I don't make it out of here…"

Mother quickly held up her hand and gestured for Bob to stop talking, "For God's sake," she said. "Don't be like that. You're going to be alright!"

Bob ignored her appeals and carried on, "Mum, I need you to listen," he said croakily. "If I don't make it out of here, I need you to do something for me."

Mum's bottom lip crumpled, and I imagine tears stung her eyes. She (and the rest of us in the corridor outside) leaned in closer, "Oh, son," she managed. "Of course, I will. What do you need?"

Bob gave her a weary look and swallowed hard. "There's a big oak tree," he said. "At the end of our back garden." Mum nodded furiously, "Ok son. What about it?" she replied.

"Has a rock wall beside it," he said. Mum was still nodding. "At the base of that wall, you'll find a huge rock."

Mum urged him on, "Right son. Oak tree, rock wall, big rock." Bob coughed a little and continued.

"You won't be able to miss the big rock, it's black volcanic glass. Has no business in our garden," he said. Mum pulled a disposable hanky from her cardigan sleeve and wiped her nose.

"Promise me," Bob continued. "Find that rock. There's something buried under it that I want you to have."

"What's under it, son?" she asked, hanging onto his every word.

Bob's composure disappeared, he turned his head towards the small window audience in the hospital corridor and gave us all a lopsided smile. He could no longer keep it going and I immediately burst out laughing. In that very moment, the tone for Bob's stroke recovery was firmly set. Minutes later, mum would find out why the Shawshank Redemption movie is still in my top ten list of all time films.

Bob stayed at the Western General for a number of weeks and his recovery was a slow, patient process. He was eventually transferred back to the stroke unit at the Borders General Hospital where they put him in a small side room on his own for a couple of days. An elderly lady required the side room because the female wards were full, so my brother was moved into the general ward. It would be in here where he'd realise just how lucky he'd been. The three other stroke patients, in the ward, were unable to do anything for themselves and Bob spent most of the time helping these guys out. The nurses took pity on him and, once the elderly lady patient had gone from the side room, Bob was moved back in.

It would be a few weeks later, when he wasn't dragging his leg or falling over, that he would finally get to go home. I'm mightily proud of my brother. The Golden Child dealt with it admirably and never lost his wicked sense of humour throughout. Get busy living or get busy dying. I'm glad my brother opted for the positive life direction – it's really all this family knows.

In May 2017, Eric and I went on holiday to Albufeira in Portugal. Sam, one of my very best friends, came along with us. It was supposed to be four of us on the trip but that's a different story. Maybe for the next book. She almost didn't go herself until we persuaded her otherwise.

The resort had its own pool and for days Sam had been informing us that, in her younger years, she used to do backflips into the water.

Casually and with a devilish grin, I asked, "What do you mean used to? Should be able to still do it right?" It was a veiled dare and before I could add substance to it – she was off her lounger and hurriedly walking to the deep end. Early morning so not many people around. I grabbed my phone and recorded the show.

She'd executed the backflip perfectly. Minimal splash as she entered the water. Eric and I were suitably impressed. A few seconds later, bubbles appeared on the surface of the water and Sam shot up like she was auditioning for the next season at SeaWorld in Florida. I fully expected her to be standing on the nose of a dolphin called Dandelion, who would delicately drop her off at the side of the pool and then demand a fish reward. I was laughing uncontrollably. When her face collided with the side of the pool, I wiped laughter tears from my eyes and sat upright. The recording ended when I dropped my phone and rushed over to help.

Sam, holding her nose as we walked back to the loungers, said, "I can still do backflips! How awesome is that! Did it look good?"

"Let me see your nose," I demanded.

"It's cool. I've broken it like five times already in my rugby playing days."

"Let me see it. Are you ok?"

"Yeah, I'm fine. It's just throbbing a wee bit."

When she bent over to pick up her beach towel her nose was, in fact, not fine and neither was she. The colour drained from her face, and she sprinted off, as best she could in her flipflops, to the poolside toilet. Eric said, "God's sake. You'll need to go see if she's alright!"

As soon as I got to the toilet doors, I could hear Sam gagging. I felt a mixture of emotions. Concern obviously, for my friend, but a hospital trip while I was on holiday? I knocked on the cubicle door and secretly decided that if medical attention was required, she was going alone. I'd even phone her a taxi. The door opened and she appeared wearing a fake 'nothing to see here' smile.

"For the love of Christ woman, yer nose is spread across yer face!" I said... sympathetically.

"I feel alright now, thought I was going to pass out there for a second."

"Do we need to go to the hospital?"

"Nah. I'm alright. Honestly. It'll be fine."

We made our way back to the sun loungers for a day of bathing. The sun was out and there wasn't a cloud in the sky. I urged Sam to put more sunscreen on and passed her a beer. Throughout the day, I periodically tossed little pebbles at her just to make sure she was still with us. It's true. I'm like... the best friend... ever.

That same night and dressed in her pyjamas, Sam took her bashed up nose to the supermarket because she'd ran out of wine. Typical 'show must go on attitude'. If her ear was hanging off, she'd ask you for a stapler and carry on regardless. We've been friends for well over three decades. She's not only a great mate – she's my sister from another mister. Family... but not actually related. Same deal as aunty Betty.

When we got back home from Portugal, mum still had the hand tremor. She made an appointment with the doctor and so it began. Three months later, and just like that, she had Parkinson's disease.

Chapter 17 – A New Hope

When I originally came up with the idea of writing this, it was supposed to be a personal compilation of funny wee stories, from the time my mum was diagnosed with Parkinson's to present day. Nothing more. I was going to print my insipid drivel and along with the rolled up ancestral tree, pass everything to the generation below my own and say here, this is what we have gathered so far, keep it updated and tell the next lot to do the same. Mum and I had literally sweated blood and tears for this information, so it had to be preserved.

Somewhere along the line, in a random sister conversation, I happen to mention my 'writing little stories' when Lorraine barged in with a tirade of comments,

"Where's the context though? You can't just write these short stories and expect it to be something. Need to give the readers an idea of what's going on and who it's going on with."

Alright, Barbara Cartland. Calm yer jets. Who said anything about a published book?

I had no intention of writing a book. In my early twenties, I'd already tried. Shipped out a couple of manuscripts, dipped my toe into the published author pool – the water proved to be far from lukewarm. The consensus was, sure, the style of writing was passable but the storylines… 'required work'.

Perhaps my personality traits were more of a hindrance than a help.

Fun fact number one – I have a low boredom threshold so getting this far has surprised many people. Even my mother. A recent conversation is described below and for the jury, marked as exhibit 'A',

> Mum: This is the fourth telephone call in less than an hour. What do you want? I'm trying to watch Downton Abbey.

Me: [ignoring obvious disgruntlement] You know when granny worked as a civil servant – do you know what she actually did for a job?
Mum: I've paused mid episode for this? Why are you asking?
Me: Just trying to get the details right. For context you know?
Mum: You still working on this story? I thought you'd have given up on it by now.
Me: Your support is overwhelming. I believe I may cry.
Mum: Your sarcasm is overwhelming. I believe I may hang up.
Me: Can you just end my pain and answer the damn question?
Mum: She worked in various government offices. Not sure what she did for a job though.
Me: Fucks sake. I went through all of that for nothing.
Mum: Stop swearing.
Me: Your input is greatly appreciated.
Mum: You're welcome. Anytime!

Fun fact number two – I have, over the years, racked up a sizeable amount of half-arsed ideas but very few have ever come to fruition. The reason being… please refer to fun fact number one.

Fun fact number three – As previously explained, I have little or no patience. Not exactly a healthy attribute for most things in life. I'm working on it.

To summarise, I'll come up with a hare-brained scheme, give it my full attention until the low boredom threshold kicks in and then move on to something else due to a lack of patience. My school report cards, and the teachers comments therein, are entirely accurate. I'm willing to bet some of those directives were written through clenched teeth. Phrases like 'complete bell-end' or 'spawn of Satan' probably sprung to their minds instantly but were discarded for more politically correct remarks such as 'needs to concentrate more' or 'apt to talk too much'.

I am what I am. Someone should write a song about that. Wait…

I'm sadly lacking in the empathy and sympathy departments. Growing up, and throughout my life, I was never lavished with either of these qualities. Getting a hug from either of my parents? Meant you were secretly being frisked. If you done anything incredibly stupid and hurt a body part, my parents would ask 'is it gushing blood?' or 'is there anything hanging off?'

If you answered no to both these vital triage investigations, then you were considered fit for duty. Sometimes offered an Elastoplast for your 'efforts'. The fact your wound required ten sutures and the blood loss, considered moderate by general medical standards, didn't factor. Mum said a plaster would suffice and you went on to wear that patch of honour like a Victoria Cross medal.

You'd suffer periods of light headedness throughout the day and succumb to a mild infection because the plaster would inevitably slide off your wound at some point. You were too busy being knee deep in muck, without a care in the world, to even notice the protective covering had decamped.

Mum would rip you a new arsehole when you got home because you didn't keep the plaster on, then proceed to clean your wound like it was a dirty front doorstep. Full-on elbow grease, beads of sweat visible on her forehead while she muttered, under her breath, about how wonderful a single, childless life would be. I'm sure she never meant any of it. Thank God some Scottish fella invented penicillin. Pre-antibiotics? I'd have lost body parts for sure.

Allegedly, I do have some good qualities. Couldn't think of any personally but when I questioned family and friends, the overall theme was that I was far from the arsehole I consider myself to be.

I'm a natural problem solver. Instead of shelling out quotes like "aw that's a shame" or "how awful" (empathy/sympathy), I'm more likely to pitch in with actual solutions in a real effort to lighten the situation, making it easier and more manageable to deal with.

I don't ever sweat the small stuff and worrying about 'what ifs', in my opinion, is a waste of time and energy. Let's just deal with the issue as and when it happens (my mother = exact opposite). "It'll be fine" is my natural endorphin. This simple quote shakes down most anxieties, I throw it around like a chef does salt and pepper. Things in general are, and usually will be, fine. If not, there's a viable solution to every problem.

Regrets? By definition this word means sadness or disappointment. I absolutely will not live my life rooting around in the past, mulling over choices I made years ago that ultimately determined where I am now. I tried and failed. I moved on. I'm neither sad nor disappointed. Who knew!

My family are number one on my list of priorities. If any required a left nipple or an eyeball (for whatever reason) I'd pop some serious painkillers and rummage in the cutlery drawer for a suitable utensil. They'd do the same for me... possibly.

Approachable and non-judgemental were also popular assessments. Compliments I accept with dignity. It's only when you ask others how they portray you, do you find out where you sit in life (I'm rarely offended so their comments came thick and fast). By far and away the most common attribute assigned to me was... direct. I am direct.

Over the years, I've learned that my directness isn't everyone's cup of tea. Some people can't handle the reflection in the mirror I provide and would rather skirt around in the grey area to avoid it. It's cool. I get it. If I offend anyone with being direct, then I've ultimately made you angry or upset. This wasn't ever my intention, so perhaps it's a situation you needed to address a long time ago and haven't because the middle, non-productive route was safe, comfortable? Can you imagine a world without the procrastination space? Where everyone just blurted out actual truths and opinions? With no offence meant or taken? The time saved alone... monumental.

Sure, not all the reflections I dish out are 100% accurate in every case but my goal was to open the gate, cut through the crap and encourage a new train of thought to pass right on through. One that you couldn't see for the self-made trees. What you do with the locomotive is completely your prerogative. Re-invent your life perhaps? Or did it make you want to grab a lightsabre and play the role of Darth Vader to my Luke? That's a chance I'll always take in life. Hell, I'll even offer you my wrist for the overhead slash when the times comes. Just the things I do. You're welcome.

I'm fully aware of my direct and to-the-point superpower. I've walked into plenty of family functions where mum has felt the need to pull me aside at the entrance doors and remind me of the decorum I should exhibit. Now and again, her words had a pleading feel to them. I'd slap her gently on the back saying, "Don't worry mother, I got this," and she'd raise a suspicious eyebrow. At random intervals, during these family gatherings, she'd throw me 'the look' thus indicating I was, or had already, taken it too far.

That last paragraph is quite possibly the reason my family are marginally worried regarding the contents of this book. Don't worry guys… I got this. It'll be fine.

Finally, a note to all who survive me. If the following quote isn't in my obituary, I will squeeze my forthright ass out of your bedroom wall and in my apparition form, proceed to haunt you all for eternity.

I am terribly sorry if you didn't like my harsh honesty, but I didn't care much for your sugar-coated bullshit either.

Chapter 18 – The Empire strikes back

If you haven't watched any of the Star Wars original trilogy, then good grief. Where have you been? Consider this an education. When you get into the nuts and bolts of this film, I often wonder if George Lucas delved into the lives that people led after WW2 for ideas and movie plot lines. Take my granny/mum adventures for example.

In the mid-1990s, my mum found her real father and then later, a brother she knew nothing about. There's no death star arrangement or anyone frozen in carbonite, that we're aware of, and I've yet to see any signs of 'the force' in either uncle Tom or my mother.

In fact, the only weapon I've ever seen her wield is a slipper. She didn't exactly swirl the slipper around her head and perform the perfect gymnast floor routine, simultaneously. None of that. The plastic-soled munition was simply dangled off her big toe and we knew that a can of whoop ass was imminent. The simple, yet effective, action was enough to make us disappear into the background and start behaving.

I'm fairly certain William Harold Schaeppi wasn't running around wearing a black, plastic bag cape and breathing like he smoked sixty cigarettes a day either. He did live in a galaxy far, far away though…

Maybe my granny (Alice) recognised his dark side qualities emerging and purposely left him at the dock because the ship that arrived was just too crazy to board. Part of the Rebel force maybe, and not the British Secret Service? If you all weren't aware of how my mind works, you do now.

Chapter 19 – The Return of the Jedi

At some point, I do have to switch from context to the actual short stories from my journal. I've done a fair amount of rambling on about my family and how we cope with adversities on this journey called life.

When mum's Parkinson's disease came along, it was just another pothole in the road. Yeah, it rattled our kidneys and made us curse the lack of road maintenance, but you know what? We carried on. Dealt with it. Still dealing with it.

You'll realise by now; we don't do grim or sombre. In funeral terms, we'd be a humanist affair. Celebrating a life lived, rather than a death mourned. It's not to everyone's liking but neither is Marmite and if you believe I give a flying hoot, or live my life based on other people's judgements, then you're sadly mistaken. I spread my wisdom like you would Nutella on warm toast. Plentiful and occasionally, wildly inappropriate.

My nephew Lewis has Asperger's syndrome. A form of autism, possibly a result of his premature birth. During his primary school years, he suffered a god-awful amount of bullying. Other kids, who were completely unaware of the syndrome, poked fun at him. In doing so, they had brought to his attention that he was different and for the most part, he didn't care.

Ensconced in our family unit, there was no differential. At the age of four, he was reading you stories from books. History was, and still is, his favourite genre. When you gave him a cuddle, he went stiff as a board. Asked him for a kiss? He reacted like you'd thrown used toilet roll in his face.

I remember 'Santa Claus' left him a huge encyclopaedia for Christmas and a couple of history books from WW1 and WW2, the delight on his face was indisputable. Getting him to actually believe some old dear, dressed in a red suit, slipped down your non-existent chimney, delivered these gifts and countless others to children everywhere on earth, in one night, was a tad ambitious. He never bought it. The questions were endless. In the end we responded with 'no comment' and eventually, we pleaded the fifth.

At Halloween, Lorraine made him a 'tin' helmet and that topped off the full khaki soldier uniform perfectly. She even gave him a couple of face scars and a sling for his 'broken' arm in later years, when he was going for the 'walking wounded' look. He loved it.

In High School, that's where his shields were finally pierced. Puberty kicked in and suddenly things mattered. From the outside, there was no issue. With Asperger's, if you want brutally honest answers, you don't ask vague questions like "how was school today?" Cue me and my hatred of the vague. We worked out the correct form of interrogation (the desk lamp shining right in his face was hilarious but non-productive) and finally the truth spilled out. He wasn't visibly upset but knowing him inside and out, we were fully aware of the impact. I mentally opened the chocolate spread jar and grabbed a butter knife – wisdom incoming!

"Lewis, who on hell's earth tries that hard to fit in when you're naturally born to stand out?"

I could see him digesting it. Contemplating. I grabbed him in for a cuddle, met the rigid board.

"For God's sake, put your arms around my spare tyre waist and hug like you mean it!"

I heard him chuckle and that was it. The battalion had stormed the bridge and making for the portcullis. The dark side eliminated.

At the time of writing this (could be a decade before it ever gets published), nephew Lewis (NL on text messages) is sixteen years old, freely gives out hugs and never misses an opportunity to tell you that he loves you. He also has a crew of pals that I believe are called bruddas (brothers) and, other people's conjecture? Shrugged off with consummate ease. The balance truly restored.

Chewbacca, punch in the co-ordinates and take us to lightspeed. Destination; A compilation of short stories about

Parkinson's disease. Don't assume it's a grim affair. Alternative therapy is more accurate.

Chapter 20 – No animals were harmed in this story

I opened mum's living room door and 0.002 seconds later she announced,

"I need a new handbag."

There was no 'hello' or 'how are you'. Just this one-line statement. Like she had sat all morning, waiting for us to arrive, saying it over and over in her head so she wouldn't forget.

"Yours get stolen?" I asked.

"Nope."

"You give it to the charity shop by accident?"

"What? No."

I picked up her current handbag and dangled it from my finger,

"Oh wait! It's not been stolen. It's right here; condition suggests that no replacement is necessary. How weird is that?!"

She sighed. "Why is everything a circus with you?"

I put the handbag down. Ok, I'll indulge her,

"We're fine by the way, the drive here was most excellent, minimal traffic and nice to see you. Mother dearest, please enlighten us. Why do you need a new handbag?" I walked into the kitchen and put the kettle on. From there I heard her say,

"Can't carry the bag in my right hand anymore. Yesterday, at the bus stop, people were looking at me funny."

"Are you making a point soon?" I gathered the cups, took the milk from the fridge.

"My hand is shaking so bad it looks like I'm carrying a ferret around in my bag and I'm no getting lifted by the police for animal abuse!" she'd said it quickly, embarrassed almost. The kettle popped off. I heard Eric chuckle as I walked back into the living room.

"You have a ferret? Where you get that? Pet shop?" It was my attempt at reducing the high level of drama that was brewing.

"No, I don't have a ferret!"

"That's alright then. Police won't find anything in the shake down. You'll be fine." I walked back to the kitchen. "Tea or coffee?"

"Will you take me to go buy a new handbag? I just need to go brush my hair." I turned around and saw her scuttle past the kitchen doorway.

"Here's a suggestion" I said, "If you're interested?" She was already in the bathroom, looking for her comb. "What? Yeah sure. Go for it," she replied.

I couldn't resist, "Don't you mean, go ferret?"

"Pauline!" she was trying not to laugh.

"Why don't you just carry your handbag... wait for it... in your left hand?"

Eric and I heard her gasp. She appeared at the bathroom door, one side of her hair perfectly groomed, the other side... clearly not. I smiled.

"I've never carried a handbag in my left hand. That's just wrong." She disappeared back into the bathroom. Eric and I traded looks. I leaned against the kitchen door frame, with my arms crossed. If ever something was teed up perfectly, this was it.

"How do you know it's wrong, if you've never done it?"

When she came back to the living room, the hair was in perfect order. She picked up the handbag and put it in her left hand. Walked around the living room, clutching the 'offensive' article, trying it out.

"God no! Feels like I've put my knickers on inside out AND back to front!" she dropped the bag like it had spontaneously combusted. The prosecution rested. I had nothing more to offer. I took the car key fob from my jeans pocket and said,

"Get your coat then." Before I'd even finished the sentence, she was making for the front door.

An hour later, I was finally drinking a cup of coffee and mum had a new shoulder, crossover handbag.

Chapter 21 – The cousin from Australia

Before I pull at this yarn, I do need to explain a couple of things. My mum drinks very little by way of alcohol. There was a time she could hoover it up like a sailor on annual leave but these days, not so much. At Christmas time she's been known to partake in a small glass of bubbles but even then, it's down to the occasion and very rarely does she ever finish it. This night was very different...

Mum had come to Edinburgh, under the guise of visiting Eric and I for the weekend. "It'll be lovely spending the weekend with you both," she proclaimed. More accurately, it meant she wanted to go shopping in the stores that aren't available in her hometown of Galashiels, with door-to-door 'taxi' rides and three-square meals that she didn't need to cook.

I loathe and despise shopping. More so when you're trawling these stores with the woman who brought me into this world. Every item, on every shelf must be touched at least once. Clothing is always tested for durability (she'll hold both ends of said article and firmly snap the material). The entire store will be inspected. Even if she's there with the intention of buying a bar of soap, you'll find yourself in the garden section and she'll be opening shed doors, wandering in. The urge to push the door closed and lock her inside is always strong.

Of course, you'll leave without the soap, then it's onto the next store for a repeat performance. Five hours into the horrifying ordeal, she'll buy something too big to take back home with her on the train and now she's bagged herself a more pleasant car trip down instead.

On this weekend, our cousin Linda and her friend from Australia were here for a visit. They stayed at Lorraine's house. After dinner, I drove mum and Eric around to see them. When we got there, a bottle of prosecco was doing the rounds and since it was a special occasion, mum took the glass on offer. I made a cup of tea.

Several glasses of bubbling fizz later, the conversation was in full swing and stories from the 'good ole days' were, naturally, hot topics. We hadn't seen Linda in over forty years so there was a lot to cover.

I'm not sure how many drinks mum had but getting her back in the car was a chore. From the backseat, she babbled incoherent nonsense and at one point, even had a two-sided conversation with herself. It was mildly amusing.

When we got back home, she latched onto the living room door handle in a bid to stabilise herself. I grabbed her arm and said,

"What are you doing? Let go of the handle."

"I can't," she mumbled.

"You can, just let go. The door isn't going anywhere."

"I can't."

"You need to. Unless you want to stand there all night?"

"I can."

"What? Let go of the door?"

"No... I can stand here all night, is what I meant."

I started unpeeling fingers from the handle. She protested. I leaned into her ear and, through clenched teeth, said,

"Let go of the fucking door handle or I'll tip a basin of cold water over your head."

A mischievous glint appeared in her eyes, "Go on then," she said.

"Are you kidding me? What are you? Like twelve years old?"

She laughed and snorted. "You wish!" Being unsure of the reasoning behind that particular blurt out I carried on.

"Let... go... of... the... handle or I will lose my shit."

I could see the calculation going on behind her eyes. The fight diminishing. I was still picking at her fingers by way of a backup plan.

"I'll let go but only because I want to, not because you told me to!"

"Sure. That's an excellent decision. You go for it."

She let go and fell backwards a little. I caught her arm, guided her towards the sofa. She launched herself down on it. I searched in her overnight bag for pyjamas and medication. Handing over a filled glass of water, I offered,

"Here. You'll need to take your medication."

"I'm alright. I don't want anything to eat."

I held the medication in my cupped hand, "It's not food. It's your drugs."

Mum peered down at my feet. "Is the floor sliding away?"

"Never mind the floor. Take your meds."

"Are you offering me drugs now? I don't do drugs."

"You do, for your Parkinson's."

"I take drugs for the guy on television?"

I sighed. "For the love of Christ woman, will you just, for once, do as you're told?!"

She tossed the medication in her mouth and slugged the water. I'm certain one of the tablets disappeared between the seat cushions, but I had little to no fucks to give at this stage.

I passed her the pyjamas and said, "You need to put these on."

"It's too early, I'm not going to bed."

"Newsflash! It's almost one in the morning, and you ARE going to bed. Get your jeans off, come on."

She unbuckled the belt at her waist and out of the blue, started giggling. It was a full-on belly laugh twenty seconds later. I lifted her legs, grabbed the bottom of her jeans, and started pulling. The leather sofa was hindering our progress. Traction, non-existent. A moment later and still laughing, she was half on, half off the sofa, hands flapping above her head searching for an anchor. That's when my last nerve called it a day and finally shredded.

I spun her legs around, dropped them on the sofa. Shoved a cushion under her head and tucked a blanket around her chin. She was asleep before I turned out the light.

Chapter 22 – Touché

Mum called me on the Thursday night and announced she was coming for another weekend visit. I tentatively dipped a toe in the 'mood water',

"Lorraine is having a barbeque on Saturday night; it's supposed to be sunny. You alright with that?" It was a loaded question. Our 'tin nights' are rare. I can count on one hand the scarce number of days, in the Scottish capital, where the ball of fire in the sky is to our favour. We, siblings, grasp these freak opportunities and gather spontaneously. I've witnessed Jackie and Bob make it to Lorraine's house, an hour after receiving the tin night text. Considering they live an hour and a half away and probably stopped for provisions, it's impressive. Much alcohol is consumed. Occasionally, even neighbours join in. AKA mum's definition of pure hell.

"Sure. I need to go to IKEA if anyone will take me?"

Whatever she wanted from IKEA, she wanted it real bad. That much was clear. I was shocked, tried not to let it show in my response. She knew a trip to IKEA would shrink my very soul.

It's a store where they actively encourage child participation, the mini shopping trolleys are evidence of this fact. Akin to supplying pre-cut lengths of rope to the Boston strangler or flashing your organ donor card to Hannibal Lecter. I witnessed a kid pull a set of curtains down from the display, wear the ensemble (pole and all) like a batman cape and proceed to launch his small frame into a metal floor basket of scatter cushions. No one batted an eyelid. I would much rather excavate my own kneecaps, with a toothpick, than enter the Scandinavian revolving doors of mayhem.

"Great!" I replied enthusiastically. "What train you getting and what time will I pick you up?"

"You alright with that?" mum asked.

"Yep. Absolutely!"

Let the battle of wills commence. I know a disguised touché when I hear it. To anyone else, this whole conversation is completely normal, benign. It meant something very different in this dynamic. Little did she know… I had formulated a plan.

I called Lorraine immediately, told her mum was coming up. "Eh? Did you tell her we're getting the tin out?" she asked.

"I did. She wants someone to take her to IKEA. This is our penance."

We settled it in the usual grown-up fashion the very next day. Lorraine lost. She'll learn someday that choosing paper never wins, certainly not three times in a row.

While I put my feet up and rested for this evening's fare, Lorraine chummed the old dear to IKEA. Judging by the text messages I received from Lorraine, amid trawling of the aisles, avoidance of the mini trolleys and unruly kids, it was a 'pleasant affair'. She was being sarcastic and protesting but I didn't care. An hour later, she called me,

"Mum face-planted outside IKEA."

"God's sake Lorraine. Did you push her? Was it all too much for you? Tad savage in my opinion."

"I didn't even see it happen, she was walking behind me, just heard the landing."

"She alright?"

"Says she is, more embarrassed than anything else."

"What time are you cranking up the tinnage?"

"Bob says he and Donna will be here about two o'clock," she replied. "When you come round, can you bring a bag of ice and a couple of limes?"

"Sure, I'll see you in a bit."

When we arrived, Lorraine was flipping burgers and giving a full account of this afternoon's visit to the concrete. Mum was trying to get comfortable in the foldaway deck chair; at regular intervals, and throughout the story, she said things like, "it was embarrassing," or, "never been more embarrassed in my life."

Apparently, mum had missed the last step when they were leaving the store and, "full-on timbered." She didn't even have time to put her arms out and dampen the fall. Lorraine picked her up and sat her on the step until she'd regained some composure. IKEA members of staff began appearing from all over. A potential compensation claim will do that.

"Hi! I'm Bruce and fully trained in first aid," he looked at Lorraine, pointed at mum and said, "Who do we have here?"

Lorraine explained what happened. Bruce carried on,

"Oh dear! Are you still in one piece? Does anything hurt?"

Mum shook her head and quickly replied, "I'm fine! Just give me a minute." She was rubbing her shoulder, Bruce noticed and in his best teacher-attempting-to-reason-with-a-child voice said,

"Are you sure? Do you have pain in your shoulder? Might be worth a wee visit to A&E for an x-ray, no?"

Mum was annoyed. She knew Bruce was only trying to help but her wounded pride let rip, "For God's sake. I'm ok!" she blasted.

Bruce wasn't convinced. He gently coaxed Lorraine to the side and when they were out of earshot, he whispered, "I think your mum is in shock. You want me to phone an ambulance?"

Ever the diplomat, Lorraine replied, "Bruce, it's not shock. If she needs to go for an x-ray, I'll take her myself. We're good."

He persisted, "It's shock alright. Look, her hand is visibly shaking. It's a classic sign."

Lorraine put her hand on Bruce's arm, "That, my friend, is Parkinson's disease."

"Oh! I didn't realise! Sorry. I get carried away sometimes!"

"It's fine. Can you stay with her while I bring the car around?" Lorraine asked.

"Sure. Consider it done!"

When they got back home, Lorraine suggested the x-ray again, but mum had shot the idea down in flames. Several times. I found an empty chair and poured my first glass of chilled rose wine. Was busy admiring the condensation forming on the outside of the glass when I felt the need to confirm mum was ok,

"Now... mother... before I slurp this pink nectar, are you quite sure you don't need someone to take you to the hospital? For your own peace of mind?"

She gave me 'the look'. The only thing missing was a slipper dangling from her big toe. I settled into the patio chair and sipped the alcohol delight. The sun was shining. Music was playing in the background and the general, hilarious chit-chat was ongoing.

Not quite sure of the actual time but at some point, mum began complaining about a sharp pain in her side. In all honesty, I was too hammered to notice it at first. Bob and I were busy discussing Scottish independence. Unclear as to why that topic had even been selected but we were in full flight when Lorraine tapped me on the shoulder.

"Think mum needs to go for an x-ray."

When you're three sheets to the wind, it takes a while for information, such as this, to sink in. Once it did, I fashioned an intellectual reply, "Eh? How come?"

Lorraine, who was in a similar state of alcohol ruin, gathered her thoughts and continued, "Says her side is sore and she's struggling to breathe," she'd slurred her way through most of this sentence, but I got the gist of it. Sort of.

"Fuck's sake," I drained the last of the wine in my glass (typical Scot), got up from the chair and staggered into the house. Mum was sitting on the sofa, TV remote in hand and she was busy flicking through the channels.

I pointed my thumb towards the outside party area, could feel myself swaying and blurted out, "Lorraine says you're struggling to breathe?"

Mum looked up, "Yeah. It's sore when I breathe in. Probably nothing to worry about." With hands on my hips, I rolled my eyes like a petulant child and made my way back outside.

"Does anyone have the number for NHS 24?" I'm fuzzy as to who supplied the information, but I heard someone say '111'. I picked up my mobile phone and dialled the number. Had to close one eye to see the numbers on the keypad. Slurred my way through a 'conversation' and the result was that a mobile doctor would come out and 'take a look'. I hung up and made my way back inside. Mum was engrossed in an episode of 'Murder She Wrote'.

"There's a doctor coming to see you." I blurted out.

"A what? Who called for a doctor?" she was visibly aghast.

"I did. So… there!" It was my punitive attempt at closing down the exchange. In my drunken stupor, I stumbled back outside and left mum alone with Jessica Fletcher.

Once I announced the impending arrival of said General Practitioner, there was a flurry of activity. Cans of beer were suddenly 'hidden' from view and Lorraine decided it was a great time to recycle the empty bottles. I flopped back into the chair and grabbed my empty wine glass. Eric refilled it and the political debate carried on.

Twenty minutes later, the doctor appeared. She was a lovely lady. I believe I offered her a glass of wine which she, sensibly, declined. We all piled into the living room behind her. She asked mum a series of questions, got her stethoscope out, asked Lorraine about the fall earlier in the day, received a garbled response, chuckled a little and then carried on with the assessment. Desist with your judgement please. It was a sunny Saturday night in Scotland. Like a lunar eclipse or a sighting of Haley's comet by way of rarity.

The nice lady doctor insisted mum go for an x-ray at the Edinburgh Royal Infirmary. She explained that it wasn't an emergency, and we should make our own way down there. How that was going to happen was a mystery. I'd watched the entire scenario unfold with one eye closed and a voice in my head saying, 'party is over dude, sober up'. The doctor left: we called a taxi.

When we arrived at A&E, only one person was allowed to accompany mum into the department. Eric nudged me with his elbow and pushed me forward. He and Bob made their way back to the waiting area as mum and I were escorted inside.

I remember hitting a wall of noise. It was absolutely heaving. The A&E department of the Royal Infirmary is a complete square of numbered booths on the outside, with an administration centre in the middle. We followed a nurse to one of the booths. To be fair, there's not much of this ballgame that I remember. Details are sketchy. Mum was sitting in the chair opposite me. There was a hospital bed between us, filling the void.

For once, mum looked relaxed. She had already considered this hospital visit as a 'just to confirm nothing was wrong' experience. Normally, I would have agreed and taken it all in my stride but, in my inebriated state, I had doubts.

I'd love to say that ten minutes later a nurse opened the curtain and asked mum to board the wheelchair she had provided. I have no idea how long we were sitting there. I think I woke up when the nurse arrived. Mum shuffled over to the wheelchair, and I followed them both to a side room.

In this side room, I remember an elderly woman, also in a wheelchair, and she was flanked by two younger ladies. Bookends. I'd decided they were bookends. One of the younger women began stroking the back of the old woman's hair and offered comforting words like 'it'll be alright'. Mum and I watched the kind gesture unfold.

I leaned over, stroked mum's arm and through a drunken haze mumbled, "It's cool! This is cool! Absolutely nothing to worry about!" I was being an arse. Mum tapped the back of my hand and laughed a little. She was humouring me; I was too stewed to care or be annoyed.

Another nurse appeared at the door and called mum's name. I instantly woke up.

"That's us mum!" Again, I have no clue what was going on, but I felt obliged to act like my comprehension level was completely normal. Mum was duly wheeled out of the side room; I followed on behind.

"It's just your mum we need for the x-ray, make your way back to the booth and I'll bring her back when she's done," the nurse said.

It was an easy instruction and the nurse had said it as she was dragging mum backwards in the wheelchair. Mum was smiling a 'don't worry, I'll be fine' message but seeing her disappear behind the automatic doors, without me, was just plain weird. I turned around to face the central administration desk and quickly learned, I had absolutely no idea what booth we'd previously vacated. Fuck.

I zigzagged my way to the hub in the middle. Getting a nurse, in this area, to acknowledge my need for answers, was a trifle difficult. I get it. I'm as pissed as a fart and completely unaware of what's happening around me. I started talking to myself. Come on Pauline, get this act together.

Finally, someone took pity and directed me to the correct booth. I perched myself on the end of the bed and pulled the mobile phone from my pocket. I text Eric a cryptic, unintelligible message. As I hit send, I found myself moving backwards. I looked around the room. It took me a while to realise, it was my own doing. If you lean on a bed with wheels, it will move until resistance is met. I'm glad it was the back wall of the booth. Could've ended up in the hospital car park otherwise.

When Eric and Bob appeared like superheroes, from the madness, I was instantly relieved. They had somehow managed to evade the eagle-eyes at the reception and made their way inside. I could feel my bottom lip crumple. Eric directed me outside and Bob stayed behind.

"You never saw her getting dragged away though, Eric! She just looked like a frail, old woman in pain!" I was inconsolable at this stage. Tears were streaming down my face. My arms started flailing around and a couple of times, I stumbled backwards but the slurred words just kept on coming. Eric intervened,

"Your mum is going to be ok. You know that. There'll be nothing on this x-ray and in the morning, this will be something that we'll laugh about. Trust me."

He was offering a modicum of perspective and deep down, I knew he was right. A moment of silence followed. I was mentally sucking it up. Getting a grip. Having a word with myself. I took a deep breath and, using the sleeve of my jacket, wiped my nose. We bumbled our way back to the A&E doors and slipped past the security detail once more.

Bob was sitting on the end of the bed when we eventually got back to the right booth. Eric and I did two full circuits of the department before reaching our destination. We even managed an impromptu visit to a random elderly lady in another cubicle, with a dislocated finger. I think she was pleased to see us…

Every room, every curtain looks the same! Not easy when you have one eye closed, and a skinful of alcohol.

Mum wasn't there. I pulled up a chair and was about to throw myself upon it when she appeared from behind the curtain, swiftly followed by a doctor carrying a medical chart. A true 'Stars in their Eyes' television moment. Tonight, Matthew, we're going to be Kenny Rogers and Dolly Parton. Missing the dry ice fog behind them, warm applause, and glittery outfits, obviously.

Instead of belting out the timeless classic that is Islands in the Stream, the doctor reported nothing untoward on the x-rays. Mum had maybe torn a shoulder muscle in the fall. He handed over a prescription for pain killers and bid us a good evening. We called another taxi to take us all home.

I woke up the next morning feeling slightly ropey, managed to cook breakfast for everyone without losing the contents of my stomach and in the afternoon, drove mum home. From nights like these, memories are made. I'm just glad I have a vague recollection of it. Touché mother. Touché.

Chapter 23 – Everyone likes a visitor

I did say I would impart my meagre knowledge of PD throughout this book. Here's another piece of the disease puzzle. Dopamine. Where for art thou?

Parkinson's disease is caused by a loss of nerve cells in the part of the brain called the substantia nigra (it's ok, you don't need to remember this). Nerve cells in this part of the brain are responsible for producing a chemical called dopamine. What is dopamine? I hear you ask. Well…

Dopamine acts as a messenger between the parts of the brain and nervous system that help control and co-ordinate body movements. If these nerve cells die or become damaged, the amount of dopamine in the brain is reduced. This means the part of the brain controlling movement cannot work as well as normal, causing movements to become slow and abnormal. Hand, leg tremors, etc.

The loss of nerve cells is a slow process. The symptoms of Parkinson's usually only start to develop when around 80% of the nerve cells in the substantia nigra have been lost. So, Mr Dopamine? Where did you go?

It's not known why the loss of nerve cells associated with Parkinson's disease occurs, although research is ongoing to identify potential causes. Currently, it's believed a combination of genetic changes and environmental factors may be responsible for the condition. Genetics? Gulps…

A number of genetic factors have been shown to increase a person's risk of developing Parkinson's, although exactly how these make some people more susceptible to the condition is unclear. Parkinson's can run in families as a result of faulty genes being passed to a child by their parents. But it's rare for the disease to be inherited this way. So, not genetics then? Or rare genetics? *Stares blankly at screen for a minute*

The upshot of all that PD information? Medication and lots of it. Four times a day. Since the tremor is in her right hand and mum is right-handed, she has trouble getting tablets out of the blister packs. She didn't tell us, of course. I'd probably hoovered up a week's worth of medication, from underneath the coffee table, before common sense prevailed. I made her buy three Dossett boxes, which I duly fill on the weekend visits. I'm her medication bitch. Someone had to take it seriously.

I was busy filling the second Dossett box, maximum concentration level was engaged, when mum said, "Did I tell you that I had a couple of visitors yesterday?"

I poked a tablet out from the prescription, watched it roll across the coffee table and drop off the side. Suddenly, I was fully aware of the difficulties involved with this process. I looked over at mum; she was trying not to laugh at the medication escapee. I got up from the sofa and retrieved El Chapo from the living room carpet,

"Visitors, you say. Anyone we know?" I sat back down.

Mum chuckled. "Oh, I'm confident you don't know these folks," she said.

I was busy scanning the twenty-eight Dossett box windows; looking to find the right spot for the would-be deserter that I had clamped between my thumb and forefinger. I'd lost my place; the schedule was disrupted. I began a 'head' count in each of the windows,

"What were they here for?" I asked.

Mum replied, "Probably just came over to say hello," she shrugged, "I don't know really."

I was back on track with the medication and began popping out more tablets. Twenty-eight multiplied by two... equals... fifty-six. Ten tablets in this sleeve means I need five of those, plus these two I had left over from last week...

I looked up at mother, "Eh? Let me get a handle on this. You had visitors, who you don't know, that just came over to say hello?"

She looked smug and said, "Yep, that's right."

Either I had lost the ability to concentrate on two things at once or this conversation made absolutely no sense. I stopped with the medication arithmetic and pushed my glasses to the end of my nose. Peered over the top of them and looked at mum,

"These cryptic, half arsed chats are bursting ma heed!"

She laughed and picked up her mug of tea. With the hand tremor and before the cup had even reached her lips, tea had trickled out onto the carpet and over her t-shirt. She started wiping herself down with the other hand.

"Karma… it works in mysterious ways," I sniggered. "So, these visitors. You don't know them?"

Mum was dabbing at the carpet with a disposable hankie. "Never seen them before in my life," she said.

"And you just let them in the house?"

"Well… sort of," she replied.

"What time of day was this?"

"About eleven o'clock maybe?" she had answered it like a question. More confusion from me.

"Eleven o'clock maybe? That's your answer? Couple of randoms turn up at your front door and you don't even know what time it was. Inspector Morse would have a field day with this scenario."

"Who said anything about them turning up at my front door?" again with the smugness. I rolled my eyes and sat back. Mum was smiling away to herself.

"Ok, I'll play the game mother." I pointed to a living room window and said, "They come in through that?"

"Oh! You're close!" she said. "But no cigar!"

"Are you shitting me with this? You're one floor up. Did they have a ladder?" I laughed a little.

"There wasn't a ladder. They didn't need one," she'd answered it quickly and I could feel my eyes narrowing. The mystery. The intrigue.

"If the visitors didn't come in through the front door, the only other entry points are windows. Unless it was Santa fucking Claus!"

She sipped her tea and said nothing. I looked over at Eric. "Are you helping out here buddy?" He, also, was trying not to laugh.

"Maybe it was another window?" he offered. I spun my head around to look at mum. She was pointing at him in a 'you got it, correct answer' type of deal and said,

"Bedroom window. They were at the bedroom window."

My brow furrowed instantly. "Wait a minute... Complete strangers came to visit you? Through your bedroom window?"

"Yep, that's right. They never actually came in. Just hovered around," she said, matter-of-factly.

"Like from the movie Salem's Lot? When the wee boy lets his 'possessed by the devil' pal in the patio doors?" I'd said it jokingly, wasn't expecting a reply.

Mum laughed out loud. "Yes, exactly like that!" She put her cup of tea down on the table and quickly looked between Eric and I's stunned faces before she went on to tell us what happened.

Around midnight she had 'seen' an elderly woman, and a wee girl, at her bedroom window. Ghosts, she'd called them. Just floating around outside, saying hello. There was no freaking out. No hysterics. They were, "actually pretty nice," she'd said. Apparently, they 'hung in the air' for a couple of minutes, then bid her a good night before they sloped off, I presume, back to their creepy lair. Mum thought it had something to do with the 18th century lamp post in the square across from her bedroom window. I was sure it had everything to do with the assortment of drugs I was sifting through and portioning out. It was a... surreal moment.

Two weeks later, the spooky two-some had returned. Mum was in the living room talking to Lorraine and Lewis about her night-time 'friends', while I was in her bedroom, rearranging the furniture. A change is as good as a rest. Her bed now faces the opposite wall and not the window. Betty and Victoria, visitors of the undead ilk, have never been back.

I'm all for visitors and friends when they bring a supportive aspect to the mental health table. These transparent 'pals' offered nothing but floating outside a bedroom window. Beat it. Jog on. Take your see-through hovering elsewhere.

Chapter 24 – Pensioner 'abuse'

Parkinson's disease is a progressive disorder and because of that, mum is subject to cognitive testing every six months or so. Handwriting, balance, memory tests, etc. Occasional scans of her brain. Apparently, she has one! A computerised tomography (CT) scan uses x-rays and a computer to create detailed images of the inside of the body.

Mum had an appointment at the Borders General Hospital to have the contrast dye injected into her arm and slide through the rotating ring of noise. Sounds like a pleasurable experience. Says I, who's never had one. I've booked a half day's annual leave from work, drive down from Edinburgh to Galashiels, take her to the hospital for the 2:30pm appointment. Easy.

The plan went tits skyward at the very start. I was supposed to finish work at 12pm but was still on a telephone call ten minutes after this time. Finally ran out the office door at 12:14pm. Naturally, I missed the bus home. Technically, not my fault. The bus driver saw me running along the pavement in his wing mirror but slammed the entry doors shut and hit the accelerator. I mumbled an assortment of expletives under my breath and one clearly out in the open. "Wanker!"

Eleven minutes later, I was on another bus home. Still no concern at this point. I was mentally adding up the schedule. Twenty minutes to get home. Forty minutes to get to Galashiels (without traffic). Ten minutes to get from mum's house to the hospital. It'll be fine.

Sod's law. I got home just before 1 o'clock, Eric and I jumped into the car, and I wheel spun out the car park. The traffic on the A7 was horrendous. There's only four, maybe five (if you know the road) areas where you can safely overtake on this road. The six cars in front of me were completely fine with the thirty-five miles an hour speed we were currently travelling at. I eyed the clock at regular intervals.

I hate being late. For anything or anybody. Probably a throwback from the 1980s. A time where mobile phones didn't exist, and the only form of communication was the landline at home. You called your friends on it, arranged to meet at 7pm with a ten-minute grace period. If you weren't there at ten past seven, your friends fucked off and you'd have to walk back home. Respect.

These days, it's completely acceptable to get a text message from friends saying they are running late and an hour later, they appear with an air of nonchalance, without any apologies. Like we should be greatly appreciative they even turned up at all. It's maybe my age but man… I still think that's rude.

At 2pm, we'd made it to Stow. A small village, seven miles north of Galashiels. I could see the driver of the car directly in front of ours, pointing out the side window at the scenery, the passenger busy taking pictures of it on their mobile phone. Typical.

Mum called me, she sounded frantic. "Where are you? I'm supposed to be there ten minutes before the appointment!"

"Just in between Stow and Galashiels, we'll be there in ten minutes. Stop panicking woman! It'll be fine. See you in a bit." I lied. I was angry with myself and this situation. For the next seven miles, I took several deep breaths and finally accepted we were going to be late.

When we got to mum's, she was sitting on the sofa, coat on, handbag on her knees. I'll never forget the look of disappointment on her face. I waved an arm towards the front door, "Come on then. Let's get this show on the road!" it was my desperate attempt at restoring some optimism. Mum was silently raging. On the drive to the hospital, no one said a word. I considered getting my excuses in early but decided against it. She was in no mood to listen.

The upside of arriving late to any appointment, we had barely sat down in the waiting room area, when mum's name got called. I got up to help her out of the chair and we walked through to a little side room. A nurse went through the process and five minutes later, I was sitting directly outside the scanning room. I could hear someone telling mum the dye was going into her arm, I sat forward in the chair and craned my neck to look inside the room. Could see a nurse helping mum onto the bed that sat in front of the scanner. I settled back into the chair. Started reading posters on the wall opposite. Twenty minutes later, she appeared from the room looking slightly dishevelled.

I stood up and asked, "How was that then?"

"Think I've peed myself," she whispered. A nurse came out the room, touched mum on the elbow and said,

"Mrs Kennedy, that's completely normal. It's the warm sensation caused by the dye we injected." I could tell mum wasn't convinced. She desperately wanted to check the gusset of her trousers but informed us both it could wait until we got outside. The nurse laughed.

We collected Eric from the waiting room and made our way to the car park. It was clear, mum was still stewing in her own juices. We all got in the car, and I was reversing out of the space when mum, from the backseat, said,

"Wait... I can't get the seatbelt thing in." She was fighting with the clip and getting more annoyed at her shaky hand. I put the handbrake on, got out, walked around to the passenger side, and opened the door. I leaned over mum and that's when she let go of the belt. The metal clip flew up and hit me on the chin. The anger inside me bubbled some more. My turn to give her a stern look.

She tried to look sheepish as she said, "What?"

"I'll fucking what ye the now!" I roared back at her.

Mum smiled. I grabbed the seat belt, dragged the length of it down over her chin, forced the clip securely in and slammed the car door. When I got back in the driver seat, I heard the end of a mumbled sentence from the backseat,

"... treating me like I'm five years old."

I looked in the rear-view mirror and asked, "What was that?"

Mum pointed a finger in my direction and said, "You! Treating me like I'm a child!"

"Listen. When you quit acting like one, I'll stop treating you like one."

Mum snapped. "This is outright pensioner abuse!"

Let me tell you something before I finish this story. I can count on one hand the number of times I've truly lost 'my shit'. It happens very rarely because I naturally nip situations like this one brewing, in the bud. However, on this day, mum had every right to be angry with my tardiness, but this silent treatment was doing my head in. I'd much rather she ranted at me, and we'd have argued it out before now but here's where we've landed with it all. Me... losing my shit.

With my eyes still fixed in the rear-view mirror I blasted, "How about I stick my foot right up your arse and really drive that accusation home! Give it some gumption!"

Eric stifled a laugh from the front seat just as I heard a car horn behind me. I shifted my eyes left in the rear-view mirror. Mum was smiling at my gumption comment but past her, I could see the car behind us. In a car park the size of ten football pitches, I was allegedly blocking the only exit route. Either this dude had checked the 'not required' box beside the reverse gear in his list of vehicle optional extras or he was just being a tool. The horn sounded again, I thrust a forefinger in the rear-view and shouted,

"And you can fuck off 'n all!" I started the car engine and rammed it into first gear.

The car radio kicked in and D: Ream were telling us that Things Can Only Get Better by way of song. Timing. Classic timing. I burst out laughing, followed by Eric and then mum. Mr I-am-completely-incapable-of-reversing-my-vehicle blasted the horn for a third time. Long and hard. I rolled down the driver side window, thrust my arm out, raised a middle finger in his direction and hit the accelerator. Fuck this day.

Chapter 25 – The mobile phone charade

Before I begin this story, couple of reference points first. When mobile phones were first introduced, I opted for a flip phone version. I'd considered it 'cool'. It would be months before someone called me on it and I got the chance to flip it open, pull the aerial out the top of the phone and actually talk to someone. There was no predictive text back then either, so if you told someone to 'Duck off', you had number 3 issues…

Even sending a text message, back in those days, required a series of accurate button pushing. One wrong move and you were halfway to launching a ground-to-air missile off the Gulf of Mexico. An hour later, you'd have written a total of fourteen words and the text message was ready to send. Over the years, you knew what letters were under the numbers on the keypad (without looking), got quicker at it and suffered a certain degree of arthritis in your thumb (later in life) because of it. Changed days now.

Like everything in life, you build up an allegiance with a certain manufacturer. I'm an iPhone person. Could probably find employment in Apple's technical department such is my knowledge of their equipment. You put a Samsung in my hand? Well… I'm like a sweaty sixteen-year-old boy trying to unhook a girlfriend's bra with one hand in a dark room. Mother has a Samsung so you can see where this is going.

Mum had been throwing hints around that she needed a new mobile phone for two months or so. I had been swatting them off with comments such as 'If it's not broken, don't fix it' or 'A new phone and the hassle that comes with it, isn't always the answer'. Statements that would normally appease the situation but on this day, she wasn't having any of it.

"You've noticed the tremor is in my left hand now, right?" she said. I had noticed but why was that an issue? Mum carried on,

"The phone I have now is too small and I'm struggling to select the contact names with either hand." It was a fair point. "Even holding the phone is difficult," she added. Another valid proclamation. The comebacks were mounting up. I done what any self-respecting iPhone user would, I got up from the sofa and changed the subject.

"Anyone want a cuppa?"

Mum sighed, "Did you hear anything I just said?"

"Tea or coffee?" I was ignoring her on purpose. Had no intention of entertaining the new mobile phone idea. Maybe she'd moan to another sibling, they'd naively help her out and my inclusion in this Samsung Galaxy hell would be over. That was the plan.

"Go on then. I'll have a cup of tea," was all she said. I notched up a silent win from the kitchen and fist pumped the air. Next weekend, we'd probably do this dance again but for now, peace had been restored. I opened the fridge to get the milk, there wasn't any.

"Mum. Do you need to go for a food shop?"

"Yeah, sorry I forgot about that. Need a few things. I wrote a list," she said. "Can you take me now and I'll get some milk?"

"Sure," I said. "Let's go."

We travelled up the escalator and into Tesco. I got a trolley for her, and she pulled the list from her handbag. We went inside and that's when she made a beeline for the Tesco mobile shop, at the far corner of the store. Never witnessed anything like it in my life. Like the first strip of hair from a buzz cut. She was off like a shot. I'd been duped. My cup of tea offer was all the opening she required. There was no milk, and she knew it. I sighed heavily and looked skyward. Meanwhile, Jan was giving Linford Christie a run for his money. She made it to the mobile phone shop, some 100 meters away, in 9.91 seconds flat. Her cunning plan was mildly impressive, but I was in too much of a rage to be proud of her achievements.

Another thing I need to mention. Mum had bought a Samsung tablet maybe four or five months previous, from the same Tesco store. Stuart was the young lad who had helped her with the purchase. At the end of the sale, Stuart had unwittingly said, 'if you have any problems, just come back in and I'll help'. It was mere sales jargon – straight from the customer service training manual. The poor lad had no idea what he'd let himself in for. Of course, mum had taken his offer of help literally so even with the smallest problem, she was back in. From the eleven or twelve subsequent visits, tablet in hand, they'd become 'friends' in her opinion.

When I reached the mobile phone store, Stuart's eyes were feverishly darting around in his head. I suspect he was looking for the nearest exit route or maybe it was some form of post-traumatic stress. Either way, he'd failed miserably. Jan was standing at his desk and digging around in her handbag for the existing mobile phone. I instantly felt sorry for Stuart. He looked like someone who'd been kneed in the crotch. This was my fault. I'd been caught napping. Blind-sided if you will. Ten minutes ago, I was fist pumping the air in her kitchen…

Jan appeared completely oblivious to the havoc that she'd just created and said,

"This will be the easiest sale you've ever had son! I know exactly what phone I want." She pointed to a batch of mobile phones; security cabled to the front display. "That one on the left – I seen it advertised on television," she declared. I looked over to the display. Maybe this wasn't the nightmare scenario I had envisioned. I pulled the empty shopping trolley away from the desk opening and encouraged Stuart out from behind it. He had doubts, I could see it. I shared the same doubtful moment with him.

Stuart slowly made his way out from behind the desk and walked over to the display. He had the appearance of a war veteran, in the video game Call of Duty. Someone who was fresh out of ammo and fully expecting a deluge of open fire. Jan was right behind him, old mobile phone in her hand – like the worst wing man ever. I sensed a thankful respawn incoming.

Stuart cleared his throat and pointed at the phone on the left, "This one here?"

"That's the one!" Jan said. She picked it up, held it in her hand. "It's bigger than I thought, looks smaller on the advert?" The comment was thrown out as a question and we expected

Stuart to dive in with dimensions, phone stats, memory sizes, etc. but absolutely nothing came out. Stuart was a broken man. I gently nudged his arm and offered up my pearls of wisdom,

"Stuart? The quicker we get this done fella, the easier it will be for everyone." Suddenly a light appeared, and he instantly bounced into action. The respawn complete. Mobile phone and package selected; we made our way back to the desk. Jan sat down.

"We just need a few details from you Mrs Kennedy and we'll have this done in no time," Stuart said. You could tell he was back in the game and with a full arsenal of weaponry. "How long will this take?" I asked. "Ten minutes or so," was his reply. I took Jan's shopping list and with the empty trolley, left them to it.

When I returned to the mobile phone store, a queue of perturbed customers had formed behind the chair Jan was still sitting on when I left. Stuart and another member of staff were hovered around a computer screen. Both Jan's shaking hands were telling a story of their own, she was stressed and anxious. Stuart and the unknown staff member were busy discussing Vodafone...

"Sorry," I said. "Why are we discussing Vodafone? She's with Tesco mobile, right?" Stuart was showing every sign of fucked-off-ness and his reply suggested the simple personal detail gathering I had left them with, was now the bane of his very existence,

"There's something wrong with your mum's PUK code – it won't let us transfer anything over to the new phone," he said. "I asked your mum if she's clicked on any email links from other mobile phone companies and she mentioned something about Vodafone?" I looked down at Jan, who was suddenly wishing she was somewhere else.

"You got an email from Vodafone? What have I said about clicking links in emails?"

Jan recognising my rising anger level said, "I told you about the email from them, said there was a link in it, but I didn't click it!"

I stared her down and pointed in Stuart's direction, "So why does he think you have then?"

"It was that email that came from the bank, remember? But you sorted that out did you not?"

The bank? What was she talking about? Suddenly the penny dropped, and I looked at Stuart sympathetically, "Just forget whatever she said about Vodafone," I said. "That's not the reason for the PUK code error. It must be something else."

"Ah! Ok. Let's check out the other reasons for the error then," he mumbled. I threw Jan a look and cursed my shopping trip around the store. I heard sighs from the irritated string of would-be customers behind us. I was off my game today, that much was clear. Forty-five minutes later, we walked out the store with Jan's new mobile phone, her food shopping, and a burning desire to be anywhere but this godforsaken situation.

When we were back in the car, I felt weirdly calm. A calm angry if you will. It was a new emotion for me. When I thought about the Vodafone confusion, it actually made me smile. Driving out the car park, I turned to Jan in the passenger seat and asked, "Needing milk, you say?"

Jan stared out the car window and then up to the sky. "Looks like it'll rain today," she said.

"I see. We're glossing over this travesty with weather chat, are we?"

"Yes" she replied. "Yes, we are."

"The Vodafone thing? You want to explain that?" I asked.

She was about to answer and abruptly stopped herself. Considered her reply, then simply said, "I thought it had something to do... with that... banking app thing." Jan was digging a hole for herself, I let her, she deserved it. "Yanno... that... thing... from the app... thingy." I purposely said nothing. Forced her to carry on,

"The email... you know... app upload or whatever... clicking the link?" She lifted her hand; did a mouse click in mid-air with her finger. "You click on it... so the app thing comes on?" I couldn't help smiling. Turned to look out the car window so she couldn't see.

129

"I know you know what I mean!" she vented. Jan was still clutching the new mobile phone box in her hand; the frustration was palpable. She tried an apology, "Sorry! Alright? I'm sorry!"

"Vodafone but? Where did you get that from?" I'd asked the question completely straight faced. Jan immediately gasped,

"I never said it!" she claimed. "Stuart… in the phone shop… he mentioned Vodafone."

"So… it's his fault?"

"I never said that either." Jan was muttering something incoherent under her breath. She gained some composure and carried on. "Listen… he was harping on about PCU codes or whatever it's called and other stuff, then he said Vodafone and I remembered the email."

"It was a Virgin Media email mother, toss all to do with Vodafone!"

"Same difference," she muttered.

"The two aren't even in the same postcode!" I yelled. "You do realise Stuart is laying in a dark room right now, with a wet flannel on his forehead?"

"Will you wheesht! He's had worse than me, I'm sure."

My turn with an unintelligible remark, "I doubt it." I was too deep in the argument now to look for the rescue helicopter, I carried on. "Is this what happens when you reach a certain age in life? Is it?"

"What?"

I turned to face her, "Become completely unaware of innocent bystanders in your quest for new technology?!"

Mum tutted loudly, "It's his job!" she squealed.

As predicted, and over the next two months, the telephone calls with regards to usage of said new phone were relentless. 'How do I save a photo?', 'Do I have to push the button at the side every time to switch it off?', 'How do you turn the volume up?' Sometimes she even called by mistake, and I'd hear her putting the kettle on or asking herself where she'd put the television remote.

As luck would have it, Eric's mum also has a Samsung, so he was able to help with the smaller issues. When it was a 'Jan-made' problem ('I must've clicked something and now the screen is tiny – how do I fix that?'), Eric resorted to Google and the Samsung trouble-shooting pages. I am truly thankful he has the patience of a saint. Left to me? Jan's new mobile phone would be lying in a roadside ditch; she'd be working a Nokia burner and continually moaning about her aching thumb. Sheesh.

If anyone in the hierarchy of the Tesco mobile phone store in Galashiels is reading this novel, I duly recommend Stuart for employee of the month. The year even! Damn straight – not all heroes wear capes. Dude is a legend. Stuart, my parting advice to you – always remember that your present situation is not your final destination. The best is yet to come young man. Expect Jan to visit you real soon! Be kind, as always.

Chapter 26 – The medication increases

Two years into her Parkinson's diagnosis and mum has tremors in both hands. Mr Lefty hand has decided to join Mr Righty in the shake fest. Although women are 50% less likely to be diagnosed with the disease – PD generally progresses quicker in women than it does in men. Like some perverse consolation prize for the reduced probability of developing the disease in the first place. The wooden spoon in Six Nations rugby, if you will. Please also refer to Scotland and their rugby trophy cabinet for further clarification. It's choked with engraved kitchen utensils of this nature.

After her six-month check, it was decided that her medication should be increased. Specifics incoming!

Co-careldopa, the main prescription, is a dopaminergic medicine. It contains two ingredients, levodopa and carbidopa. Once in the body, levodopa is converted into dopamine, which helps to restore the level of dopamine in the damaged area of the brain. The medication helps with shaking (tremors), slowness and stiffness. These are called 'motor' symptoms because they affect the way you move. As with most medications, there's a string of side effects:

- loss of appetite, feeling or being sick (nausea or vomiting)
- feeling dizzy when you get up from sitting or lying down.
- problems sleeping (insomnia)
- uncontrollable twitching, twisting or writhing movements (dyskinesias)

It's a tricky drug for the body to tolerate and mum has been subject to every side effect on the list above. The dosage of the Co-careldopa had to be increased gradually, over seven weeks. Mum's neurologist handed her a 'simple' chart that would 'aid the process'.

Let me tell you, I've read that chart multiple times, and I still, to this day, don't understand it. I arranged a séance with Albert Einstein, introduced the elementary schedule and requested that he peruse the information contained therein. He told me to sling my hook in a creepy, haunting tone. We were on our own with it. I grabbed a slide rule and summoned all I could from my higher maths at school. Three hours later, I surfaced from my calculations like a twenty-year-old from an STI clinic. Shocked and violated.

"Do you understand it then?" mum asked.

"Sure! Piece of piss this!" I lied but there was no sense in adding to the gloom. Mum was already worrying over the medication rise and both hands were shaking viciously. I pushed the communal reading glasses up and started popping tablets out from the new prescription.

The second and forth doses of the second week should include 12.5mg extra. In the third week, only first and third doses should have 12.5mg extra. Fourth week, first, second and third for two weeks. Sixth week, all doses should contain the additional 12.5mg. If you have 25mg tablets, these can be easily halved.

Easily halved? I carried the tablets to the kitchen, got the chopping board out and a sharp knife. When I cut the first one, the two halves disappeared instantly (still don't know where they are). Wrong knife angle. I tried again. One half disintegrated into a fine powder and the other, hit my eyebrow (that's the last I have seen of it). I swore under my breath.

From the living room I heard mum ask, "Is everything going alright in there?"

"Absolutely," I replied. I put the knife down and eyed a cloth at the kitchen sink. I slapped it over the chopping board and got another tablet out. However, third time wasn't a charm. The right half turned into a powder, but the left remained intact. Result! My celebration was short lived though. Yes, it remained in its solid form, but it bounced up from the cloth and for a split second, it was airborne. I watched it land in the kitchen sink and scurry down the plug hole. "Fuck sake!"

I opened the cutlery drawer and eyeballed a pizza cutter. Surely not? Number four tablet was quickly prepped for surgery on the cloth. My gut instinct was correct. The tablet was too small to pin down and cut it like you would a pizza. Chopping down on it didn't work either. I would find one half of it, three weeks later, in the box of teabags. I stormed out the kitchen. "Get your coat on," I demanded. "We're going down to the pharmacy!" Mum looked shocked but said nothing.

When we arrived, an all too cheery member of staff asked, "How can I help you today?" I offered up the bag containing the 25mg tablets and asked if they could be swapped for 12.5mg instead. It was a simple request. We'd get the 12.5s, go back to mums and figure this shit out. The chemist wouldn't even notice the box had been opened or that the tablet count had reduced by four.

"Do you have a prescription for 12.5mg tablets?" she asked with a smile.

"No, that's why we're here."

"Ah! That's a problem then," she said. "You'll need a prescription for the 12.5mg ones."

"I just collected these ones this morning. I think the prescription said 12.5mg tablets originally but the pharmacist said it had been filled with 25mg ones instead," I replied.

"Did they ask you at that point if the 25mg tablets were ok?"

"I just took the bag and left," I said. "I couldn't answer the question in reference to the 25mg tablets at that point because I didn't know."

She took the paper bag and said, "Hang on a minute please, I'll go check."

Mum started fiddling with bottles of nail-polish on a nearby stand. She could sense the underlying tension and was looking for a change of subject. "What do you think of this colour?" she asked waving a small bottle of blood red in my face.

"This for your nights out, at the club, when you and Betty are getting down and dirty?"

"I don't know anyone called Betty," she replied. I sniggered and mum put the nail-polish back on the stand. She was touching the purple-coloured ones, when happy, smiley staff person came back to the desk,

"Right! Think we're getting somewhere now," she said. "The pharmacist filled the prescription with 25mg tablets because we didn't have any 12.5mg in stock." A weird silence followed her statement. She was waiting for me to accept their prescription fill decision, take the 25mg tablets back and leave the store. She didn't know me and the stare-off continued. Mum had moved to the pink coloured bottles in a bid to blend into obscurity. Happy staff broke the awkwardness,

"Just a thought but the 25mg tablets – cut them in half maybe?" she was shrugging her shoulders as she offered the advice.

"I tried that."

"It didn't work?" she was surprised.

"It's the reason we're back in here."

She scoffed a little at my comment. "Should be easy enough, no?"

"We'll wait right here if you want to try?" I offered. Perky chick was annoying me. Mum was now amongst the shades of blue nail polish at the very bottom of the stand. If it was possible for her to lay flat on her stomach and commando crawl out of the store, she would've.

"We don't offer a tablet cutting service," she replied through a snort.

"So... tell me... how do we get 12.5mg tablets?"

Her shoulders visibly sagged; the smile was fading. "I'm not sure," she said. "Wait here, I'll go ask." I understood. It was a tricky question. She'd need the commander-in-chief to get involved. I looked around the store. Mum was in the shampoo aisle now. I could see the top of her white hair moving down it. An elderly gentleman was standing beside me, holding a prescription line in his gnarled hand. I wondered how long he'd been there. Another member of staff called him forward and I moved out the way. The old dear drilled me a stern look. He was clearly displeased with the interruption to his day.

I started peeling sunglasses from another stand at the desk. I tried a couple of pairs on. The label at the bridge of the nose caused me angst. It's a complete impossibility to gauge the look with a big, plastic, unyielding label draped over your nose. Why? I was trying to hold the label up on my forehead and peering in the tiny mirror, when another woman, behind the desk, caught my eye. I quickly took the sunglasses off and threw them back on the stand.

"Are you the lady looking for the 12.5mg prescription?" she asked.

"Yes, that's me."

"I think it was me who gave you the prescription this morning?" Not sure why that was important, but I entertained it, "Ok?" I answered.

"I did ask you this morning if 25mg were acceptable. Do you remember?"

"I do."

"You said yes?"

"I did then but I know better now," I replied.

"So... what's the issue?" she asked. Her question was dripping with cynicism. She had chosen ridicule as her weapon of choice, believing this tone would ultimately cleanse herself of any wrongdoing. I narrowed my eyes, found myself requesting strength from God and adopted the same attitude with my reply,

"Well... it's 12.5mg tablets we need. That's what the prescription was for?"

She nodded, "That's right."

"And you guys decided on the 25mg tablets?"

"Correct." She was in full agreement.

"Forgive me for stating the obvious but... that's the issue." My revelation had obviously irked her. She stepped back and mocked my intelligence further, "25mg tablets – just split them in half and there you go! 12.5mg dose!"

This female...

"You can't – I've tried." My reply was sharp, no nonsense but she persisted and lifted a packet of paracetamol from the shelf behind her. She pointed to the medication image on the front of the painkiller box and dragged a perfectly manicured fingernail down the middle channel of the picture,

"See here. This isn't your mum's prescription obviously but the 25mg tablets should have a line down the middle like this."

I nodded, "They do."

"Great!" she replied. "You just put a knife down that very same line, and they will half easily." A mental image of me grabbing her by the scruff of the neck and hauling her over the counter that stood between us, drifted into view. I swallowed hard to dispel it and with every ounce of self-constraint I possessed, spewed forth an obnoxious response,

"Would I be back in here, wasting my time and yours, if that was the case?"

She steadied herself and I was fully expecting the disdain to continue but all she said was, "I'm afraid we don't have any 12.5mg tablets in stock." I was disappointed with her come back. We'd already danced to this excuse.

"So... why fill the prescription with 25mg tablets?" I asked. She flicked her eyes quickly left, then to the right. Trapped in a hypothetical corner and desperately in need of an escape route, that's when she yelled "George!" Shouted so loudly, I flinched a little. We traded smart ass glances until a small, grey-haired man, in a white coat appeared at her side. They turned to face the cabinets behind the counter and started mumbling to each other. Mum tugged at my arm, pointed at the two white coats behind the counter and asked, "What's going on here?"

"Fuck knows," I replied. "Clearly it's a private conversation."

"Stop swearing," she said. "I need to get back home and take my one o'clock medication."

"I massively appreciate your input mother, but you're only sprinkling more pain over this hell."

She didn't answer. We began staring at the back of George and Mildred's heads. A couple of minutes later, George shuffled over to the counter and said,

"Big mix up. Apologies. Our fault." If he was going for sincerity, he'd missed the boat. My composure was dwindling. The need for a resolution was strong and over-bearing. We'd been here long enough.

"George, is it? Err... thanks the 'apology' man but these 12.5mg tablets aren't going to sort themselves out, are they?"

He promptly ran a weary hand through what little hair he had on top of his head; pulled the original prescription out of his pocket. "I can get these in for you next weekend. Is that alright?" he asked.

"Next weekend? Like what the f...?" mum nudged me in the back before I could finish the sentence.

"It's the Scottish Borders, we only get a delivery once a week," he shrugged. As if it was completely out with his control. I held my hand out, palm upwards,

"Give me the prescription," I said quickly. "Hand it over." George was mystified. He looked over to Mildred who hadn't moved from the spot beside him. She clearly had sod all to do by way of work this day and was hanging around for the money shot. It was gossip she wasn't going to miss.

"The prescription has already been filled by us," he said. "There's no other chemist that will be able to give you these 12.5mg tablets. Even if they have them in stock." His statement was delivered with a huge amount of self-pride. This dude...

"Wait a minute, George. Let me get this right," I said angrily. "You dish out 25mg tablets incorrectly because you have no 12.5s in stock and in doing so, believe you've done us a favour?" He opened his mouth to reply but I ploughed on,

"We are here today because I *naturally* tried cutting the medication in half," I gave Mildred a 'fuck you' stare mid rant, "Of course I would, half of 25 is 12.5 - huge thanks for pointing that out by the way." I took a deep breath and looked back at George, "Now you're telling us that we'll have to wait another week for this pharmacy to get 12.5mg tablets and that no other chemist can make right, your mistake, even if they had them in stock? Is that an accurate description of today's events?"

George and the scandal hunter traded sheepish glances. It wasn't a rhetorical question – I fully expected an answer. He eventually conceded, told us to wait a few minutes and made his way to the back of the store. I glowered at the one left standing alone behind the counter. She got the drift and quickly bumbled away.

I turned to face mum. "For the love of the Baby Jesus," I said. "Is this actually happening?"

"Just calm down," mum replied. She was churning out the advice today, but it was easier said than done. The old guy with the gnarled hands walked past us with his prescription bag and offered a sympathetic smile. He nodded to the back of the store, in Mildred's direction and said,

"Bloody chemists, eh?"

I smiled. "Aye, nightmare." It was all I could muster by way of a reply. He wrestled with the entrance door, and I quickly walked over to help. He doffed his cap in appreciation as he made his way out. I'd made a friend at least.

Five minutes later, George appeared at the counter. "I've had a word with the pharmacy down the road and they have 12.5mg in stock," he said. "They will give you the medication and we'll sort it out between ourselves." I saw a vivid mental picture of me walking backwards, flipping him the bird with both middle fingers right before I asked, "Great. Are they arranging that now?"

"Should be, yes," he replied. George pulled the 25mg tablets out of his pocket and said, "Here, you can take these ones back if you want?"

"I believe they've caused enough trouble for one day – consider it a gift, George." I tugged at the bottom of mum's coat and encouraged her to the front door. She was already late for her one o'clock tablets, and I still had the medication hellfire matrix to figure out. I didn't have a headache just yet, but it was in the pipeline for sure.

I fully understand and appreciate the chemist was only trying to help. Perhaps they weren't aware of the difficulties in halving this medication and filled the prescription with the higher dose instead, as they normally would.

In my opinion, it would have been infinity easier, if they had just said we don't have 12.5mg tablets in stock and I'd have taken the prescription elsewhere. In retrospect, maybe I was the problem? Trust me. I've been 'the problem' on many occasions and enough to know it should be thrown into the mix for ongoing consideration.

Chapter 27 – COVID-19

You all seen this chapter coming. I hummed and hawed about the inclusion of it in the book. There are some things you must drag out of your memory because the need outweighs the want, this is one of those times. The pandemic had such a massive impact on everyone, so here's my recognition of it.

For a good portion of covid, mum was in the shielding category, as was Eric. I packed up the work computer and our dining room table at home became 'the office' for a period of fourteen months. Eric, to this day, refers to my remote working as his mental health saber (more Star Wars analogies). He'd have struggled to make it through otherwise.

However, mum was completely isolated. Naturally, we attempted face time conversations, in a bid to gain some normality. I quite often had full-on discussions with the side of her face, maybe her chin or forehead, the ceiling of the room in which she sat, the television, the floor or wardrobe doors. On rare occasions, we'd see her face, briefly. Always whenever she dropped the phone though and it landed camera side up, defying Sod's Law. There are only so many times you can say things like – turn it around, no not you, the phone I mean, push the button that looks like a telly screen with an arrow wrapping around it, need to lower it down a wee bit, stop crouching, I meant lower the phone, before you simply give in and accept whatever image is on the screen when mother clicked answer.

I broke coronavirus restrictions, on numerous occasions, just to make sure she had food in the cupboards. If someone wants to hand me a fine for doing so, then I accept whatever comes my way. I'd drive down to Galashiels, leave shopping bags of goodies at her front door then go back outside, stand underneath the kitchen window, and call her from my mobile phone. She'd open the window, hang out and we'd chat a while.

I often got back in the car feeling emotional and close to tears. This was at a time when no one was permitted to travel between towns and cities, but I cared not a jot. Mum needed company outside of her own, life support and something to eat. There was no traffic cop ever getting in the way of that. There are things in this life that go beyond the scope of the law – humanity for one.

Even procuring the food items, for the parcels I left on mum's front doorstep, wasn't easy. Standing alone in lengthy queues outside supermarkets. I'd find myself sparking up conversation with complete randoms in a bid to pass time and skip over the circumstance we all found ourselves in. One time, I remember it being glorious sunshine for the hour's wait outside, very pleasant, and then five minutes from the entrance doors – it pissed with rain. Welcome to Scotland, a place where four seasons in one day is a likelihood rather than a mere possibility.

Inside the store, a woman's voice, from over the airwaves, would remind you of the queue still waiting outside and I'd start jogging down the aisles like I was in an episode of the television show Supermarket Sweep. The wet t-shirt version of it (if one exists). Trying to avoid head-on trolley collisions with other customers hurrying around the store, grabbing what they could. The pasta and toilet roll shelves were always empty – still confused over the reasoning behind that detail.

Further into the lockdown, I would text Lorraine and we'd covertly, arrange to meet up in the supermarket car park. Like a Tinder date or some weird special ops mission. We'd join the horrendous string of people waiting outside and my sister and I would have a face-to-face catch up, while the store employees corralled everyone towards the entrance doors. I missed my family. It was desperate times.

Eric and I would watch Nicola Sturgeon with her daily pandemic report on the television. The word 'unprecedented'… man… It was thrown around as some lame-ass excuse for the utter devastation that surrounded us. Quite why politics were involved in this extraordinary circumstance, I will never fathom out. Surely, the directive and stats should have come from the Chief Medical officer or scientists themselves and in doing so, their unbiased recommendations would have been more influential, perhaps. Thus, targeting the whole audience instead of potential voters?

Boris bumbling his way through the daily covid update also made for excruciating viewing. The four governing nations of the UK, each making different covid judgements and all claiming their way was the best way. Occasionally, they'd even slag each other off on national television. When they did, I was instantly transported back to my school days, at the back of the bike sheds, watching kids squaring up to each other. Guaranteed an afterschool-rammy would be organised where someone was 'gonny get it' because their dad was, quite simply, bigger than everyone else's.

A united nation? Sure, if pulling in opposite directions at a time when we needed to pull together is being united? Then yeah, I guess we nailed it.

Listen… I'm the least political person you'll ever meet and my opinions here, are just that. It's my point of view. Feel free to disagree. Shout at the page if it makes you feel better. Call me an arsehole. You won't be the first or the last.

At lunchtime, during my remote working and when the daily stats were released, I was overcome with a huge sadness, every time. The covid deaths were astronomical. Treasured family members, gone. Countless people who left this world, most of them without a final goodbye or a respectful funeral service. A stark reminder that life is a gift. Be sure to hug your family and friends. Let them know how big of a deal they really are.

My absolute hope is that we've learned from this terrible experience and will be better prepared, should it or something similar ever knock on our doors again. From a personal note, my heart truly goes out to everyone who lost loved ones during this time. God bless them all.

For mum, the covid tornado ensured that no medical professional would physically see her in almost two years. The Borders General Hospital reduced the frequency of the six-monthly Parkinson's check-ups on site and moved the neurologist, holding these clinics, to the back arse of nowhere. For a progressive disease, I'm not entirely sure who decided that was a good idea, but it defied all kinds of logic, in my opinion.

The new directive probably came from an insanely overpriced think tank, subcontracted by the upper echelons of the NHS, who knew diddly-squat about PD or the need for steady monitoring. Sure, I could tiptoe around this delicate subject, as if I were barefoot in a field of thistles, but I'm direct… remember?

When the covid restrictions were finally relaxed and home visits permitted (albeit restricted in numbers), the progression of mum's Parkinson's disease was a stark reality. Mr Right Leg had now joined both hands in the growing list of shaking body parts. It was quite shocking to see but in true 'let's cover up this bullshit with humour' fashion, I insisted that she purchase a starter drum kit and we'd put this newfound characteristic to good use. Our Lorraine played a mean recorder in school. We'd get a band going. Call ourselves the Three Tremors. Headline Glastonbury. Sunday night, Pyramid stage, obviously.

Mum wasn't even aware that her right leg had gate crashed the tremor party. Perhaps her subconscious had entered the fray and quashed the new shaky leg predicament from her thoughts. The brain's natural self-defence mechanism stepping up to the plate? Or maybe she did know and in true 'old dear' style, ignored the jittery intrusion and hoped it would go away.

Didn't get passed ole Hawk-Eye Pauline though. "What's going on with that?" I asked pointing at her limb.

"What?" mum replied.

"Can you not feel that shaking?"

Mum stared down at her leg, full concentration mode engaged, and thirty seconds later the tremor subsided. I felt as if I'd been privy to a Jedi mind trick. This isn't the tremor you're looking for, but the calming effect was short lived. When she lifted her head to tell me there was nothing going on and that I was talking 'pure rubbish', her leg began quivering once more. Like a mischievous brat.

I shook my head in surprise; "What the fuck did I just witness?"

Mum chuckled, "Och I do it all the time, with my hand, at the bingo," she said. "If I concentrate hard and stare at it, the tremor stops for some reason. If I didn't, I'd be shouting for houses I haven't even won."

To all non-bingo goers and for explanation, if mum didn't fixate on keeping her hand tremor under control, she'd mark off numbers not yet released by the machine and call a 'bogey'. This action is very much frowned upon by the bingo fraternity.

I've been diplomatic in that last paragraph. Mum actually said that if she didn't apply this serious level of hand focus, other people in the bingo hall would probably slit her throat for continually shouting 'bogies' (unrelated to actual snot) and they'd carry on playing while she bled out on the floor. A tad barbaric and quite possibly over dramatised but she'd said it with such conviction, I fully believed her claim. I've always considered bingo to be a placid affair, a social catch up with the added advantage of maybe winning a monetary prize. You learn something new every day.

What follows next is a classic example of sarcasm misuse and a warning to all who use it in their day to day lives…

"How long you been doing the Shakin' Stevens impersonation?" I asked.

Mum frowned a little, "Does he have a wiggly leg?"

"Well, he had a lot of moving parts but yeah, his legs were all over the place."

The avoidance of the initial question continued, "Does he have Parkinson's disease?"

I sighed, "I can private message him and ask if you want?" My reply was oozing sarcasm and I figured it was enough to shut this line of questioning down, but no. Mum looked surprised,

"You can message Shakin' Stevens?"

"Fuck no. How would I know him or what diseases he has or doesn't have?"

"You said he had a lot of moving body parts," she fired back at me.

"Yeah," I said. "When he was on Top of the Pops? Hands, legs, head, everything was going on when he used to sing."

"Oh. Right. For a minute there I thought you and he were pals," she replied.

"Nah, I have too many celebrity friends already," I said. "It's not easy being this popular. Downright burden some days."

"I didn't even know you had celebrity buddies. Anyone I'd know?" I raised an eyebrow and felt immensely proud that mother had joined the satire-fest,

"I met JK Rowling once," I replied. "On Princes Street."

"I bet she's a lovely woman. Did you suggest a wee coffee somewhere?"

I put a finger to my bottom lip, feigned contemplation and said, "Maybe 'met' is too strong a word for it." I flapped my hand in mum's direction, "Ach, she was rushing a bit, had no time for coffee," I said.

"So, you just had a chit chat on the street then?"

"She was asking how you were getting on with the Parkinson's and all that."

Mum smiled, "Aww bless her for asking. That's nice, eh?"

"Wholesome," I said.

Mum laughed, "You didn't even meet her, did you?"

"In all honesty, I've no certainty that it was even her. I saw a woman on the other side of the street that kind of looked like her," I answered. "Didn't have my glasses on either, so in retrospect, it could've been anyone."

"This imagination of yours, I've no idea where you get it from."

"That's because you went home, from the hospital, with the wrong kid," I replied. "I was the only new-born who lay silent in the row of cribs, so you lifted me instead. Admit it woman. Go on! Rid yourself of guilt."

"God's sake! Our Lorraine claims that she was adopted, and now you, with this?"

"Once is a coincidence, right?" I asked laughing.

Mum slapped the top of my arm, "Hoy you! *Yer heid's beef that's no bin paid fur!*" she said. "That's how rumours bloomin' start!"

I smiled and winked, "They have to start somewhere."

Mum's disease had progressed into her leg and, no doubt, Mr Lefty wouldn't be too far behind. As if the fallout left behind by covid wasn't enough to be dealing with. I instantly hated Mr Right Leg and the inconsiderate timing. Selfish bastard.

"How long has your leg been like that?" I asked.

"A couple of months maybe," she replied.

I rattled my lips, slapped a hand over her shaking kneecap and declared, "The power of Christ compels ye! Be gone with this shaky fuckery!"

Of course, my cleansing process had no effect on the tremor, but it made us laugh. Mr Neurologist, time for you to get off the bench and start warming up sir. I'll be securing an appointment, and you'll see us both, very soon. No doubt, getting to your janitor's store cupboard will be a logistical nightmare but we appreciate a challenge. Get the kettle on my good man (assuming you have one in your new office environment). Just milk in mine.

Scottish slang - I have no literal explanation of this term. A Google search does produce a whole host of common Scottish sayings, but this one isn't listed. When I quizzed mum, she told me that it was just something her granny always used to say when someone was being outrageous. What it has to do with your head and free or stolen meat products? No clue. I have it on good authority, Glasgow readers will be in the know. I gently tip my cap to all Glaswegian's and their exclusive forms of communication. Further evidence that I was plucked from this fine city too young.

Chapter 28 – A shaky leg to stand on

Not only did Mr Shaky Right Leg arrive unannounced, but he also presented with new physical challenges. In true pensioner spirit, mother carried on as normal. Ignored every fresh symptom and reaped the consequence of her actions. I shall take this opportunity to explain.

All comes down to thinking and decision making. Your mindset when choices are made. Does the effect of your chosen action, ever figure into the equation? If you apply even a basic dual process theory, the two types of cognitive processes are type one: *more intuitive* and type two: *analytical*. Mother is more intuitive. I'm the analytical one. Now, type one processing, in this example, tends to be much quicker, automatic. Obviously type two is more... well... systematic, diagnostic.

Let's take pulling on trousers, with a newfound tremor in your right leg, as a physical example. From a nerd/geek perspective (type two), I've already mentally declared this simple action, in the natural standing position, is no longer a viable option. The type two in me, evicted a multitude of cuddly toys, from her bedroom chair, so that mum could sit on it and with consummate ease, pull on her trousers. A simple, yet effective, aid. A pre-emptive measure if you will.

Mum duly ignored the empty chair, in fact, she even re-instated the small family of fake fur and eyeballs upon it. It would be a few Sir Isaac Newton, gravity confirming, nose dives to the bedroom carpet before she finally surrendered to common sense. Not before she collected a couple of forehead eggs along the way. Mum attempted shoddy cover ups, sweeping her fringe to the opposite side. Forgetting I was the one who cut and styled her hair. I felt obliged to flick the top of her head, with the comb, when I discovered the crudely hidden bump,

"Ooooya!" mum said rubbing her hair. "What was that for?"

"Do you honestly think I came down in the last shower?" I asked. "Why can't you just sit the fuck down to put your trousers on?" Mum reburied her hand under the hairdressing cape around her shoulders,

"Force of habit," she said.

"Are you auditioning for the next series of Star Trek?"

"Eh? What?"

"If this carries on, you'll have the Klingon forehead perfected," I answered.

Mum chuckled, "It's not like you to exaggerate."

In the month that followed, I noticed various bruises and scrapes appearing on her arms. Mum, naturally, had an answer for everything. "Oh, I knocked it on the kitchen cupboard door" or (my particular favourite) "I don't know where that came from." Classic if all else fails – plead ignorance.

Sitting beside her on the sofa, I poked a bruise on the top of her arm with my finger and asked, "What happened here then?"

"You need to stop poking it for a start," she said abruptly. Mum lifted her arm in the air and inspected the mark of purpleness, "I think I caught it on the towel rail in the bathroom."

"Uh huh," I replied. "What about this one on your kneecap?" I was about to poke that one as well until she slapped the back of my hand. Stung a wee bit.

"Who are you now? The bruise police?" she asked.

"Wait… There's an actual department, of Police Scotland, dedicated to contusions?"

Mum shook her head and laughed, "It's true," she said, "We are incapable of having a normal conversation."

"I guess it depends on your interpretation of normal," I answered. "It's like cleaning… everyone's definition of it is very different."

"How did we get from a chat about bruises to cleaning?"

"Everyday occurrence for us," I said.

It wasn't just the falls and the scratches and the bruises. Watching her trying to stand up from the sofa was a sight to behold. The analyst in me, suggested she move to the far end of the sofa and use the arm of it to pull herself into the upright position. For I am certain, the sofa arm was predominately designed with that very function in mind.

Instead, mum employed various methods in a bid to streamline the awkward process. Finally, she 'mastered' a forward propulsion technique using a grip on the underside of the sofa cushions. Don't ask me to explain further. It'll be an Olympic sport in years to come. Both the dexterity and upper arm strength involved, are awe inspiring.

Now on her feet, a moment of steadiness is required. She'll spend this time swaying in the non-existent breeze, ask herself why she even got up from the sofa, gather her composure, and then shuffle off in the necessary direction.

Walking involves balance and co-ordination of muscles so that a person moves forward in a rhythm. A stride or gait (hark at me, getting all technical). Mr Right Leg, the lack of dopamine, death of brain cells and a list of other Parkinson's disease attributes, pissed all over her normal walking function. So... mum adopted a shuffle. A highly inefficient process that takes longer and tires her out quicker. It was either the shuffle or we super glued roller skates to her feet and pushed her from behind.

Naturally, the skate idea highlighted a few concerns. Pavements, of the downhill nature, was the main one. Mother didn't care much for the "I'll just let go and collect you at the bottom of the hill" reply. A perfectly solid idea was immediately squashed. I revisited the drawing board,

"What about a trolley?" I asked.

Mum looked confused, "A shopping trolley? The ones in the supermarket, you mean?"

"Fuck no. We'll not get it out of the carpark," I said. "Security would lynch us."

"What do we need a shopping trolley for?"

"Dear God. I wasn't talking about a shopping trolley," I said. "You know. A trolley thing. For walking with?" I was holding onto imaginary handles and working a pushing motion at this point for effect.

"Some of these even have built in seats. Handy for a wee sit down if you needed one," I continued with the hard sell. "We could pimp that bitch right up. Get some lit wheel trims on it. Add a sound system. Furry dice." I was too engrossed in my walking aid ideologies to notice the look on mum's face deteriorating. When I did, I instantly felt sorry for her. "What is it?" I asked.

Mum stared out of the living room window, she was thinking, analysing the verbal diarrhoea I had just spewed forth in reference to the walking aid. I was convinced that we'd be searching for trolleys on Amazon, she'd be waving a debit card in my face, feeling excited about the purchase, and making sure I'd clicked the next day delivery option.

She turned around to face us and very simply declared, "Am no' ready for that."

Chapter 29 – Home Sweet Home

Following on from the 'am no' ready for that' mic drop, my thought process headed straight for other avenues of the help variety. Mum wasn't too keen on any form of support, so all my search efforts had gone under the radar. If I happened upon a solid idea, that could potentially be a goer, then we'd work on a presentation and slowly introduce it into weekly mum chats. Throw it out there as a naive suggestion and she'd be completely unaware of the ninja attack being formulated in the background. Like the sales folks who are conveniently placed around the aisles of Costco. The ones that you'll attempt to shuffle past, avoiding all eye contact, feeling supremely proud of your efforts but somehow, you're still drawn over to their booth, accepting a sample of the 'new', keenly priced, maple syrup pancakes and are now shoving a two-kilogram box in your shopping trolley. It's an artform.

Assisted living accommodation = maple syrup pancakes. Strike plan activated. Research done. Costco booth set up. Baited fishing line in the water. All we required, was an active participant. As it happens, Mr Shaky Left Leg chose this very moment to introduce himself and in doing so, gave us the green light. Perversely, it was an opening for engaging Stikedawn Assisted Living protocol. We had no option but to roll with it.

Mum and I stared down at her left leg, she was first to comment, "It's not as bad as the right leg, I don't think?"

"No," I agreed. "It's still giving it large though. When did that start?"

"I'm not sure," mum replied. "Monday or Tuesday maybe? Only noticed it when I was trying to put my slipper on."

"You have to chase it around the bedroom floor?"

"Chase what?" mum asked.

"You know," I said, pretending to put a tremoring foot into an invisible slipper that keeps getting pushed away. "Your slipper?"

Mum chuckled. "It must be tough for you."

"What?" I asked.

"Living a normal life with the stuff that's rolling around in your head."

I flapped my hand in her direction, "Ach. You get used to it," I said making my way towards the kitchen door. "I'll make some tea. That shit cures all ails."

In truth, the tea production was an excuse to disappear from mum's view and develop the assisted living accommodation strategy. I just needed an ambiguous one-line conversation opener to kick start this bitch. Thankfully, a concept transpired while I was stirring the cloudy brown liquid and staring down at the contents moving inside the mug.

"You think you'll still manage the stairs outside?" I asked, nonchalantly, from the kitchen. Mum answered straight away, "Don't see why not." I batted away her completely reasonable reply and pushed forward, "New shaky leg won't hinder the process?"

"I'm still getting around the house ok," mum replied. This wasn't going very well. It was little wonder that I do accounts work for a living. I persevered, "Didn't you struggle with the stairs when your right leg first started playing up?"

"I use the handrail now though. That works," said mum. Of course, she did. I was thrashing around like a complete amateur and the conversation was suddenly turning conspicuous. Staged almost. I was trying too hard to be something other than direct. I should have aborted the mission and tried another day. 'Should have' being the operative words.

Get a grip Pauline. Focus. "Be nice to live somewhere without the hassle of the stairs though, right? Wee change and all that?"

Mum ultimately stole my direct trait and threw the whole lot back in my face with her reply, "I don't know where I'm getting this notion from, but is there something you're trying to tell me?"

Fuck sake. I picked up the cups of tea and made my way into the living room. "Biscuit?" I offered. As I walked back into the kitchen, my brain was in overdrive. How dare she oust me with my own personality. Weirdly, I felt proud and couldn't stop the wry smile that crossed my lips. Point blank it is then – my natural environment,

"I was looking into assisted living accommodation in Galashiels the other day." I collected the biscuit tin from the cupboard and turned back towards the living room. "Some of these places look lovely."

"What?! A home?!" mum hollered. "You're putting me in a home?!" I almost dropped the biscuit tin in the outburst. To be fair, I expected some pushback, but she had roared it so loudly, I almost made a Pauline shaped hole in the kitchen door. Before I could defend myself or the assisted living accommodation, mum was getting her opinions out first,

"No way, in hell's earth, am I going into a home!" she blasted. "You promised Pauline! You promised I wouldn't go in a home! Am no' ready for that! Nowhere near ready!" I stood open mouthed, clutching the biscuit tin to my chest like a bullet proof vest as the rant continued,

"Old folk's homes?! I mean come on!" Mum held out her arms to the side, "They hate pensioners! I've seen them on telly documentaries. Mistreating the old dears. Breaks my heart!"

I tried to cut in, "Wait… it's not…" Mum pointed a finger in my direction, she wasn't done yet, "Don't you stand there and tell me these places aren't like that!" I put the tin down on the coffee table and slowly backed away with my hands in the air before I responded, "Whoa! You need to bring it right down to a simmer here. What the fuck?"

Mum still wasn't finished, "I'm not going into a home! You can't make me. I'm telling Jackie on you; she'll take me in and look after me!" I sighed heavily and began nodding slowly, "Really? I see. You've chosen the thoroughly mature route then?"

I could see tears forming in mums bottom eyelids but her need to fight back was strong, "I know one thing. I'm not going down the old people's home route!" she said furiously. I looked directly at her and conjured up my best reasoning face,

"Who said anything about an old folks' home?" I asked. "Come on. Who?" Mum looked away but I could tell the tears were about to flow down her cheeks. She didn't respond so I carried on, "Assisted living accommodation… well… it does exactly what it says on the tin." Mum snorted and mumbled something akin to 'aye right', which I duly ignored.

"These documentaries you've watched on telly? Of course, I'm not denying there's places out there, like that," I said calmly. "The fact you believe I'm going to research the worst old folk's home ever and then purposely sign you up to it. Is quite frankly… disturbing!" Mum shot me a wild look and she was about to retaliate but thought better of it. It was clear, I was in no mood for these ignorant hysterics.

I took a deep breath in and continued, "I get it. You think old people's homes are tiny rooms, with no windows and a mattress on the floor. You believe their version of an evening meal, is to open your creaky bedroom door and throw a boiled egg in, making sure it bounced off your forehead!" Mum smiled a little, wiped her eyes and sniffed.

"Assisted living accommodation," I offered. "Isn't like that. Not the ones I've researched anyway. I admit, bouncing an evening meal off anyone's head, wouldn't be something they'd freely advertise on their websites but what I did read, well… sounded alright!" I finished my outburst still glaring at mother and was utterly surprised when she began chuckling. An hour later, mother had got her shit together and as part of a recon mission, we drove past some of the assisted living places I'd researched. I'm mightily glad her opinion of them changed – I'd already filled in the application forms, for all these gaffs, three weeks earlier. Just the things I do.

As a side note – I'm not entirely sure whether this whole assisted living accommodation discussion went down much better than I anticipated, and more so at the exact point when mum threatened to grass me up to Jackie about 'shoving her in the worst ever old folks' home' plan but the end goal was achieved. I really do have to wonder though. Jackie taking you in and looking after you? Let's please all agree and as a family unit, that my oldest sister is more likely to be the one launching a boiled egg at your dome. Facts are facts people.

Chapter 30 – The 1514 conversation

Let me set the scene for this 'episode' and you fine people reading it. Saturday morning, down at the old dear's gaff for the usual visit. Mum has a huge corner sofa, Eric is sitting at one end, and in a clockwise direction, mother is next (wedged into the corner of it), nephew Lewis is next to his granny and Lorraine is at the end (diagonally opposite to Eric).

In the car trip down, I'd already called shotgun on the single tub chair that inwardly faces the sofa. It's the best seat in the living room and much sought after, hence the requirement for the shotgun call. An agreement we made months previous which negates the need for constant bickering over it. There's a big coffee table in the middle, with a fruit bowl in the centre of it and place mats around the edge.

My mother has an uncanny knack of filling every corner, nook, and cranny of her home with items of, dust gathering, furniture. A pot plant sits on top of everything with a flat surface. There is no open plan or minimalist feel here. The only benefit to all these sideboards and bookcases, that I can see and from a logical standpoint, is the carpet hoovering time is significantly reduced.

The mail dropped through the letterbox and, instantly, the living room fell silent. Like a scene from an old western movie. Cowboys standing at either end of a sandy street, hands hovering over their side arms, waiting for the shit to go down. Saloon doors clacking in the background and an occasional tumbleweed rolling by.

There's a nervy feel to it. I'm in the tub chair, searching the faces of those on the sofa that are doing the same to me. I know my dibbed seat is the one closest to the living room door so, naturally, I should be the one to get up, and collect the post that's just been delivered. Such a simple, naïve task.

I also fully understand the consequence of this harmless action. For the very minute my arse leaves the tub chair, and I am suitably distanced from it, here endeth any right I have to it. Another unwritten rule. Pushing or general manhandling is not allowed. It used to be, until that nasty affair where I had to reconstruct a bookshelf from its broken parts, and a pot plant lost its life during the fracas.

The stare off continued. I witnessed neck and hamstring muscles being stretched. Knuckles were cracked. The goading would commence shortly. I had every right to be fearful, the situation was fraught with danger. I searched for an out, my gaze fell upon Lewis and an instant solution popped right in. I pulled diplomatic rank and asked nephew Lewis to get the mail for his granny. Of course, the unwritten terms and conditions were challenged at this juncture, but mum told everyone to pipe down. Next week, an adjudication officer would decide whether I had dishonoured any of the shotgun regulations but for now, I still had the dibbed chair of choice.

Lewis gave the post to his granny and sat down. He and Eric started talking about football. Mum opened, what looked like a Matalan catalogue and began flicking through the pages. I chose this opportunity to ask Lorraine about the Hawick Common Riding and the whole 1514 thing. During her time as a journalist for the local rag, she had, over the years, become quite knowledgeable regarding all things Common Riding.

"It's the year 1514 that's on the Hawick Common Riding flag, right?" I asked. "Battle of Hornshole and all that?"

"Battle is a strong word," she said. "It was more of a skirmish."

"Right," I nodded. "So, it had nothing to do with Battle of Flodden then?"

Lorraine was busy looking for something to watch on the television, "Maybe as a result of Flodden," she answered.

"What you mean?"

Suitable telly program selected, she picked up her mug of tea and said, "Loads of Scots were killed at Flodden and that pretty much left the Scottish Borders vulnerable due to lack of available living bodies."

"Right," I said.

"Why are you asking?"

"Just knowledge," I said. "For the book." Lorraine took a sip of her tea and replied, "Yeah Flodden was in 1513, after it though, young Hawick guys caught wind of some English raiding party at Hornshole and they charged out there," she said. "Done them over like kippers at night apparently, stole their flag and there began the Hawick Common Riding."

"Just like that," I said.

Lewis decided to join the battle conversation, "There was probably more to it than just that aunty Pauline," he said.

"What? More than a moonlight sneak-up and flag pinch you mean?"

"Is that even considered a battle?" he asked. Lorraine drew her eyes from the television and refocused on the discussion in hand, "I never said it was a battle. Think I described it more as handbags at dawn," she replied.

I interjected, "Hold the phone! You said they had kippers for weapons. Wasn't any mention of handbags."

Lewis chuckled, "They just run up to the English blokes, slapping each other in the face with fish and that, aye?"

"According to your mother, they were all thrusting Louis Vuitton and Chanel around in their faces," I said laughing. "Woman needs to make up her mind."

Lewis smiled, "Maybe it was kippers in Flodden. Handbags at Hornshole? he suggested. Lorraine chuckled and took a sip of tea. We had already taken this conversation too far. The normal Kennedy 'sliding doors' moment. Make up a nonsense version of actual events and see where the humour goes but it was about to get much juicier when mother, out of nowhere, and still flicking through the catalogue said, "I was there you know."

With this statement, mum had instantly joined the alternate rendition without even realising it. Loads of things happened, simultaneously. Eric and Lewis looked at each other and said "Eh?" out loud. Lorraine sprayed a mouthful of tea, some of which came down her nose and most of which landed on my arm. I was busy wiping the ejected caffeine drink off my sleeve when I asked for some clarity, "This in a previous life mother?"

Lorraine beetled off to the bathroom, laughing as she went. Mum lifted her head and said, "Eh? What?"

"At the Battle of Flodden," I queried. "Was it kippers or handbags?" Mum looked confused. Lorraine came back from the bathroom, sat down, and took a sip of her tea when mum said, "I've no idea," she answered. "I'd have to ask Jean, she might know."

Eric and Lewis said, "Eh?" out loud again. Lorraine sprayed more tea, this time landing on the carpet. Mum licked her finger and flipped to the next catalogue page. Completely unaware.

"Jean was there as well?" I asked. "Was she in the handbag or fish battalion?"

"Yeah, Jean was there. It was her suggestion that we go," mum said holding the catalogue page closer to her face and following it up with, "Oh, those bathroom towels are nice."

I flicked my eyes right, saw Lorraine wiping her nose and rubbing tea spittle into the carpet with her foot. "So, you met Jean in a previous life? What's the chances of that?" I asked.

"I can't remember where I first met Jean," mum said. "Where's that?"

"Where's what?"

"This previous life place you're talking about," mum urged. Eric and Lewis again with the "Eh?!" Totally in sync but, this time, their outbursts had a more incredulous feel to them.

I shook my head, "Did the pair of you meet up in some ye olde inn, steal a couple of horses and haul your ass east?" I asked her. "Followed the rebel crowd and joined the battle?"

"We went on the bus," mum replied. Calm as you like. Lorraine got up from the sofa and disappeared into mum's bedroom where I could hear her snorting with laughter. Eric and Lewis were quietly chuckling. Shoulders bouncing up and down. Mum was still completely oblivious.

"The bus you say. Who knew public transport was even available in the 1500s," I said calmly. Mum looked over the top of the catalogue as Lorraine came back into the lounge and sat down,

"It was a tour thing. Up north," she replied pointing a finger towards the ceiling. "Was a field near Inverness." My eyelid twitched. Lewis furrowed his brow and turned to face mum,

"Eh? Granny you must be some age now," he said. The Matalan catalogue folded in half, like a wilted flower, in mum's hand.

"Seventy... something," mum replied. She looked over in my direction for help,

"Four," I said. "You're seventy-four."

Everyone looked at Lewis, "So, you're talking about the Battle of Culloden," he said. I couldn't help feeling aunty-proud of this lad's knowledge of history. "How does that even work?" Everyone turned their heads to look at mother. Like we were watching a tennis match.

"How does what work son?" mum asked.

Lewis stopped mid text to a friend, put the palm of his hand on his knee and turned his body around to face his granny,

"Well... How can you be in two different battles, that are nearly two-hundred-and-fifty years apart?" he asked. "Previous life or no, that's no right." His capacity for asking questions, while keeping a straight face, was improving. It was another proud aunty moment.

Mum's turn with the "Eh?!" reply.

"How many previous lives are you wanting like?" Lewis asked chuckling.

Eric bounced in with a sarcastic retort, "To be fair," he said. "It's no like this entire conversation is the epitome of continuity."

"Yeah, the Battle of Culloden," mum said. "That's where Jean and I went. It was fascinating. We had a great day out."

"And absolutely nothing to do with the Hawick Common Riding," I declared.

"No," mum said. "Flodden probably influenced the Common Riding. That was a couple hundred years before though. We got our arses kicked in that battle. Lost a huge number of Scottish men." She snapped her fingers in the general direction of everyone in the living room. "What was the name of that place, couple miles outside of Hawick?" she asked.

Lorraine answered with the merest hint of irony, "Ehhhhh... Hornshole?"

"Yeah, that's it!" mum replied. "There's your reason for the Common Riding."

Destination eventually reached. Via a side road of humour, a Matalan catalogue, and some nice bathroom towels. Apparently.

Chapter 31 – Medication increase – part deux

Around March 2022, there was a general feeling that covid had finally taken the hint and slinked back into the hole from whence it came. People were returning to some semblance of work order, and I was trying desperately to get over my annoyance of the NHS Parkinson's department radio silence.

I need to tread carefully here; I have friends and family who are currently employed by the National Health Service establishment. In the height of the pandemic, Eric and I were there, every Thursday night, hanging out the living room window, favourite saucepans in hand, banging out noise, along with the rest of the neighbours. We'd see people driving past in cars, tooting their horns. It was evident, in our neck of the woods, people were genuinely full of admiration for nurses everywhere. Well… as genuine as you could be with a non-stick pot and a wooden spoon.

Eric's mum is a nurse, and she'd quite often furnish us with gut-wrenching stories of families with tragic losses or the unrelenting daily pressures the NHS staff endured. She'd unload and we'd listen, nodding in all the right places. I like to think we helped some, in our own little way.

I do understand that the NHS, as an organisation, well… she's a big ole ass to turn and set back on her original course. Titanic-like. It will take an inordinate amount of time, co-ordination and require a renewed surge of productivity. A huge ask and more so when you demand it from an under-staffed crew, who are already exhausted and still apprehensive about discarding their life jackets. Hardly the perfect brownie mix, but it's either that or our treasured health service splits in half, sinks to the bottom of the Atlantic Ocean floor, leaving Aneurin Bevan turning in his grave.

Out of desperation, I took a chance and called the Borders General Hospital. Let's see if we can't get an update on the mysterious new location of the Parkinson's disease clinic (since it no longer resides in the central Borders hospital grounds) and maybe a wee appointment, with the neurologist, for mother. If you don't ask…

"Yes, there's still only one Parkinson's clinic a month," said the woman who answered the telephone when I called.

"And where's that being held now?"

"It's in Hawick," said she.

"Great," I replied. "How do I go about getting an appointment for my mum?"

"It's in Hawick though."

"Yes… you said," I replied.

"But your mum lives in Galashiels."

Awkward silence followed. I wasn't clear on the conversation direction. I plucked a stock answer out, "Yes. Yes, fully aware of that."

"And the clinic is in Hawick," she reiterated. A myriad of replies washed over me. I opted for courteous. Strangely.

"Yes. Thanks. I'm clear on the logistics. Can you tell me if there's any chance of an appointment for my mum?" I asked. "Only she has a new tremor in her leg and…" I was interrupted (biggest… pet… hate… ever),

"So, before we carry on, there's no problem with a clinic appointment in Hawick?"

I went down the route of answering a question with a question (number six on the list of my personal pet hates), "Should there be?"

"Well, I know it's not very convenient for some people," she offered, "appointments are getting cancelled because of it."

"But… I called you guys… looking for the appointment?" My question brought on more silence followed by a nervous laugh, "Yes so, it's not an issue. I understand," she said.

I felt an immediate, strong desire to have a proper rant. A full-on vent of my personal frustrations. Mentally, I heard myself saying listen lady, there's no one seen my mother in over two years or the new shaky leg symptom. I opted for key words like progression, obvious, current medication, help, lack thereof. I expressed concerns that the only medical professional she'd 'seen' during the last twenty-six months, was a fucking

Google search doctor and in no world was that right. I ended my hypothetical tirade with an understanding of the pandemic, the emergencies prioritised because of it and my appreciation for every NHS effort made in the wake of it. All of that, went on, inside my head and the whole blow off took like, eight seconds. This situation wasn't her fault.

What actually came out was, "Great. So, an appointment then. What's the chances?"

A couple of months later, our Jackie took her for a day trip to Hawick and the neurologist checked out Mr Shaky Right Leg. Jackie had firm instructions to pay attention at the appointment. It was an important visit and I required precise details for this section of the book. Obviously, mum's new shaky leg was top priority but material for the story ran a close second.

What transpired was a folded sheet of paper, with three handwritten comments on the reverse of it (none of which were legible) and another Co-careldopa prescription.

"What the fuck is this?" I asked… with warmth.

Mum looked like she'd been dragged through a bush backwards. She held her hands out and shrugged, "That's all I was given," she said.

I slowly unfolded the sheet of paper, "I swallowed my pride for this clinic appointment so there better be winning lotto numbers on here, at least." Mum chuckled but I saw no humour in my comment. Being truthful, when I clocked the paper, my initial fear was another medication chart of algorithmic formulas that would serve no purpose but to insult my diminutive intelligence. I opened it like you would a birthday card, knowing it contained a £50 note, outside (for some reason), in a 60mph wind and fighting with the envelope adhesive. In other words, close to my chest and full of dread.

The handwritten notes on the back of the paper, remain a mystery to this day. Hugely important information disregarded because the writing looked like a spider had wandered into an ink spill and onto this paper. I flipped it over quickly. Nothing charty or matrixy on there with regards to the medication increase. Just a whole bunch of information about Parkinson's disease. It was… anti-climactic. Bland but re-assuring. I turned to mum, "So, what did they say?"

She sighed, "Nothing much really. Just did a couple of tests, with my leg and walking, things like that."

"Did you ask any questions? Did Jackie ask any?" I was grilling her. Mother opted for a sarcastic response,

"No, Pauline. Nobody asked anything. We all just sat there in silence and said nothing." Both her hands were shaking furiously. She was worried. I changed tact.

"Let me see the new prescription," I said. Mum passed it over. Another 12.5mg of Co-careldopa, four times a day. There was no mention of it being a gradual increase or when it should start. I opened my mouth to ask but mum, reading my mind, supplied the answer,

"As soon as possible they said." Her reply hung in the air for a couple of minutes. It wasn't anything that we didn't expect but no matter how prepared you think you are, there's always someone or something willing to smack you in the face with a huge dose of reality. Mr Right Leg was an arsehole. I disliked everything he stood for (no pun intended).

I gently nudged her arm with my elbow, "Listen, it is what it is," I offered. "And if these new meds have no impact, we'll look into that Irish dancing thing for you."

Mum frowned. I did a mock leg shake and pretended to 'Michael Flatley it' right up in front of her. "You'll nail that for sure, won't even have to work at it." She didn't want to, but mum laughed, "No idea where you dig this stuff up," she replied.

I made a cup of tea before we took the prescription line down to the pharmacy. Hopefully they'd have the 12.5mg in stock, we'd hang around in the store (trying not to look like we were casing the joint) and ten minutes later be making our way back to mum's house with the white paper bag. A week later, I collected the damn drugs and added the extra medication to her Dossett boxes.

It was a tough couple of weeks that followed, understandably so. The first three years of her diagnosis, mum had grown accustomed to small medication increases, so no concerns or worries over it. Pre covid, mum was chowing down on 50mg of the Co-careldopa a day. This second medication hike, some two years later, meant she was up to 150mg a day. Fifty milligrams per limb – the 'cost' of doing 'business'.

As previously explained, this medication is a combination of two ingredients, levodopa and carbidopa. Levodopa is converted into dopamine, so helps with the level of dopamine in the damaged area of the brain. Carbidopa prevents the levodopa from being broken down into dopamine in parts of the body other than the brain. For those of you losing interest in the technicalities – if levodopa is ingested by itself, it breaks down in the bloodstream before it crosses to the brain (the important destination). Carbidopa is the piggyback, getting the levo to where it needs to be and reduces any side effects along the way. Neither drug slows the progression of Parkinson's disease, it just treats the symptoms of it. Toleration of the medication, without the luxury of a gradual increase or side effects aplenty? Easier said than done.

Fatigue, as an example. For the next three weeks, getting mum to answer any telephone call was a challenge. Images of her lying face down in the hallway would, quite often, interrupt my working day. As the day progressed, doubt turned into anger. I'd start to question her level of selfishness regularly and follow that up with derogatory swear words. When she eventually answered one of the many telephone calls, we'd argue, naturally, and then she'd brush off my angst with consummate ease. Just a 'nanna nap', she'd call it. This particular comment would serve no purpose but to infuriate me further.

"You can't just answer the damn phone when it rings though?" I asked her.

"I was sleeping," mum said. "Funny that, I could hear a phone ringing, but thought it was part of a dream."

"You're an absolute tool," I said.

"I'm aware of it," mum replied.

"Well, that makes everything ok then, right?"

"Listen," she said, "there are people walking this earth that have no idea they are tools. At least I know."

"Dear God, this is a new kind of fresh hell," I said. "Answer the fucking phone when it rings. People have concerns over your wellbeing. Quit being an arsehole."

"Right you are then," mum replied.

Dizziness – another side effect. Mum would continually play it down, claim to have gotten up from the sofa 'too fast' and then wait until the 'wee funny turn' had passed. Quite often she'd hang onto the kitchen sink for several minutes or stand in the middle of the living room, pretending to have 'forgotten' what she'd got up for. Lies. Theatrics. All of it. Sleight-of-hand magic tricks, so we'd look the other way until the room stopped whirling.

During the pandemic, I broke my little toe. Cobbled a self-care package together where I strapped it to the neighbouring one and carried on regardless. Even ignored the 'pure purple' stage. On one of mother's dizzy bouts, she stepped back a little and I watched in horror as the heel of her slippered foot came down on my DIY taped up digit. Well… you can imagine how that went down.

It would be in the third week, during a telephone call with the old dear, where I finally intervened and drew a halt to these farcical proceedings. Her David Copperfield antics were impressing no one.

"Are you alright?" I asked mother upon noticing her slurred speech.

"Marvellous," she replied. "Any reason why you're asking?"

I chose my next words with the upmost care and compassion, "Cause you sound absolutely fucked out your head." A ten-second silence followed. Mum broke it with her reply, "How?" (I appreciate this word, as a question, looks and sounds grammatically incorrect but trust me, it's a Scottish interrogative term; closely related to the word 'why').

"Have you been on the Special Brew?" I enquired.

"What?"

"You sound cake holed."

"Drunk?" mum asked. "How?" Although she was slurring her words, there was no confusion. Still as sharp as ever. Compos mentis.

"Are you even aware of your current speech impediment?" Mum's answer to this question, launched a series of misconceptions, outright frustration by both parties and ended with the normal casting of aspersions.

"I lost a bridge," mum said.

"Eh?"

"Can't find it," she went on. "Probably in bed."

"What is?"

I heard mum sigh. "The bridge," she said exasperated. "I checked the kitchen bin, before you ask." My personal bewilderment continued, "Before I ask what?"

Mum groaned, "Yes," she said. "Before you ask me where I had it last."

"It?"

At this point, I mentally heard my mother saying for the love of Christ but instead she opted for, "Are you even listening to me?"

"Funny that, I was about to ask you the very same thing," I said. "How did we get from you sounding drunk to raking in the kitchen bin?"

"I'm not drunk!" she squealed. "My teeth Pauline! I was talking about my teeth!"

After her denture outburst, I should've played the sensible card and just said something like 'ah' or 'ok' but what actually came out of my mouth was, "Your teeth are drunk?"

Mother quickly mumbled something under her breath and then slurred her way through an open reply. "You know, there's some days I really do question whether you even came from my loins."

"Just some days?" I asked chuckling. "Dammit, I aim to get on your nerves every single day. One simply must intensify one's efforts."

She didn't want to, but mum started laughing, "Do I really sound like I've had a skin full?" she asked.

"Yeah," I replied. "Some folks would pay good money for the slur-age you have going on there."

"Should I be worried?"

I shrugged my shoulders, "Fuck woman, how would I know?" I asked. "Fairly certain your worry horse will already have bolted though. Let me phone Jill the Parkinson's nurse and I'll call you back."

I always feel like I'm harassing Jill whenever I text or call her, but she continually assures me that it's 'no bother' and likely to her own detriment. Sometimes I do wonder if I've ever called her mid episode of a television series, that she's waited two months to binge watch. She's maybe even swore out loud when my number or 'Kennedy arsehole daughter' appeared on her telephone display. Worse yet, perhaps I'm not even saved in her contacts. In my imagination, I always see her fumbling with the pause button on the telly remote control and taking more than a few seconds to gather her nurse composure before she hits the answer button. I explained all when she did.

"When we saw your mum at the clinic, it was obvious that she required a medication increase and important that she started the new dose as quickly as possible," Jill said. "It's all about the tolerance of the drug and in your mum's case, there was no time to find out exactly what she could or couldn't handle by way of side-effects."

"So, mum sounding like she's busted all of her pension down at the local off licence is normal then?" I asked.

Jill laughed a little, "Yes," she said. "Unfortunately, it's a side effect but it should get better in the next couple of days."

"And if it doesn't? Doctor's appointment after that?"

"Definitely," Jill replied. "I'm confident the slurring will improve over next couple of days though. Tell your mum not to worry, I know what she's like." I laughed a little, "Too late for that Jill but thanks again for your help."

I called slurring Annie back, "Jill says it's nothing to worry about mother."

"You think I'll be alright for the bingo tomorrow?" mum asked. It was evident that any worries or fears she had, weren't from a medical standpoint anyway.

"Sure," I said. "Your slur doesn't affect the word bingo when you shout it, right?"

"Nobody actually shouts bingo when they win," she said dryly.

"You'll have to find your teeth before you go," I said. "Maybe try the kitchen bin?" Mum told me to 'go away' using sweary words of that ilk and in a somewhat aggressive manner.

Credit where it's due, Jill was correct. Mum's slurring lasted for two days and during this time, I royally took the piss at every opportunity. Safe to say, I was even marginally disappointed when her speech returned to normal, as this ultimately forced me to come up with alternative stuff to grind her last nerve with. Mum located her teeth, sloped off to the bingo and won £16. Small wins all round.

Chapter 32 – Covid & Mother

The inevitable happened, covid ripped through the occupants of the bingo hall. Amidst the social distancing and hazmat suit wearing, the virus latched onto whoever it could. Mum, who had pretty much self-isolated and shielded for the best part of twenty-two years (slight exaggeration), finally succumbed to 'the bugs'. During a Thursday night telephone conversation, mum had naively said her throat was a bit sore. By Friday afternoon, it was fairly obvious she had 'the vid'. I said nothing.

Saturday morning, Eric and I arrived with a box of antigen test kits. We met resistance, of course, but once we wrestled the old dear to the floor and Eric eventually had mum in a decent headlock, I unsheathed the cotton bud and jammed it right up her nostril. A single tear escaped from the corner of her eye, but I felt no remorse. Obviously, this is how we should've tackled it. How it actually went down was a very different scenario.

"I'm not sticking that up my nose," said mother.

I rejected her matter-of-fact statement, "It's funny, you're saying that like you have a choice."

Mum snorted and replied, "I do and I'm not doing it. End of."

"You have to, and you will," said I.

"Nope." Mum shook her head slowly, "I don't have the virus."

I twirled the cotton bud between my fingers and stared at the tip of it, "Says who?"

Eric was busy laying out the rest of the test kit like he'd found new employment at the local crime scene investigation unit. All he was missing was some protective eyewear and latex gloves.

"It's just a sore throat," mum declared. "It'll be alright in a couple of days."

"Fine," I said, "if it's just a sore throat, this test will be negative and everyone's a winner."

"No. Put it back in the box. I'm not shoving anything up my nose," said mother.

I took this small period of calm to select, from the mental vault of Pauline, a trusted form of manipulation. I call reflective moments, such as these, my 'reasoning with mother when she's being a dick'. I opted for reverse psychology; it has never failed me.

"Right," I said pretending to push the cotton bud back into the paper sleeve. "No bingo on Wednesday for you then."

Mum inhaled sharply, "Wait… how?"

"Suspected covid. Can't go anywhere with that," I replied. "Eric, hand me over that test box and let's put this crap away. Anyone want a coffee or cup of tea?"

I was 'packing' the various test items back into the box when mum quietly asked, "I can go to bingo with a negative test?" I nodded and stood up with the test kit in my hand, "Sure, but it's too late now," I declared.

"How's it too late?" asked mother. I turned and made towards the kitchen in a bid to keep up the pretence but mainly so she couldn't see me smiling.

"Stuff's already back in the box and you don't want to shove a cotton bud up your nose for 10 seconds," I said. "So… the game's a bogey." I'd almost made the kitchen door when mum finally caved into the raw power of direction, "Alright," she said, "give me the cotton bud."

Fifteen minutes later, the test result confirmed there would be no bingo, for at least a week and with this grim recognition, the room fell silent. I'll not lie – I was still secretly marvelling at modern day science and slightly in awe that a virus could be detected, in the comfort of your own home, using these plastic implements. Mum pulled me back into reality,

"Am I going to die?" she asked. Her bottom lip instantly crumpled. I could see tremoring hands trying to find each other so they could clasp together. "Because am no' ready for that," she said.

I wasn't prepared for this line of questioning or her declaration of not being ready to become another covid statistic. Mum's pleading gaze searched the room for an answer. The situation was fast becoming too morose for my liking. I pitched out the first thing that swept into my mind, "Fuck me, that's a bit dramatic," I said in a tone slightly higher to that of my normal voice. "Is dying from lack of bingo an actual thing?"

From outside, a woodpigeon favoured this exact moment to fly into the living room window and everyone heard it thud on the glass. I literally watched the feathered arsehole slide down the entire windowpane and disappear from view. The chalk outline of said kamikaze bird would remain on the outside of the glass for three weeks, before the window cleaner, tidied up the scene. Lewis and I frequently studied the dusty imprint real close, you could see actual feathers, an eyeball, and a beak. A form of art created from velocity, pigeon bad eyesight and a rogue gust of wind, perhaps. Whatever the reason, I hoped the little guy was alright.

Mum held her arms out at the side and then brought them forward to point both hands in my direction, "Again with this charade," she said flatly. "Every time."

I felt the need to defend my original comment, "I'm certain, lack of bingo play has never been mentioned on any certificate as a cause of death, but I'll gladly debate it." A faint smile appeared on mum's lips but didn't stop her shouting out, "Covid Pauline! Am I going to die of covid?!"

I shrugged, "Probably not today," I answered. "If you're looking for my best guess."

"That's your answer?" mum fired back at me. It was clear she had concerns, most likely the reason why she didn't want to take the test. Deep down I think she knew, and this release of pent-up frustration had now firmly landed on my 'shit to deal with' list. I inhaled slowly through my nose before delivering the words of reason,

"Listen here," I said. "It's a slightly weird, underhand compliment that you believe I went to medical school and have all the answers." Mum attempted to intervene at this juncture, but I held my arms out to the side, and ploughed on,

"Full disclosure? I have no fucking idea when you will leave this mortal coil or if this virus will be your downfall," I shook my head. "Not one clue do I have!" Even to my own ears, it sounded harsh, but it was truthful, and she needed to hear it. I hadn't even contemplated the notion of her dying from this test result... until now. So, my whole outburst was, perhaps, saturated with my own fears. The room fell silent again. I stood up and reverted to type, "Who wants a coffee or tea?" I made for the kitchen, internally cursing my distinct lack of compassion.

Eric, with his powers of perception, took over, "Jan," he said, "you've had all your vaccinations, right?" Mum sniffed and nodded her head. He continued, "So, maybe thinking about a covid death isn't the best plan of attack, you know?"

"You're right," she replied. "Just a bit of a shock."

"Course it is. Christ, when we had covid three weeks ago, I thought Pauline was joking when she said her test was positive but, guess what? The two of us, we're still here," he said. "Alive and kicking."

I finished making the cups of tea, dropped the teaspoon into the basin and wrapped a tea towel around the bottom half of my face. I picked up mum's cup – wandered back into the living room. When she lifted her head and saw me, mum chuckled. The tension lifted and normality was restored. For that day, at least.

The next week or so... (puts index finger to bottom lip and contemplates the appropriate wordage) peculiar is how I'd best describe it. A complete range of weird shit went down. If you require further clarification, it was the full gambit of strangeness, if you please.

Mum lost her voice for the first couple of days and felt generally unwell. Flu-like symptoms. I was calling her every day, just to confirm she was still with us. Safe to say, I was getting on her tits. Some days, she even told me so and occasionally in less-than- flattering terms, but like a bar of wet soap thrown on a rhino's back, it just slid right off.

Day four and on the usual lunchtime 'let's bust the old dear's balls' telephone call, it all got a bit... kooky. After five rings, she answered the call then followed it up with complete silence. For ease, I've portrayed this part of the story, in script form.

What you see hereafter, is based on actual events. Nothing changed for dramatic purposes.

Me: Hello?
Mum: *[silence]*
Me: How's it hanging the day mother?
Mum: *[more silence]*
Me: *[Using my best ghostly haunting voice]* Is there anybody there?
Mum: *[even more silence]*
Me: Helllllllllllloooooooooooo?
[Ten seconds later, the line went dead. I hit redial and mum answered again]
Me: Hello?
Mum: Pauline? Is that you? I need to go; someone is trying to call me on this mobile phone.
Me: Yeah, that was... *[Call disconnects]*
[I hit redial and after listening to the engaged tone for the first three attempts, mother successfully answered on the fourth]
Me: What in the holy fuck is going on here?
Mum: *[using a slightly aggravated tone of voice]* Pauline, you need to stop calling me for five minutes! There's someone trying to get through. God's sake! *[Call disconnects]*

I pulled the phone from my ear and stared at the display of it. Maybe someone else was, indeed, trying to contact her. Or maybe she was interviewing for a new sex chat position. I shrugged my shoulders and was about to hit redial when it started raining. I pulled my coat hood up and walked back to the office with a self-made promise that I'd try again after work.

On the bus ride home, I redialled her number and mum picked up immediately,

Me: Ah! You're still with us?
Mum: Who is this?
Me: Mother Teresa.

Mum: Who?
Me: Are you kidding me with this?
Mum: Is that you Pauline?
Me: If that's what it said on your display when the phone rang... then... yes, it's me.
Mum: Eh?
Me: *[swallows back mounting frustration]* Yes. It's me. Pauline.
Mum: Thank God for that.
Me: Compliment accepted.
Mum: Eh?
Me: Never mind. What you been up to today?
Mum: This phone. It's driving me nuts.
Me: How come?
Mum: Was ringing for ages.
Me: Did you answer it? Speak to whoever was calling you?
Mum: Mostly, there was no one there.
Me: Where?
Mum: I told them to stop calling me in the end.
Me: Interesting. You told me to stop calling you. At lunchtime today.
Mum: Did you call me?
Me: *[tries not to say 'are you kidding me with this' again]* Yeah, several times.
Mum: I don't remember talking to you.
Me: Well, you didn't really.
Mum: What? Call you?
Me: *[tries not to say 'for fucks sake' out loud and instead, smiles at complete random sitting in bus seat opposite]* No. I called you, but you didn't say very much.
Mum: Hello?
Me: Hello? Can you hear me?
Mum: Is there someone talking in the background?
Me: Background? Maybe it's other people on the bus you hear?
Mum: What bus?

Me:	The bus I'm on. Going home? From work?
Mum:	No. Wasn't that. Sounded like something else.
Me:	Moving swiftly on. Are you feeling better?
Mum:	Yeah, fine. Should I not be?
Me:	*[Oh... my... fucking... God]* Well, you're probably still covid positive. Figured it was worth a check in.
Mum:	I'm fine.
Me:	Your throat sounds a lot better at least.
Mum:	What was wrong with my throat?
Me:	*[Stopped myself from swearing out loud on public transport]* Right. The bus is pulling up to my stop (it wasn't). I'll phone you later, ok?
Mum:	What for?
Me:	Shits and giggles.
Mum:	Stop swearing.

Before I could say my goodbyes or question her weirdness during our chat, mother hung up. Opposite fellow bus traveller gave me a sheepish 'goodness that conversation didn't end very well' look. I smiled and flicked an imaginary middle finger their way. Nosey bastard.

"Just had a strange conversation with mum," said I to Eric, who was busy slicing tomatoes and adding them to a salad bowl when I got home. "You'll have to narrow that field down," he replied. "You forget, I've witnessed the chats you and your mum have."

I took my coat off and started walking down the hallway towards the bedroom, "Can't put my finger on why it was odd," I said. "She sounded like she was miles away. Confused maybe." When I got back to the kitchen, Eric popped a slice of cucumber in his mouth and mid chomp, asked, "Confused?"

"Yeah, it reminded me of you," I said. "When you first wake up, you know? Like that?" Eric smiled, "Christ it was bad then. When you called her, had she been sleeping?"

"I never asked her. Didn't get a chance to really."

"Phone her back in a couple of hours," Eric said, "should be an easier conversation to have when you aren't on the bus." It was a reasonable suggestion.

Me: Aloha!
Mum: Did you call me earlier?
Me: Loads of times.
Mum: What for?
Me: Just to see how you were. Some folks consider that thoughtful… you know?
Mum: Uh huh. What's that thing where you… *[apparently that was the full question, silence followed thereafter]*
Me: Where you what?
Mum: Chess. Like in a game?
Me: *[oh boy, here we go again]* Chess? Yes… that's a game. Although Bobby Fischer might believe otherwise.
Mum: *[tuts loudly and groans]*
Me: *[attempts to hurry the chat along, searching for a point]* With chess pieces and a board?
Mum: Yeah.
Me: What about it then?
Mum: I forget where I was going with this. Nope. It's gone.
Me: *[sighs with relief]* No matter. It'll come back to you at some point. You alright?
Mum: Yeah. I think so.
Me: Only think so?
Mum: Yes, I just said that did I not?
Me: Sure. Yes. Yes, you did. *[attempts a subject change]* What culinary delights did you feast upon this evening?
Mum: You see with chess?
Me: *[good effort on the change of subject]* Ah, we're back to this. Yes. Chess?
Mum: Moving in front?
Me: *[not one clue, did I have on where this was going]* Yep.
Mum: *[silence]*
Me: Hello? Yes. Chess. Moving in front?
Mum: Like fifteen moves or whatever.
Me: Yep, totally. What about it?

Mum: I'm thinking.
Me: *[silence]*
Mum: Ok. Well thanks for phoning. Will you be here at the weekend?
Me: *[patience gauge almost at empty]* Wait. What?
Mum: I need shopping. Milk and things.
Me: Yeah. We'll be down. Hopefully you'll be covid free by then.
Mum: What day are we on?
Me: Tuesday.
Mum: Bingo tomorrow then.
Me: Ah. No. You won't be doing that.
Mum: I always go on Wednesdays.
Me: *[trying one's darnedest to soften the incoming blow]* How about we start wiggling free of these bingo routine shackles? Huh? You like that idea?
Mum: Yeah fine. Except Wednesdays. That's bingo day.
Me: *[failing on all kinds of levels today]* Bingo will probably be cancelled this week. You know. With the vid outbreak and all.
Mum: I'll be there.
Me: *[it's like a hostile gang of youths have thrown me an open container of disposable straws and demanding that I should 'clutch them' while they all stand back, laughing at my demise]* Bingo isn't really a game that you can play on your own though, is it?
Mum: I won't be going on my own.
Me: It'll probably be cancelled but we'll see, eh?
Mum: This is Tuesday, right?
Me: Yep. Tuesday.
Mum: I've asked that already? Struggling to keep up.

Brief interlude. All you readers will need it – trust me, I'm in the know. Maybe use this time to get a cup of tea, drink neat alcohol, inhale a kilo bar of the finest chocolate or use this well-deserved respite to simply question your current selection of reading material.

In offering this time-out, I have, perchance, shot myself in the foot. Doing so, instils a personal fear in me that this book will now lay on a bedside cabinet with a folded corner at the top of this very page and gather dust thereafter. Never to be picked up, or even opened, again because who in their right mind would choose to read the rest of this tiresome conversation? I have 'gifted' you all a hypothetical opening. A moment to save yourself. It's obviously too late for me.

However, may I take this opportunity to humbly thank you for spending your hard-earned cash and selecting our story from the shelf. You've not only shown my family and I huge recognition, but you've also helped Parkinson's disease and other motor system disorder groups, throughout the UK. On behalf of these lifeline groups, massive appreciation, and respect, right back at you. Not all heroes wear capes.

For those of you with masochistic tendencies or those who have simply (and mysteriously) adopted the typical Scottish flavour known fondly as 'I've paid good money for this, I will read it to the end or so help me God', then the intermission is over. Brace yourselves.

Me: Let's play a wee game. You up for that?
Mum: Chess?
Me: Fuck no.
Mum: Stop swearing.
Me: What year we in?
Mum: 2022.
Me: What year was I born? Pauline. Third offspring?
Mum: Emmm... 1971.
Me: What was granny's first name?
Mum: Was I right?
Me: With what?
Mum: The year thing?
Me: Yeah, spot on. I'll let you know if you're wrong. This needs to be a quickfire deal though. You understand?
Mum: Sure.
Me: What was granny's first name?

Mum: Who? My granny you mean. Or yours?
Me: *[fuck]* Ehhh... yours.
Mum: Gran. I called her gran.
Me: *[stifles laugh]* No. Her actual first name?
Mum: *[laughs]* Oh right. Ehhh... Margaret.
Me: What day is it today?
Mum: Tuesday?
Me: You guessing? Or is that your answer?
Mum: Sod it. That's my answer.
Me: Who's the current president of the United States?
Mum: We really doing this?
Me: *[senses the slightest hint of mum's displeasure but ignores]* I'm asking the questions here.
Mum: I don't want to play this game anymore.
Me: Can you just answer this one? There's only one more after it.
Mum: Is there something wrong with me?
Me: I'm asking the questions.
Mum: You think I'm losing the plot, right?
Me: All I know is that answering questions, with a question, is considered rude.
Mum: *[heavy sigh]*
Me: Come on.
Mum: *[said slowly, through gritted teeth]* Joe... fucking... Biden.
Me: *[pretends like that was completely normal behaviour for mother]* T'riffic. Last one. When was the last time you took your medication?
Mum: Emmmm...
Me: Or had something to eat?
Mum: That's two questions.
Me: Classic avoidance.
Mum: I just ate a Mars bar.
Me: Anything of the cooked variety? Vegetables? Fibre? Anything containing vitamins?
Mum: *[silence]*
Me: Hello?
Mum: Wait. I'm thinking.

Me: What about your tablets? Check your box. Where we up to with those?
Mum: A cheese and onion sandwich. At lunchtime.
Me: *[obvious delay in communication]* And your box?
Mum: It's in the recycling.
Me: Eh?
Mum: Or maybe isn't. Think I only ate one.
Me: What the fuck?
Mum: I put the box in the fridge.
Me: Your Dossett box?
Mum: No. The other sandwich.
Me: *[slaps own forehead]* Where's your Dossett box?
Mum: It'll keep better in there.
Me: Earth to mother! Will you stop with the fucking sandwich chat?!
Mum: My tablets are here.
Me: Right. Have a look at the windows. Tell me which ones are empty.
Mum: What you mean?
Me: The box with your tablets? Which ones are empty?
Mum: There's loads of tablets in it.
Me: Should be empty spaces though?
Mum: What you mean?
Me: Well, the entire first column should be empty?
Mum: There's tablets in all that row.
Me: Columns were talking about. Rows are irrelevant.
Mum: Columns, rows, whatever.
Me: *[patience gauge is now flashing a red light]* No. Not whatever. This is important. Is the first column of windows empty?
Mum: You mean up and down? Not going across?
Me: Yes. Up and down. Is the first up and down empty?
Mum: There's no tablets in the first up and down.
Me: *[wipes brow]* So you've taken all of Monday's tablets?
Mum: Must have. If the windows are empty?
Me: Is that an answer or a question?
Mum: You said there wasn't any more questions.

Me: You know this isn't some kind of torture campaign, right?
Mum: Says you.
Me: What about the next column? How many empty windows do you have?
Mum: This window thing is confusing me.
Me: The windows that you open four times a day to take your tablets? We can call them something else if you want.
Mum: Ah. Those windows!
Me: *[patience gauge – below empty and hovering between 'despair' and 'fuck this shit']* So, with that, how many empty windows do you have under Tuesday?
Mum: Emmm… Tuesday up and down, they're all empty.
Me: I see.
Mum: Is that right?
Me: *[sucks air through teeth]* Well it's only 6:30pm and you're supposed to take your last meds at 8:30pm soooooooooooooooo.
Mum: Oh… Wednesday up and down is empty, Thursday is full, Friday is…
Me: Wait. What?
Mum: There's nothing in Wednesday either, there's tablets under the up and down on Thursday. Friday is…
Me: This is Tuesday though?
Mum: Yes, you said. Bingo day is tomorrow.
Me: Can I just haul this conversation back into 'the now'? Bingo aside and talk about medication?
Mum: Uh huh.
Me: *[takes deep breath]* To confirm, the column of four windows, under Monday, are all empty?
Mum: Uh huh. Yes.
Me: The column of four windows, under Tuesday, all empty?
Mum: Yep.

Me: *[my crazy hand gestures start around this point]* Moving onto the next column, Wednesday. All four windows are empty?
Mum: Yep.
Me: Thursday? Four windows under that day, what you got?
Mum: Stuff in those windows. All full.
Me: *[Help me OB1 – you're my only hope]* Right. All the other days, after Thursday, they're the same? Tablets in all the windows?
Mum: That's right.
Me: *[audible loud sigh]*
Mum: What about Friday?
Me: Huh?
Mum: There's tablets in all the windows under Friday.
Me: Yeah. I know. We're done with the window and tablet counting.
Mum: So, I can put this away?
Me: How many times have you taken your tablets today? Can you remember? It's ok if you can't.
Mum: I didn't think I'd taken any today but there you go!
Me: Why would you not?
Mum: What?
Me: Take your medication or think you haven't?
Mum: Maybe I did then.
Me: If all of this is a pure wind-up, I'll wish your next shite to be a hedgehog.
Mum: Wind-up?
Me: Never mind. Just thinking out loud.
Mum: I've not missed any tablets then?
Me: No. Nothing missed. I might have to call you back in a bit though. Try not to fall asleep.
Mum: Okay dokey.

Believe it or not – I've actually condensed this entire conversation. The chess reference went on for a soul-destroying length of time that I can't explain or fathom out why it was even introduced. It's a game she's never liked nor played. The column versus row part of the discussion? Ruined me.

Eric, who'd only heard my side of the hour-long exchange, quite rightly said, "You just need to roll with it and make allowances. Your mum has no idea. This is like a normal day for her." I couldn't hold a single thought in my head. It would be fourteen cigarettes, two bottles of lager, four packets of crisps (various flavours) and a moment where I rested my forehead on the fridge door, before I called Jill, the Parkinson's nurse again.

"Hey, Jill. Hope you don't mind me calling you again," I said. "Bit worried about the old dear you know?"

Jill quite possibly fibbed and said, "Not at all. Happy to help. What's up?" I explained that mum had covid, tested positive on the Saturday past and then supplied a rough outline on the shit that had just gone down. "So, it's more confusion you'd say?" she asked. "Still aware of her surroundings and past or present events?"

"Yeah, she answered all the questions that I fired at her," I replied. "My granny had Alzheimer's and a bit of dementia knocking around, so I know the difference."

"You don't feel that it's any of those then?"

"Just going with my gut instinct here Jill, you know," I replied. "If that counts for anything?"

"Sure. Do you know if she's missed any of her Parkinson's meds?"

"If anything, she might have double dosed. I'm not sure though and neither is she. Would that cause confusion?" I asked.

"Hmmm. Can sometimes cause dizziness, fatigue maybe. It's tricky to answer because we don't know if she's taken too much or too little of it," Jill answered. "Definitely needs to see the doctor, if only to rule out any urinary or ear infections."

"Both of those good confusion instigators then?"

"Yes definitely," she replied. "Maybe even try and get the doctor out to see her because she has covid? Your mum needs to get a hold of the PD medication intake as well."

"Right," I concluded. "Doctors appointment and I'll make sure she takes the right tablets going forward."

"At least until the confusion subsides," Jill said. "Anything else, just ring me as always." I was about to ask her what television program she was watching, the season she was on and whether I had interrupted the finale but decided against it. "Thanks Jill, pleasure as always," is all I said, before hanging up.

I afforded myself the luxury of four dark chocolate digestive biscuits and hoovered up a cup of tea before I called mum back. If it wasn't a 'school night', for sure I'd have thrown ice cubes and lime wedges in a tall glass of gin & tonic before I hit the redial button.

Me: Hello? Are you there?
Mum: There's a thing on television.
Me: That's usual when you have it on, right?
Mum: It's on. The television.
Me: Astonishing, we really must follow up on that television thing. Anyway, so I called Jill.
Mum: There's something walking around on it.
Me: Jill. The Parkinson's nurse. You know?
Mum: I know Jill and it's not her, no.
Me: No. She'll not be on television because I've just spoken to her.
Mum: I think it's gone now.
Me: *[What? My patience and sense of humour? Quite possibly]* Anyhooooooo. Moving on. Jill says it might be a good idea to get you a doctor's appointment. What say you? On that?
Mum: *[says not a word]*
Me: I see how it is.
Mum: Nope. It's definitely not there.
Me: *[My will to continue this conversation? Yes. Accurate]* What's not there?
Mum: I got off the sofa to see but it's disappeared.
Me: Any chance you could focus on what I've said. Here. In this conversation?
Mum: I am.

Me: Cool. Jill was saying I should get you a doctor's appointment, so I'm going to phone them tomorrow.
Mum: It was just a bug.
Me: I believe the covid virus has been scientifically proven to be a tad more formidable than 'just a bug'.
Mum: Like a daddy long leg or something.
Me: *[Oh brother]* Are you still talking about the television?
Mum: Will you be down this weekend?
Me: You hear me talking, right? To you? On this phone?
Mum: Yes Pauline! For fuck's sake! I'm no daft!
Me: *[again with the swearing]* So I'll phone your doctors tomorrow and see if I can get you an appointment.
Mum: For what? I'm not going to the doctors.
Me: Unusual that you are showing resistance.
Mum: Just wasting everyone's time.
Me: *[said calmly but with a twitching eyelid]* Doctors. You know. That's their job. They check over sick people. Pensioners are probably their bread and butter when you think about it.
Mum: You don't understand! You never will! Our generation is very different!
Me: Generational? This here? *[pointing downwards]* This moment and what's going on with you? Has fuck all to do with the generation gap.
Mum: See! Told you!
Me: *[takes a deep breath and mentally formulates another plan]* Ok. You're right. I am aware of nothing. My generation? We don't know anything.
Mum: It's like chess. When you think.
Me: Right. We'll be down at the weekend. I'll phone you tomorrow at 8:30am.
Mum: Ok. Why?
Me: That's the time for your first lot of medication.
Mum: Bingo as well mind.
Me: Sure. That too. Talk to you tomorrow.

When the call ended, I found myself staring at a black mark on our living room wall, above one of the framed pictures hanging upon it. I wondered why I hadn't noticed it until now. This blemish on the stark white landscape, reflected the conversation I'd just endured. It was both startling and wholly unwelcome.

I walked to the kitchen, picked up a damp sponge, stood on the arm of the sofa and gently dabbed at the stain on the wall. As if this very action, perhaps on a sub-conscious level, would somehow wipe away the last hour, taking all my concerns with it. The mark on the living room wall disappeared easily – the weird discussion? Not so much.

Chapter 33 – The Aftermath

I'm a good person to have in your corner, amid stress-ball situations. Without even batting an eyelid, I'll breakdown the cause of the issue, suck up any dramas in relation to it and in doing so, lower the general anxiety. That's the plan anyway. I've been called many things in my life (profanity, mostly) but 'stress hoover' or 'worry crutch' are labels I can get behind and appreciate. I am that annoying individual who really does work much better under pressure. Calm down. It's fine. I got this.

Let me tell you though, this telephone call that just ended? Carved an egotistical trench through my top ten list of stressful life moments and planked itself firmly in the number one spot. Leaving a whole host of emotional crap behind in the tear up. I've injected pops of humour into the conversation script, so it makes for better reading, but the reality was very different. Far and away, it was one of the worst nights of my life. The days that followed thereafter, tested me as a human being and my resolve. Everyone has limits.

The very next morning I reverted to type, adopted my usual 'fuck it' attitude and called mum's doctors. When they called me back, the doctor and I concocted a reasonable plan, she would arrange a home visit for mum under the guise of checking out the elderly folks who were part of the bingo covid outbreak. "Please don't mention that I called you for this appointment," I asked, "she's not having any of it and I just need someone to check her out." Mum, to this day, still believes the doctor turned up for the home visit out of personal covid concern for her patient. Wait 'til she reads this.

After the home visit, the doctor concluded that mum's befuddling was mysterious, but she went on to rule out any kind of infection. However, if she was still 'not of this planet' by the end of the week, then we'd have to contact the surgery for another appointment. I felt mild relief.

Thankfully bingo was cancelled on the Wednesday (fist pump) and mum didn't feel well enough to go anyway. The next couple of days in general though? Well... they were complete hell. I got into the routine of calling her four times a day, just to make sure she was taking her medication. I'd ask her if she'd eaten and every single day, she fought me on it. She even questioned my parentage occasionally which I thought was... ironic. Surely, she was on scene and, at the very least, participating when I slid into this world?

We argued incessantly. Now, when I say argued, I don't mean this namby-pamby bickering over miniscule details where it ends with a conservative handshake and the ongoing promise to remain friends. No. None of that.

I mean all-out war. Carnage of the verbal nature. Shouting so hard and loud that you unwittingly induce a 'flashing lights in your peripheral vision' headache. Of course, the telephone conversations wouldn't start out like we had murder on our minds. Initially and occasionally, there would be normal pleasantries but when those were out the way. Free game after that.

Mother, very quickly, dispatched with the boring, classic, obvious telephone openers. Favourites such as 'Hello' and 'How are you?' were tiresome. These were soon replaced with stark questions instead like 'What?' or 'Who is this?' From time to time, she even kicked off these conversations with deadpan statements like 'Every fucking day with these phone calls' or 'I'm fine, don't ask'.

For the first two days, I glossed over mum's undeniable annoyance and her irritations. Every so often, her disparaging comments would, inevitably, claw at my forthright personality trait and an internal battle would rage on. When my back teeth began grinding together, I would hear Eric's words of wisdom in my head. *Just have to roll with it. Allowances must be made.*

It wasn't easy. These chats were generally all over the place. It would, quite often, take me a full ten minutes just to ground it and gently coax her back on the right track. The things I said out loud (and abnormally) were 'Don't worry about it' or 'That's absolutely fine'. Things I desperately wanted to fling right out there (instinctively) were 'Fuck me, this is a new level of tragic' or 'I must've wronged someone of great importance, in a previous life to qualify for this detail'. It was a recipe for disaster and guaranteed to fall apart at some point... as it happens, Friday morning, on the third day mum adopted a 'slightly' abrasive nature when she answered my 8am phone call, "What Pauline? For Christ sake! What?!"

Now, two days prior to this exact moment, I would've brushed off her shitty opening, with surprising aplomb, and then wallowed in a huge amount of self-pride thereafter. Not today though. Not here, standing outside my place of work, in the heavy rain, where a crowd of less than sociable members of the public had gathered and a stray from said entourage was now in my personal space, asking whether I had a cigarette, or eighty pence change for the bus that they could borrow. This wasn't the day.

I slowly turned my back on the newly procured, inquisitive 'friend' and through gritted teeth, but in a quiet, unassuming, tone of voice that contradicted my actual feeling towards this ongoing situation, I asked my mother the simplest of questions, "Who the fuck do you think you're talking to?"

Naturally, cigarette/change-for-the-bus guy assumed I had directed my inquiry at him, so that was another communication mess I had to tidy up. There are just some days where you wished you'd bitten your tongue right off and said absolutely nothing. Smile and nodded, while you choked back your own bile. Played the better person and rose above it. Cast aside the 'bang out of order' mother vocalisations and conformed to social niceties. Diplomacy. There's that word again.

I imagined all sorts after my one liner had been delivered. First and foremost, would it be another year of not speaking to mother because she'd determine that I had taken it too far this time and it was outright disrespect? I wondered if any of my siblings would see my side, understand my outburst and back me up on it. It wasn't all grim thoughts.

My natural optimism afforded me some upsides to this scenario also. I saw another Christmas day with just Eric and I, in our PJs, feet up, guzzling chilled rose wine like it was going out of fashion, and no pressure to cook a sixteen-course meal or keep anyone but us, entertained. Ying and the Yang. I was pondering the next downside when I heard mum say, "You! I'm talking to you! Again! For the umpteenth time!"

I pressed the palm of my hand to my chest and opted for sarcasm in my reply, "Forgive me," I answered, "I literally had no idea these daily reminders to eat food and take your medication were such massive undertakings for you."

"It's alllllllllllllll the time," mum blasted. "Every hour my phone rings and it's you!"

"I am choosing to breeze over your exaggerations," I calmly replied.

"What do you want? What is it this time?" she asked flatly. Before I could think of a suitable response, my mouth was inadvertently working its 'magic',

"Gratitude for a fucking start!" I launched back at her. "Wait, how about not talking to me like I'm something that crawled from beneath a stone? Any chance with that?"

"You've no idea," she mumbled.

"On what? What don't I have any idea of?"

I had offered my mother an opening. A chance to dig deep, reconsider and explain her vocal savagery. I certainly wasn't expecting the abrupt conversation shutdown when it fell from her lips. "No. I won't," was all she said.

I sucked in a lungful of air before choosing my reply carefully, "Well. Here's what's going to happen," I spewed forth. "When I call you again, at lunchtime…," I duly ignored mum's tutting and trudged on, "can you just try answering the phone with a hello, how are you? Maybe even throw in a wee bit of sincerity?"

Mum replied with a non-sensical defence, "It's you! Phoning me!"

In the metaphorical sense, I pinched my nostrils and plunged right in there, feet first. I'd reap whatever consequence came my way. "You know what?" I blasted, "I don't need to phone you. I don't need to put up with your snide comments and endless protests but hey, here I am… doing it! Making sure you're eating and taking medication. In case you're in the least bit interested, it's called genuine concern for a person's wellbeing!"

"I'm fine," she replied.

"Ok. It would appear you're correct. I know sweet fuck all. I'm glad we clarified that."

I talked her through what medication she needed to take from her Dossett box, reminded her to eat some breakfast and told her I'd call again at twelve o'clock. When I hung up, Mr Change for the Bus was still lingering around in the hope I'd somehow changed my mind. I looked skyward for divine intervention, pushed open the office door with my shoulder and made my way back inside.

At 10am, I bit the bullet and called mum's doctor. It was either that or mum and I would eventually fall into the 'estranged family' category. I'd maybe require bail money before then. Difficult to say what would come first there. Jackie was going over to see mum at lunchtime when she finished work and if I managed to get an appointment around the same time, mum would be Jackie's problem thereafter. The confusion needed further investigation, whether the old dear liked it or not. Would love to say I felt guilty about ladling this onto Jackie but in truth, I didn't. If anyone could manhandle a pensioner into a doctor's waiting room and without any self-reproach, it was my oldest sister.

After ten full days of pride swallowing (several times), fibs (copious), patience (lots of), personal dignity (none left), swear words (numerous), requests of help from God himself (plentiful) and a fleeting moment where my self-confidence was completely non-existent, Jackie took mum back home, from the doctors, with antibiotics for a… urine infection.

A UTI, the source of mum's confused state and the symptoms of which, almost ended me as a decent human being. All because mother didn't want to 'bother' the doctor or waste anyone's time with it. Her generation though? Still the best in her opinion. I, however, won't ever understand why a person works their entire life, contributes to a National Health Service, throughout their employment, and then feels bad about using the service in later years. My poor wee logical brain does not compute. Sensibly though, I shall no longer argue over it. The kaleidoscope of colour in my peripheral vision is undeniably pretty but rather unpleasant. You live. You learn.

Chapter 34 – Last Monday of each month

Is the Parkinson's group meetings and I've persuaded mother into taking me along. Here is where I finally get to meet Jill the Parkinson's nurse and Gary who arranges these meetings which are currently being held in the chaplaincy unit on the Borders General Hospital grounds. I have it on good authority, they are here because the NHS give them the meeting space at a reduced rate. Other establishments apparently charge 'an absolute fortune' to use their empty social function rooms. Even on a weekday.

Now... I'm a logical thinker and I believe the neurologist when he says that PD doesn't claim lives. Holding the monthly Parkinson's meetings in a chaplaincy unit, designed, and built around death? Evidence of which is apparent. There's a room containing church pews and a huge wooden cross sitting on a makeshift altar at the end. A stained-glass window throws shards of different coloured light into the room. I'll not tell any fibs; I have issues with the arrangement. Still have and quite possibly always will.

The PD meeting isn't held in this room but walking past the entrance to it, is thought provoking. Those who attend these monthly meetings don't appear to recognise the irony. Or maybe the attendees do but choose to sweep their opinions under a non-existent rug because they are fully aware of the meagre group budget.

I very quickly realise that Jill and Gary, are two of the nicest people you'll ever meet. Thoroughly down-to-earth individuals who are clearly doing the best with the resources available to them.

Gary himself is a young man, who is not only battling this disease but treats everyone who walks through the chaplaincy doors with the utmost respect and compassion. He enters the room carrying two shopping bags and I'm instantly wondering what these sacks contain. No one else is speculating, it's just me. The newbie. The imposter.

Jill circulates around the room, and I'm announced as Jan's daughter, who is writing a book about Parkinson's and how, as a family unit, we deal with the complexities involved. It's nice meeting these new people, all in their varying stages of the disease.

A woman, named Eileen, talks to me first. She doesn't have PD but her husband, who lived with the disease for ten years, sadly died the year previous. She comes to these meetings to offer support to family and friends. Quickly, I'm recognising that I'm the only one who is there under that category. Everyone else has turned up on their own. No family members at their side. Perhaps these family members have already popped their heads in during previous meetings and its mum's turn to bring in some support for show and tell. I don't feel intimidated when everyone in the room turns to look my way. I simply raise a hand and wave.

The meeting continues as normal but somehow, I'm still curious as to what's in Gary's bags. I secretly chastise myself over the miniscule detail. Discussions begin in reference to the Christmas panto foray to Edinburgh. Everyone in the room appears to be excited about the impending trip. It's obviously a huge event in the PD calendar. Money set aside in their paltry budget for the once-a-year outing. Remarks are made about how well organised the trip is and that it's always a great day out. I smile. Such a simple thing that brings a huge amount of joy.

Half an hour later, a suggestion is made that everyone retires to the cafeteria for a cup of tea. I help mum to her feet, and we follow the crowd. Gary duly picks up the bags he brought in and joins the queue. Once in the café space, Gary pops the full bags on a wobbly table and it's now a hive of activity. Eileen puts the large kettle on and gathers mugs. She goes around each of the attendees and asks if they want tea or coffee. Mum chooses tea but I decline the offer. A woman called Margaret starts talking to me about the book. She asks me the title of it, and I tell her. She nods her head slowly and then informs me that it's inspired. I smile and say thank you. She goes on to ask me the contents of the story and I answer as best I can. "It's our take on the disease," I tell her. "Our opinions and how we deal with it, as a family unit." Margaret nods again. She gets it. I continue, "We use humour as our medicine. It's our coping mechanism. If that makes any sense?"

Margaret smiles softly, "Whatever gets you through," she adds. "It's brilliant. I love the book title. It tells a story without even reading a word." I thank her again for the kind words. I notice she has a walking aid and I ask her how long she's been living with the disease.

"I was diagnosed in 2015," she offers. "The first few years, I never noticed a difference. Slight tremor in my hand, nothing to write home about." I nod my head and Margaret carries on,

"Six years on and now I have the walking trolley. Just creeps up on you but you learn to live with whatever comes your way," she tells me. "I do the best with what I have. This group helps massively. I know it's only once a month but it's nice to step out and talk to like-minded people once a month. Others who understand. You know."

I'm suddenly aware of how important these get togethers are. Chatting to different people, who are in the same boat, living with a disease that neither conforms to rules or cares about the debilitating level it may reduce a person to. It's a wake-up call and in that moment. I think about other cities and towns that don't offer the same service. The ones that don't have a Gary or a Jill, who are willing to go the extra mile and take time out of their own personal lives to co-ordinate these social lifelines.

Eileen appears and passes a cup of tea to Margaret. A couple of seconds later, she re-appears with a biscuit tin and tells Margaret there's chocolate ones with wrappers! Jokes are made that Gary must've had a lottery win. Margaret quickly rifles through the tin and selects a Tunnocks tea cake. She holds it aloft and declares them as her favourite. I chuckle and tell her that she's very lucky to have a Gary who clearly looks after them all.

As she scoffs the tea cake, I find it amusing that her top lip is covered in mallow filling, but Margaret doesn't care. She's amongst friends who are doing the best with the cards they've been dealt. People quite often say to me that it must be difficult, with mum and her Parkinson's. They sympathise but truth be told, it's only when you're forced to deal with it or something similar, then it slowly becomes tolerable. Familiar. Just a part of your life. It's not heroic or brave. It's merely a curve ball that has you heading in a different direction.

As the meeting ends, I notice more activity. This time it's people rooting around in handbags or digging in trouser pockets. Eileen quickly slips Gary some cash. If it wasn't for his protesting, I wouldn't have seen the 'transaction'. "Hush now," she tells him. Mum gets up from the chair and does the same. Like a true professional, she also 'tips the dealer'. Gary accepts the donation with grace. I tuck my hand under mum's arm, and we make our way back out to the car park.

I open the car door and help mum inside, "Do you need to pay for these meetings?" I ask her.

"No, not at all," she answers. "We can't have Gary paying for the tea, coffee, and biscuits out of his own pocket every month. That's not right."

I close the passenger side door and as I walk around to the drivers' side, a lump the size of Mount Vesuvius is in my throat and tears are stinging my eyes. Before I open the car door, I inhale deeply through my nose and gather some composure. I get into the driver's side, start the car engine, and pull the seatbelt over my body, "That's lovely that you all do that." I say to mum. Not one person in that meeting was making a big deal out of it. I swallowed my surprising emotion and did the same.

These PD group meetings are an essential lifeline, offering the attendees a whole host of support. Above everything else and very evident in this bunch of people, is the knowledge that they are not alone. Friendships are born from this PD common denominator. Even in the darkest of places, life still grows, and hey... mushrooms are delicious.

Chapter 35 – The Grand Finale (or is it?)

Continuing with the full disclosure, I penned this chapter at the start of this book writing journey and now, here I am, fobbing it off as the grand finale. Writing it at the end, as a natural conclusion? I agree, perhaps a more uniform choice (if you've paid attention at all through this magnum opus of mine, I doubt 'uniform' would make the top ten of suitable adjectives) but since I continually row in the opposite direction, this book would never have made the shelf and you wouldn't be reading it – fact!

My low boredom threshold would've kicked in, followed swiftly by a distinct lack of patience, I'd have mumbled something akin to "fuck this shit" and then contemplated life as a truck driver or semi-professional poker player instead. Know thyself. Know thy capacities. I knew these last few pages would be the most difficult to get down on paper and for that reason, I started at the end. Wine helped. Gin also. Both, in moderation. Occasionally, I broached excess. Needs must.

I won't lie. There are parts of this Parkinson's disease marathon that have sucked on my very soul. In fact, writing most of it, has been less than cathartic. Wasn't really expecting the emotional roller coaster, for I'm hardly the emotional sort. But family man... they'll tug at every damn heart string, whether you want it pulled or not.

I always imagined my brain and thought process to be that of a locked metal filing cabinet. File, upon file containing all the past, depressing shit that I'd locked away in the rusty old drawers. Shoved to the back. Dealt with it. The information was always there, I just decided that's where it was staying.

For that reason, it was difficult recounting some of these earlier memories and events. When the need outweighed the want, I gingerly unlocked the 'cabinet' and rooted around in the various 'drawers' for accurate information. Blew imaginary dust from these files, peeled back the aging cover and apprehensively, looked inside. When I had what I wanted, the cabinet drawer was slammed shut and I got the hell out of dodge. Not without consequences though. It's mentally exhausting fishing in these murky ponds and then, from the outside, pretending like you hadn't. I wanted this story to be uplifting but hey... life isn't all about unicorns, fairies or some cartoon princess strolling through a forest, sharing a joyful chorus with animated deer and chipmunks. I really must stop watching the film Enchanted. Anyway, here comes the gloomy shit...

Eric and I were down seeing mum on a regular weekend visit. I was busy in the kitchen preparing a couple of meals for her to eat in the coming days. It had become a welcome habit. It gave me piece of mind that she was eating something and my mum comfort in that she didn't have to cook. I've been doing it for months now and through various text messages, we'd finally worked out what she'll happily chow down on and what she doesn't like. From the kitchen, I heard mum talking to Eric,

"Haven't heard anything from the American contingent for a wee while." It was a 'thinking out loud' comment, a conversation starter and Eric, as always, welcomed a gab,

"Oh really? You still getting Christmas cards though?"

"No, not even a card," she said. I was trying to work out from the tone of her voice whether she was concerned. Eric, reading my mind, continued, "When was the last time you heard from any of them?"

Mum was thinking, sucking air through her teeth. "Christ, now you're asking," she said. "Six, seven years maybe?" I put the knife down on the chopping board and picked up a tea towel, wiped my hands and made my way to the kitchen door,

"You and Gordon were emailing each other for a while. Not even an email?" I asked.

"I'm trying to think now," she said. "No, literally nothing. It's funny the random things that pop into your head, eh?"

Eric looked over his shoulder to the kitchen door where I was standing and turned back around to face mum. "Maybe you should send him an email tomorrow? Pick things back up again?"

"Yeah. That's what I'll do," she said. "See what he's been up to." After that, mum asked Eric to sort out her Netflix subscription and I went back into the kitchen.

As we made our way back to Edinburgh, Eric voiced our concerns, "You know... I have a bad feeling about the Americans."

"Yeah, Biden? You think he'll do a better job than the Trump fella?" I looked over at Eric in the passenger seat and we both smiled. I knew what he was thinking. No contact in six or seven years, meant just one thing. Bad news.

You'll remember how long it took mum and I to find her father, half brothers and sister? It took Eric thirty minutes and a fourteen-day free trial on ancestry.co.uk (other family history websites are available) to confirm our feelings of dread.

Gordon Lee Schaeppi, mum's younger half-brother (born in 1951), died in 2007. He was fifty-six years old. Eric found his obituary in the Chicago Tribune. In it, mum is mentioned. *He is survived by a half-sister Janice Kennedy from Scotland.* I printed the obituary and handed it to mum. The information left her in no man's land. Naturally, feelings of sadness came... and went. Can you really know a half-brother from two photographs and letters written because he felt he needed to rather than wanted? I'm convinced a small piece of my mum, deemed our research efforts, a waste of our time when she read that obituary.

Barbara Ann Schaeppi, mum's younger half-sister (born in 1950), died in 2017. She was sixty-eight years old. Barbara lived in Germany, was married but didn't have any children of her own. I believe she had stepchildren though.

William Lyle Schaeppi, the oldest half-brother (born in 1949), Eric struggled to find any information on him. We believe he re-married in 1998 but it's unclear whether he's still with us or not.

Eric also found all of mum's ten uncles and the only aunt. Twelve of them in total. Mum's aunt, Marion Eleanor Schaeppi, died at the age of nineteen (in 1944), giving birth to her second child, who also didn't survive the ordeal. The bad news just kept on coming.

Mary-jo Schaeppi (or Tydlacka before she married into the Schaeppi family), the woman who had given us the most family information in her letters from the mid-1990s, died in 2008. She was only forty-four years old. Her son, Avery Thomas Schaeppi, died in 2018. Ten years after his mother. He was twenty-four.

As far as Eric could tell, mum had pretty much outlived all her immediate family members from America. I remember in the letters that crossed the Atlantic Ocean during the earlier correspondence years, the Schaeppi family were adamant there would be no one visiting Scotland for any kind of reunion. I think Gordon maybe considered the notion, further down the line, but due to ill health it never came to fruition.

There was no one from Scotland doing the transatlantic journey either. The first (and only) time my mother has ever taken to the air, she damn near started a riot on the plane. Mum, dad, and Bob went on holiday to Ibiza. Her doctor had prescribed a heavy dose of 'calmer downers' to get her through the airplane fears, but it wasn't enough. You simply cannot unbuckle your seat belt or stand up when taxiing to the end of the runway and in a tumultuous tone ask, "What's that smoke?"

I imagined full-on passenger anarchy at that point. In my mind, I heard a series of seatbelts unbuckling, the grinding noise of a plastic fork being filed into a weapon, a guy banging on the pilot's cabin door, then shoving a flipflop bedecked foot on the jamb while he furiously grappled with the door handle. Flight attendants taking up residence in front of the cabin doors, launching packets of peanut M&Ms at frenzied passengers who were running down the aisle towards them. Inevitably resorting to tearing strips from their uniform allocation, thrusting the material into miniature bottles of honey Jack Daniels, and threatening a Molotov cocktail strike. Outright pandemonium. None of that happened though. My dad simply tugged on mum's arm and, in no uncertain terms, politely asked her to sit the fuck down and refasten her seatbelt. If you have an actual fear of air travel folks and just as an FYI, the window seat over the airplane wing…is less than ideal. Travelling to America to see half family members? Not a chance.

In case you haven't fathomed this out already, I'm an opinionated person. Whether my opinion counts for anything is up for debate. I like a juicy debate. So, here it comes... Now, when I read through the earlier letters from the mid-1990s, some thirty years later and with fresh perspective, the American's were quite simply being courteous. Don't get me wrong, I'm a huge fan of good manners. Barbara, for instance, always started her letters with 'I should have written to you before now, but time just runs away from you'. Reading this first hand and back in the naïve days, you honestly believed this woman ran the world. She was busy, living her life. Being Barbara. It made the lack of depth in her replies more digestible. When I sift through each of these letters and first lines now? It's clear, Barbara was merely being civil.

There's a massive difference between *wanting* to build a relationship with your half-sister and *feeling like you have to do it*. She was being gracious. It doesn't make the fourteen dollars she spent on postage costs, any less meaningful. If I was spending fourteen dollars on a letter being sent to Scotland, I would have included my life history (typical Scot – value for money). Barbara would've known my shoe size and how I preferred the cook on my sirloin steak. It would have been a life story, not one page of utter vagueness and continued apologies for not writing sooner. But allowances must be made. Everyone is different.

When I put myself in their shoes, receiving letters from across the pond, and half relationships? Would I have reacted differently? Listen, the Americans knew about mum, long before she did them and the fact, they hadn't utilised this knowledge in any way shape or form? Should have told us everything. But still we persevered. Out of hope.

I'm glad my mother found her American siblings and had some form of relationship with them. Not quite what she wanted but it was something at least. Other people walk this world and have no idea where they came from or where they belong. We did all we could to make it happen and this thought gives mum comfort. Sometimes you have a fancy for someone or something and it's not reciprocated. That's life.

I've recently concluded that in life and if you want something bad enough, you will pretty much give up your eye teeth to make it happen. Uncle Tom is the perfect example of that. When he knew about mum, he acted on it. He wanted it. If you weren't really bothered about it or anything? It will always remain, in the grey area, floating around. Mum wanted siblings bad and pretty much sold her soul for the cause. Barbara and Gordon? Simply being respectful and that, right there, is the difference.

In my opinion, Gordon, Barbara and Lyle missed a trick. A moment in life. My mother isn't perfect, but you know what? She's real and the sweetest, most comforting person I've ever known. She's never interfered in any of our lives. My siblings and I, we all made huge mistakes in life, but we learned from them and moved on without any judgement.

My mother would, undoubtedly, have been the best sister to all of them. Sometimes in life, a half chance is all you ever need. Everyone in this story is a victim of historical circumstance. Decisions made by your predecessors that we cannot change. You can only choose to deal with the events that happen as a result. RIP Gordon and Barbara. When we all meet again, we'll make this wrong... right. If you want to, of course? Family will always be a constant in your life. Blood is and will always be, blood.

Chapter 36 – The Honest-to-God Grand Finale

How is Jan Kennedy? Me maw? The wee wumin wi' the white hair? Very happy to report that she's still with us and health-wise, doing really well. Probably should have mentioned that a little further up! The 'parky' tremors, as we refer to them, are still confined to her arms and legs but best of all, she's finally getting out and about. Being sociable.

Nasty incident a couple of weeks ago (end of October 2022) where Lorraine and I dragged her slippered arse to A&E because she was 'quite unwell'. I did attempt to extract advice from NHS24 first but after listening to crummy music for over an hour, finally gave up and pulled the car key from my coat pocket. Mum didn't even want to put on her shoes or comb her hair before we left the house = complete vindication of our choice to hightail it to the hospital. Six hours later, having been moved to three different areas within the A&E department and now situated in the 'plaster room', a doctor appeared, "We don't know if your mum has an inner ear infection or whether she's had a stroke, but we'll get her discharged."

Cutting a very long story short, Lorraine and I protested to the NHS decision of turfing mum out and she ended up staying in for a week. Mum had trouble stringing words together, such was the confusion and every time she stood up, her blood pressure tanked. It was the first time I'd ever seen a nurse outwardly panic when the monitor bleeped ferociously and then flashed like a string of Christmas tree lights.

Naturally, mum rebelled against the 'staying in hospital' arrangement and on the very first night, from underneath the hospital bedsheet, she called our Jackie. Evidence suggests that, during this telephone call, a monetary incentive was offered up (amount undisclosed) and all my oldest sister had to do for the bounty, was to collect our mother from the health care 'restraints' and take her back home.

Jackie questioned the logistics of the plan ("How the fuck are we going to do that?" being her main concern) and she was duly surprised when mum recommended a hospital- issue towel over her head, followed by an A-list-celebrity-type hurry through the front doors. She was utterly convinced that no one would notice her disappearance.

The idea was rushed and desperate. No doubt in my mind, if mum was of sound mind, I'm certain the breakout would have included a grappling hook, ninja attire, video footage of her 'sleeping' on a continuous loop and several co-ordinated takedowns of the nurses and doctors, using stealth chokeholds or local anaesthetic injections, on the northbound, dimly lit, escape route. A full minute passed before Jackie stopped laughing and said no.

Jackie did the change of clothes drop off, and, in mum's opinion, it was all the wrong gear. Pyjama bottoms that didn't match the tops, knickers that she hadn't worn in years, blatant excuses to kick up some unnecessary aggro and bolster her 'I shouldn't be in here' rationale.

Mum attempted liberation three times in total before surrendering to good sense. With every new 'hostage' day that passed, her health visibly improved. Communication (shit talk) returned to normal, as did mum's innate ability to decline offers of help. When Occupational Therapy delivered a walking trolley to her room, I utilised that thing more than mum did. Funny incident occurred when I was sitting in the trolley's inbuilt seat, pushing backwards with my legs, chanting "wide load reversing" when suddenly I came to an abrupt halt against Gigantor, the biggest hospital porter you ever did see. #World's Strongest Man much? I chuckled. He didn't.

Towards the end of the week's 'holiday', a nasty rumour pertaining to a social care package for mum, began. Terms of said package were being knocked around, vague, still to be finalised but the plan was to discharge mum, with some form of outside and ongoing care. People coming to see her on the daily. Swinging by for ten minutes, bringing a bit of social interaction, making sure mum was eating and taking her meds. Perfecto. Before Florence Nightingale could recant the offer, I accepted on mum's behalf. We'd heard nothing in reference to the assisted living accommodation applications, so this new proposal was a welcome relief. Even mother got on board with it.

As it happens, mum was released from hospital and sent back home with... absolutely nothing. She didn't even have a discharge letter. My cynicism questioned if there was ever a social care package in place to begin with? Or was it all just 'system bullshit' to clear some beds and restore the flow? Newfound health service respect? Squashed like a bug, on a windscreen, in the height of summer.

Under-promise and then over-deliver. A tried and tested service plan where you give your patients more than you initially promised to placate them, make them feel valued and well cared for. Keep your promise, deliver on it. The size of your establishment or enterprise is completely irrelevant. It's simple advice and surely promotes five-star reviews. Doing it the other way around? Bonkers. All kinds of fucked up, in my opinion. When you have six NHS healthcare professionals, in as many months, telling you to write a letter of complaint that's when you realise the organisation is broken and perhaps, beyond repair. Austerity stuck the knife in some ten years ago; covid is slowly twisting it. Rant over.

Using true Kennedy grit, we swallowed the NHS betrayal, searched in the mud for circumstantial positives to this absolute farce and unbelievably, found some. The hospital 'vacation' had changed our mother. Like she had somehow been rebooted or upgraded. As if her hard drive had been serviced; circuits replaced. She had... mellowed. Become amenable. Mum was no longer batting away offers of help. In fact, she was now asking for it. Not right out there, in the open, clear as day but if you were fluent in pensioner language, you recognised the appeals. Fear is a great motivator.

Couple of examples, fear of falling in the shower. Don't outwardly ask someone to help you get washed. How obvious or mundane is that? Instead, just switch on the shower, leave the bathroom door open and stand in the middle of the floor holding both arms in the air. Someone (me) will stroll past said open bathroom door and ask, "What the fuck are you doing?" and there begins the showering aid without having to ask for it. During these showers, mum frequently complains that the delousing powder makes her eyes sting and then accuses me of water boarding her when I 'help' rinse the burning sensation away. A lesser individual would be offended.

Fear of being unable to change your duvet cover or bedsheets on your own. Again, dispense with the humdrum of simply asking an offspring to help or change it for you. Instead, come out with some long-drawn bullshit about how you watched a television program, the other day, where some woman was suggesting that you should change your bedsheets at least once a week and elaborate further by saying your sheets have been on for nine days.

Prior to this charade, mum would simply unbutton the bottom of the duvet cover, drag it off the bed and leave it on the bedroom floor, then claim that she got 'side tracked'. Zero intention of revisiting the job – confident that one of us would finish it for her. It's bringing sneaky to a new level and she's perfecting the art. Getting good at it. I can't help feeling both proud and impressed in equal measures. Progress. It really does come in various guises.

At some point, I will have to exit stage left, for the end is near. I'm not a massive fan of goodbyes so this 'see you later' will be brief. When the word got out that I was writing a book people would, obviously, ask me what it was about. You've probably guessed – I'm not a planner. In natural habitat terms and if David Attenborough was narrating in the background, I'd be described as 'spontaneous and flying by the seat of her pants'. Don't talk to me about stuff that's happening in three months' time. Not if you expect me to show interest. Eric is the household scheduler and I go the way he points us. So, people asking what the book was about and in my unprepared state? Clearly, an accident waiting to happen.

You start throwing the word disease around, as a book topic, you'll see various facial reactions that you weren't rightly expecting. Shock mostly and people, naturally, dealt with it differently. Me? I started adding 'hard sell' embellishments like,

"No, it's ok," or, "it's not a death sentence," and my personal favourite, vocalised out of sheer desperation that I was losing the crowd, "the story has funny bits in it." All of which… are true.

Parkinson's disease and the symptoms thereof, will continue and who knows what the next five years has in store for our wee maw. The disease will surely progress, and this family unit will do the very same. Tackle each new day with humour, sarcasm, respect and above everything else, hope. Medical breakthroughs are like Edinburgh buses – you don't see one for thirty minutes and whammo, five appear, all at once.

I'm still calling mum four times a day as a reminder to eat and take her medication. Don't need to, she could quite easily do it herself, but we've grown used to our daily chin wags, shooting the breeze, talking shit. I momentarily forgot who I was talking to the other morning and, as a joke, opened with, "Hello. How are you? You're looking well." Quick as a flash mum replied, "Pauline! Have you got me on that 'time face' again? I haven't even brushed my hair!" Priceless memories that will always make me smile.

Someday, I will no longer have the luxury of calling her, winding her up or hear her laugh. It's a good job I live in the here and now because, fuck it man, what a truly depressing thought that is. Shudders.

My final words are stolen lyrics from a song called Waves by Imagine Dragons (a mention in this book means that on your next UK tour, free tickets would be greatly appreciated). Cannot put this any better myself. We're all boarding the bus, conducted by the grim reaper, at some point. It's the only real guarantee in life. Do you need any further reason to simply live your life and cherish the time that you have? The obstacles that you'll invariably find in your path, exist only to make the journey more interesting. Massive love to all my family and friends, the real stars of this story. You're very lucky to have me in your lives [Thumbs up and smiley face emoji].

Ooh-ooh-ooh-ooh, ooh
Live in regret, or eye to the future?
I'd rather be here, thinking about the now
'Cause this breath could fade fast
And this day could be your last

La, da-da-da-da, la, da-da-da-da
So own all your tears and just roll with the waves
La, da-da-da-da, la, da-da-da-da
Life, it could change, it could change in a day
La, da-da-da-da, la, da-da-da-da
So cherish your years and just roll with the waves
La, da-da-da-da, la, da-da-da-da
Time doesn't hear, so roll with the waves

Chapter 37 – The encore

I always like to leave on a good note. Throughout this story, I continually make a point of looking forward. To the future. Go the direction your head is facing. Yes, you can rummage around in the historical ottoman to find out where you came from but that's not the road you're taking. It's not your current path in life.

My nephews and nieces, my great nieces, they all know the real Pauline. I won't ever shove any of my life under a rug. Being open and honest is the glue that sticks all of this together. I frequently tell nephew Lewis about my wishes when it's time for me to depart this world. He knows the score; he accepts the responsibility with decency and grace. More so when he's aware 'the ceremony' involves copious amounts of alcohol and minimal fuss. Right up his alley.

I appreciate and understand my granny's life choices. Alice did what she had to do. What she felt was right… in that time. Do I believe she could have handled it differently? More sympathetically perhaps? Fuck yeah but I won't ever judge her decisions. Could she have made it easier for mum or uncle Tom? Absolutely. Shoulda, woulda, couldas? All in the past. Let it be.

I will leave you with this funny story though. I debated whether to include it or not. Mum wasn't too keen. In fact, she vehemently protested to its inclusion. For that reason, I decided to shove it in. It's at the end of the book, so she'll think it's been discarded. Mother, just for you… this is my parting gift to thee.

For the record, this very instance is the one and only time I've witnessed my mother in an absolute state of alcohol disrepair. Hangin' out her arse. Melted. Reekin'. Snottered. Pissed. Steamin'. Blootered. Aff her face. Trollied. Wrecked. Call it what you will. There's drunk and then there's this one time…

Mum and dad, on a weekend, down at the dog track. This particular evening, dad had declined the invitation to her friend

Jean's 50th birthday party. Mum, with a couple of sherbets under her belt decided to accept. Dad went home. Mum made her way to Jean's house.

When mum got home the same night, that's when the party truly started. A taxi dispatched her at the house, and she staggered her way to the front door. We were all sitting in the living room when the front door opened, and she fell inside. We could hear her in the foyer trying to take her coat off. Mum finally bumbled her way into the living room and held onto the back of the armchair. I was first to speak, "You alright mother?" She looked right through me, trying to work out what the hell was going on.

"You'll never believe what I just saw," it was her opening line, somewhat slurred but I was hooked. I was mid-twenties age wise, wasn't missing this for the world. She was absolutely wrecked. If video footage was readily available during this era, I'd have been all over it. Sadly, you'll have to take my account of the events as evidence.

"I was at Jean's house for her birthday party," mum said. The grip on the back of the armchair was steadfast. If she had let go, she would've disappeared from everyone's view, instantaneously. "They made a barbeque, you know!"

I was chuckling away at the situation unfolding. "Did you have something to eat then?" It took her a while to focus on the question in hand, she answered it as best she could.

"Can't actually remember if I had something to eat but I tell you what..." Mum staggered a little and had a limpet like grip on the back of the armchair. "They made a barbeque out of four bricks and a bit of chicken wire!" It was a revelation. She'd never witnessed anything like it. I started laughing.

"Flinging on burgers and hotdogs. You believe that?" Dad was shaking his head in despair. Mum continued, "The burgers were sizzling. Actual cooking on the chicken wire! Flames licking out the side!" To anyone listening to this conversation, you'd think she'd never seen a barbeque in action before.

Mum was proper going for it, "Four bricks and a bit of chicken wire! Honestly. Never seen anything like it in my life!" Dad tried to downplay the position, but I was all for encouraging it. "Four bricks and a bit of chicken wire, eh?" I answered. "That's mental!"

"Burgers cooking away, hotdogs as well. Can you believe they were actually cooking all that shit on four bricks and a bit of chicken wire? They found everything in the shed?!"

"They had burgers in their shed?" I asked. "Did you partake in any of the beef fest?" I was trying to work out whether she had had something to eat or not. Judging by her incoherent state, I figured not.

"Four bricks and a fucking bit of chicken wire! I can't believe that!" mum rattled on. "You believe that? Cooking actual food? From nothing?" I nodded in agreement. Even in my sobriety, I was impressed. It was difficult not to be. Mum was acting like it was a moon landing or something equally exciting.

"Four bricks and a fucking bit of chicken wire Pauline! That's it! Cooking shit! On a bit of chicken wire!"

Mum staggered to the kitchen; I followed on behind. Wasn't missing any of this for the world. She made her way to the fridge, opened it, and looked inside. "Do we have anything for a sandwich?" she asked.

"Mum, there was a barbeque going on. Did you not have anything to eat?"

"Pauline, I can't remember what I did yesterday," she replied. I don't know what the fascination is but seeing one of your parents absolutely melted and searching in the fridge for something to eat, is a luxury.

"Four bricks and a fucking bit of chicken wire! Cooking burgers and hotdogs?" she bumbled on. "Jean was taking bets on jumping from tree to tree in her back garden!"

Wait… What? Generations below must know the full story. I followed her around the house after this statement. Mum carried on with the details, "Yeah. Jean made a bet with everyone about the distance between the trees and whether she could jump between them."

I was flabbergasted. What? Trees and jumping between them? "Jean was jumping from tree to tree you mean?"

Mum closed one eye and looked directly at me, "Yeah, she has two trees in her back garden, like four feet apart. Jean launched herself between the two. She made it though. I didn't think she would!" Mum put her finger to her bottom lip and said, "Think I owe someone a fiver though."

"Wow! What? She jumped between the two trees?" I asked immediately.

"Yeah! She made it alright," mum was making her way to the bathroom as she'd said it. "Trees were like ten feet apart. Couldn't believe it!" The distance between the two trees had mysteriously grown wider. If she hadn't closed the bathroom door in my face, I'd have perched myself on the side of the bath and continued the conversation. Instead, I sat on the bottom stair in the hallway and the interrogation went on through the closed door,

"So...these trees? Was it four or ten feet apart?" I heard a thud from inside the bathroom and then swiftly followed by an 'ooohya' from behind the door. I stood up and put my ear to the door. "You alright in there?" I asked.

Silence for thirty seconds then mum said, "I've just cracked my elbow off the sink! Right on the funny bone!" I heard her giggle then the toilet flush. She washed her hands and wrestled with the bathroom door handle before stumbling out, looked right through me again and made her way back to the living room.

"So, these trees mother? Four feet or ten feet apart?" Mum was back in the kitchen, fighting with the kettle lid. I took it off her and started filling it at the sink. She flopped onto one of the kitchen chairs. "What a night, Pauline," she shook her head and slurred on. "Four bricks and a fucking bit of chicken wire!"

I replaced the kettle and flicked it on. "Is it tea or coffee you want? What about these trees eh?"

"Oh?! Did I tell you? Jean made a bet that she could jump between the trees in her back garden?" She looked at the kitchen floor and with her arms wide open said, "Must've been like fifteen feet apart! She took off and jumped!" Mum had finished the sentence trying to simulate a big dipper ride with her arm at the top, then dropping it quickly into the bend.

I sniggered. "Fifteen feet apart? Wow. These trees just getting wider and wider, eh? Next, you'll be telling us they were fifty feet apart!"

"Noooooooooo. Was only like thirty feet maybe?" she paused. "Thirty-five at a push! She was like one of those flying squirrels!" Mum put her hand to her mouth and gasped. "Is that bad?" I took cups from the wooden tree mug holder that Lorraine had manufactured during a woodwork class at school and said,

"Is what bad? That you and your friends made a bet that Jean couldn't jump from one tree to another, thirty-five feet apart and doing it all under the influence?" Mum looked up at me and furrowed her brow. She was swaying in the imaginary breeze when she smiled, flapped her hand, and said, "Hell no! I just called my friend a squirrel! That's bad right?"

She had said it just as I was filling the cups. I burst out laughing and as a result, the hot water made its way onto the kitchen counter and subsequently, the floor. I put the kettle back on the stand, turned to her and said, "If that's the only 'bad' thing you see in this evening's festivities, just means you've had a great night!"

Mum was laughing. She got up off the chair and staggered back through to the living room. Stood in the middle of the living room floor with her hands on her hips and looked around the room. She shrugged her shoulders, mumbled something about hotdogs and off out to the hallway she went. We heard her fumble up the stairs and into her bedroom. I looked over at dad sitting on the sofa and said, "Four bricks and a bit of chicken wire, eh?"

Dad laughed and shook his head, "Four bricks and a *fucking* bit of chicken wire you mean?" he replied.

"Yeah!" I chuckled. "That's it!"

The End

Acknowledgements

"Remember, you'll need to do an acknowledgements chapter as well," said Lorraine, in an email, when she'd finished proofreading and editing this story. It's handy having an ex-journalist in your arsenal of help. I'd pretty much guilted her into doing it and then labelled the massive effort as 'drawing on family resources'. Brass-necked was Lorraine's more accurate description of the 'favour'. No offence taken, even if she meant it. I did enquire as to whether the second book would also be done free of charge. Similar mates rates deal? Still waiting on a reply. Anyway, here's the thank you section.

First time author, so there's no literary agent or personal assistant to thank for their hard work in the background. Unbelievably, I managed to pay all our household bills, cooked evening meals and even held down a full-time job while I worked on this story. Go me.

Big shout out to all the traditional publishers who completely ignored my emails containing the manuscript. Not even an automated response in some cases. Instead of draining my self-confidence and personal faith in the story, my natural defiance ignored the distinct lack of new author respect and subsequently, propelled me forward. Without your 'support', I wouldn't be here. My mother always says, if you want a job done, do it yourself.

To my friends and work colleagues who I, no doubt, bored incessantly with this entire process, special thanks. I truly appreciate the moments where you all stifled yawns and said things like "that's magic" whenever I discussed tragic sections of the book. Clear proof you weren't even listening. Just as an FYI – y'all know these particular actions are considered impolite?

Dominik, massive thanks for your Polish truth when I sent you the first three chapters at the very start. You fully understand that I am weird and rarely offended. Your red pen and highlighters were invaluable learning tools.

To Jill, Gary and everyone at the 'parky' group, huge thanks for letting me gate-crash your afternoon. You guys are truly awesome! Next time, I'll bring the teacakes of deliciousness. Deal?

My great friends Sam, Ames, Linda and Patrecko. Thanks for swinging by on text messages and picking up where we left off. The complexities of life keep our relationships digital but I'm forever in your debt. You always ask me if I'm still alive. Respect.

To Lynne, my hairdresser, my friend. When I'm slavering some amount of pish in your chair, you turn on the hairdryer. Subliminal communication at it's very best. You trawled through this waffle at the very beginning and supported throughout. This is me, not forgetting the ones who believed.

Uncle Tom, I fully recognise this wasn't easy. I salute you sir.

For my family, you guys… what can I say that hasn't already been said? Yes, you moaned occasionally, brushed me aside continually, ignored my story-line pleas in the family chat and said encouraging things like "are you still rattling on about this book?" Some folks would consider that disparaging, but you all know me. I thrive in that environment. For me, there's no better motivator than lack of support. Was that the plan? I'm chuckling so hard right now. It pleases me immensely that I'm part of your lives and there's fuck all you can do about it. My love for you all, is real and infinite.

For mum: *blessed are we who can laugh at ourselves for we shall never cease to be amused.*

To Eric, love you. Keep being you, pal. Incidentally, turning the hallway light out when I'm halfway down it, is still childish and immature. It's the reason why I occasionally hide at the side of the bathroom door and 'surprise' you when you come out.

To everyone who purchased the book, my gratitude is immeasurable. I hope you found yourself a 'right gid bargain' and some humorous insights along the way. Thank you.

May I take this opportunity to pass on some Pauline advice? When life knees you in the crotch and you eventually get your breath back, have a jolly good chuckle. In my experience, five years from now, you'll have a conversation in reference to a time when you were booted in the nunchucks and then laugh about it anyway. Save yourself some time.

It's that whole business when life deals you citrus fruit? Dear god, there's nothing else to do but reach for the gin. In moderation. Occasionally be excessive. One simply cannot have good fruit going to mush.

Printed in Great Britain
by Amazon

Dein Feuer in mir

Lisa O.

Copyright © 2021 Lisa Müller
Poststr. 2
91599 Dentlein a. Forst
Alle Rechte vorbehalten

Dies ist eine fiktive Geschichte. Ähnlichkeiten mit lebenden oder verstorbenen Personen sind rein zufällig und nicht beabsichtigt.

Für alle, die auf ihr Herz hören
und ihren Träumen folgen.

Prolog

Wärme durchdringt die eisige Nacht, Flammen ragen hinauf bis zu den Sternen, erklimmen das Dach. Das Knistern des Feuers ist der Takt zum Lied meines Engels, der in den Flammen tanzt. Lieblich die höchsten Töne hinausschreiend, während Glut deine zarte Haut versengt. Lass uns das Feuer der Leidenschaft entfachen! Verbrenne und werde Asche, sodass meine Haut, mein Haar, meine Lungen dich aufnehmen können und wir ganz eins werden. Ich kann es kaum erwarten, schüre weiter die Flammen an. Schneller, immer schneller, lass dein Lied erklingen und uns gemeinsam im letzten Ton vergehen!

Fast ist es vollbracht, mein Engel, bald gehörst du mir. Ich warte hier unten auf dich, wo mein nackter Körper vom feuchten Gras liebkost wird. Muss mich zurückhalten, mich selbst zu berühren, ertrage es nicht länger. So nah bei dir und doch so fern.

Ich opfere mich für dich.

Werde das Gefäß sein, in welchem du weiterlebst.

Verglühe und schwebe zu mir herab, mein Engel, ich bewahre deine Unschuld für immer in mir auf. Lass dich von meiner Liebe verzehren!

Ich sehe dich am Fenster, deine helle Haut rot erleuchtet, ein Feuerschweif anstatt der dunklen Locken. Wie eine Göttin siehst du auf mich herab, lass mich dir dienen! Ja! Sieh mich an, rufe meinen Namen, erwähle mich, ich gebe mich dir hin!

Unser Lied.

Paukenschläge deiner Hände am Fenster, der Wind pfeift die Melodie, die Flammen lodern im Chor.

Komm schon, mein Engel, sei die Sopranistin in meinem Stück, in meiner Sinfonie der Lust!

Was ist das? Eine Sirene?

Nein! Nein, nein, nein! Zu früh, viel zu früh! Ich brauche Zeit, verdammt! Sie kommen.

Das warme Licht unserer Vereinigung wird durch eisiges Blau gebrochen. Schreie, Rufe, schnelle Schritte. Ich muss verschwinden, muss dich verlassen!

Die Zeit läuft ein Rennen gegen mich und ich habe den Start verpasst.

Die Lust vernebelt meine Sinne. Ich muss klar denken!

Nicht zur Straße!

Die Lücke im Zaun ist mein Tor in die Freiheit, das Maisfeld wird mein schützender Mantel sein.

Ein kurzer Moment der Unachtsamkeit, schon bohrt sich ein Splitter durch meine Haut. Er kostet von meinem Blut, als ich durch die Öffnung dringe.

Regen peitscht in mein Gesicht, als ich in der Schwärze verschwinde. Matschiger Boden verschlingt meine nackten Füße.

Als würde die Welt mich verspotten.

Ich konnte es nicht beenden und nun ist es mir für immer verwehrt.

Meine einzige Chance: vertan!

Voller Verlangen stehe ich hier und habe keine Möglichkeit, dieses zu stillen. Maispflanzen um mich herum, nass, kalt, greifen nach mir, bedrängen mich. Mein Versteck bietet mir freie Sicht auf meine Bühne, deren Stück so barsch unterbrochen wurde.

Schwarze Uniformen rennen durcheinander wie aufgeschreckte Hühner, doch der Fuchs hat sich schon längst verkrochen.

Ich sehe die Männer, wie sie dich heraustragen.

Du lebst.

Das Gesicht noch gerötet von der Hitze unserer Lust. Schichten deiner Haut aufgebrochen wie ein in Schokolade gehülltes Dessert. Dein Lebenssaft tritt hervor, will dem heißen Körper entkommen.

Doch was ist das? Dein Anblick löst nichts außer Abscheu in mir aus. Schlapp und zerstört liegst du da, keine Anmut ist geblieben. Wo bist du hin, mein Engel? Deine Seele mag die Gleiche sein, doch sehe ich nur mehr das Biest in dir.

War deine Schönheit nur ein Spiel?

Hast du mich getäuscht? War es ein Zeichen des Schicksals?

Was, wenn du nicht die eine warst, auf die ich gewartet habe? Wenn du nicht die warst, die mich erlösen sollte?

Ein Trugbild!

Was, wenn es noch einen Engel gibt? Einen, den ich noch nicht kenne. Muss weitersuchen, muss von vorn beginnen!

Wie lange es auch dauert, ich werde sie finden!

Die letzte Schicht

»Pizza Margherita und eine Saftschorle, bitteschön.«

»Wurde ja auch Zeit! Ich warte seit zehn Minuten und habe nur eine Stunde Mittagspause. Können sie sich vorstellen wie es ist, zur Arbeit zu müssen?«

»Nein, kann ich überhaupt nicht nachvollziehen. Trotzdem einen guten Appetit.«, antworte ich ihm wie jeden Tag, an dem er zu uns kommt, um zu essen und über seinen anspruchsvollen Job zu meckern. Ich habe es schon lange aufgegeben, mich über ihn aufzuregen.

Als ich den Tisch verlasse, murmelt er noch etwas über die Jugend von heute, sein hart verdientes Geld und ich glaube irgendetwas von einem blöden Hund? Dann beginnt er zu telefonieren.

Seine aufgewühlte Stimme wird vom Kinderlachen am Nebentisch übertönt. Dort versucht ein gestresst wirkender Vater gerade seine zwei Jungs davon abzuhalten, die Pflanzendekoration zu zerstören. Ein Klümpchen Erde fliegt durch den Raum, ein Machtwort wird gesprochen und schon wandelt sich das Lachen in Schluchzen.

An jedem normalen Tag hätte ich jetzt zwei Lollis hinter der Theke hervorgeholt, um die Jungs zu beruhigen, den Vater gefragt, ob ich ihm noch ein Bier bringen kann und dann den Boden von der Erde befreit.

Aber nicht heute.

Heute ist ein besonderer Tag für mich. Es ist mein Letzter.

Also nicht der letzte Tag meines Lebens, sondern mein letzter Tag als Kellnerin der örtlichen Pizzeria.

Ich öffne die Holztür vor mir, auf der in großen schwarzen Buchstaben »Zutritt nur für Mitarbeiter« aufgedruckt ist.

Ihr vertrautes Quietschen, welches ich schon des Öfteren verflucht habe, lässt mich nun schwermütig werden. Dann steigt mir auch schon der altbekannte Geruch von Oregano und Tomatensoße in die Nase.

»Deliah, wie hältst du das nur aus? Jeden Tag frage ich mich, wie du es schaffst, ihm diese verdammte Pizza nicht in sein dämliches Gesicht zu werfen?«, fragt Nico, als ich die Küche betrete.

Er ist der Koch des »A Tavola« und außerdem mein

Chef.

»Was denn? Der? Wenn ich mich über jeden aufregen würde, der seinen Frust an mir auslässt, würde ich mit mehr Pizza um mich werfen, als du je backen könntest.«, antworte ich lachend.

»Deshalb verlässt du mich lieber?«

Jetzt steht er tatsächlich am Herd und zieht einen Schmollmund. Der Dampf, der von der köchelnden Tomatensoße aufsteigt, untermalt seine Mimik dramatisch.

»Nein, Nico, ich verlasse dich, weil ich mehr aus meinem Leben machen möchte, als schlecht gelaunten Leuten ihr Essen zu servieren.«, erkläre ich, während ich an ihm vorbei in das Lager schlüpfe.

Drei große Kartons trennen den restlichen Raum von einer kleinen Nische, in der ordentlich Taschen und Kleidung am Boden aneinandergereiht sind. Wir haben auch einen Aufenthaltsraum, doch der wird so gut wie nie benutzt.

»Außerdem hast du doch noch Nadja. Sie möchte unbedingt meine Stelle.«, schlage ich Nico einen Ersatz für mich vor, während ich mir mein T-Shirt überziehe.

»Nadja kann nicht einmal Spaghetti von Linguini

unterscheiden! Willst du mich ruinieren?«, empört er sich und fuchtelt mit dem Kochlöffel herum, sodass die gute Soße in hohem Bogen an die weiß gefliese Wand fliegt.

»Mamma Mia! Siehst du, was du angerichtet hast?«

»Ganz schön harte Worte für deine Tochter.«, antworte ich leise kichernd zwischen Dosentomaten und Mehlsäcken.

»Das sind die Gene meiner Schwiegermutter. Diese Frau ist il Diavolo!«, erklärt er und bekreuzigt sich dramatisch.

»Was tust du da?«, fragt er erschrocken, als ich in Jeans und T-Shirt hinter meiner improvisierten Umkleide hervortrete, die Arbeitskleidung sorgfältig zusammengelegt.

»Ich habe den restlichen Tag frei. Ich ziehe weg, schon vergessen?«, entgegne ich mit einem zuckersüßen Lächeln.

Nico sagt nichts, legt nur den Kochlöffel beiseite und kommt auf mich zu. Vor mir bleibt er stehen, betrachtet mich, nimmt mir den kleinen Stapel Klamotten aus der Hand und wirft ihn achtlos hinter in das Lager. Dann zieht er mich in die festeste Umarmung, die ich je bekommen habe.

»Oh Bella, ich werde dich schrecklich vermissen!«, flüstert er mir ins Ohr.

Aus meiner kurzen Schockstarre erwacht, erwidere ich seine Umarmung.

Wenn auch nicht so fest. Schon allein deshalb, weil ich nicht solche Kraft habe, wie er in seinen durchtrainierten Armen.

»Ich werde das hier auch vermissen. Vielen Dank für die letzten vier Jahre, Nico. Du warst der beste Chef der Welt.«, versuche ich einigermaßen deutlich durch seine Kochjacke zu nuscheln.

Er löst sich von mir, greift meine Schultern und sieht mir tief in die Augen.

»Du bist Teil meiner Famiglia und wirst es immer sein, meine liebe Deliah. Ich habe dir zu danken.

Jetzt geh hinaus und erobere die Welt! Wir werden hier auf dich warten und dich immer herzlich willkommen heißen. Buon viaggio!«

Tränen steigen mir in die Augen, sodass ich nicht mehr als ein Nicken zustande bringe. Mit einem traurigen Lächeln und einem Schulterklopfen verabschieden wir uns und ich gehe ein letztes Mal durch die quietschende Tür hinaus in den Speiseraum.

Der Mann telefoniert noch immer, während er seine Pizza verschlingt. Der Vater sammelt nervös sein Kleingeld zusammen, um bei Tina, meiner nun Ex-Kollegin, zu bezahlen. Währenddessen flitzen seine Jungs durch das Lokal.

Noch zehn Schritte.

Ich öffne die Tür, das Glöckchen klingelt einmal, dann erneut, als sie wieder ins Schloss fällt und das wars. Ich habe nach vier Jahren meine letzte Schicht im »A Tavola« beendet.

Die Mittagssonne strahlt mich an, das kräftige Grün der Bäume um mich herum erscheint mir wie ein Zeichen der Hoffnung. Ich bin bereit, ein altes Kapitel zu beenden. Ich bin bereit für eine neue Zukunft.

»Hast du deine warme Jacke auch eingepackt? Die mit dem dicken Futter?«, erkundigt sich meine Mutter, die mir gerade hinterher hastet, die goldene Lesebrille noch auf der Nase.

»Wir haben August, Ma. Ich bin sicher, ich werde gut ohne sie auskommen.«, antworte ich, als ich den Kofferraum schwungvoll schließe.

Ich liebe meine Eltern für ihre Fürsorge, allerdings ist

sie es auch, die mich hat bequem werden lassen.

Doch ich gebe ihnen nicht die Schuld. Sie meinten es nur gut mit mir, wollten mir meinen Freiraum lassen. Ich habe diesen Weg selbst gewählt.

Nach meinem Schulabschluss fing ich an, im »A Tavola« zu kellnern.

Geplant war ein Jahr. Herausfinden, was ich mit meiner frisch gewonnenen Freiheit anstellen möchte und dann die Karriere starten.

Schließlich wurden vier Jahre daraus.

Es hatte mich jedoch nie groß gestört. Ich mochte den Job und die Atmosphäre in dem kleinen Familienbetrieb. Bis eines Tages die berühmte schicksalhafte Begegnung passierte, die meiner Komfortzone einen Arschtritt gab.

Ich sah sie schon, bevor sie das Lokal betrat. Lange gebräunte Beine ragten unter dem Rock eines weißen Kleides hervor, welches sich perfekt an ihren Körper schmiegte. Ihr strahlendes Lächeln wurde von einem sportlichen Typen erwidert, der ihr die Tür aufhielt.

Warum war sie hier? Wahrscheinlich, weil dies das einzige Restaurant in unserem kleinen Dörfchen ist und dazu nicht gerade das schlechteste.

Aber warum ausgerechnet während meiner Schicht?

Die Säule in der hintersten Ecke des Raumes bot mir Schutz, sodass ich meine ehemalige Mitschülerin aus sicherer Entfernung beschatten konnte.

Ihre melodische Stimme hallte durch den Raum, als sie über einen Witz ihrer Begleitung lachte.

Mein Herz hämmerte gegen meine Brust.

Victoria.

Ich habe sie immer bewundert. Für ihre Schönheit, ihre guten Noten, ihren Ehrgeiz. Alles schien ihr immer so leicht zu fallen.

Wir haben uns damals ziemlich gut verstanden, auch wenn wir nie wirklich befreundet waren.

Rachel, meine beste Freundin, findet Victoria ätzend, weil sie der Typ Mensch ist, der einfach alles zu können scheint. Ich hingegen fand genau das immer großartig an ihr. Es spornte mich an. Ich lernte härter, strengte mich mehr an, nur um zu sein, wie sie.

Als sich unsere Wege nach der Schule trennten, jagten wir alle großen Träumen hinterher. Es zog uns in die unterschiedlichsten Winkel der Welt, wo wir die aufregendsten Abenteuer erlebten.

Alle. Außer mich.

Mein größtes Abenteuer war bis dahin wahrscheinlich der Salat nach Laune des Chefs, wenn dieser einen schlechten Tag hatte.

Alles nur übergangsweise.

Wohin auch immer dieser Übergang führen sollte.

Die Ungewissheit hatte mich nie besonders gestört.

Bis zu jenem Zeitpunkt.

Was würde Victoria wohl von mir denken, wenn sie mich so sehen würde? Nun ja, ich sollte es recht bald erfahren.

»Deliah, würdest du bitte?«, forderte Nico mich mit einer Handbewegung auf, die neuen Gäste zu bedienen. Ausgerechnet an diesem Tag musste Tina zum Arzt, weshalb ich für eine Stunde die einzige Kellnerin im Lokal war. Und ausgerechnet in dieser einen Stunde beschloss Victoria hierher zu kommen.

Also gut. Ich straffte die Schultern, setzte mein fröhlichstes Lächeln auf und steuerte in gespielter Selbstsicherheit auf den Tisch zu.

Warum musste sie so dermaßen umwerfend aussehen? Könnte sie nicht wenigstens Augenringe haben? Irgendein Anzeichen von Stress oder Übermüdung?

Nein, sie strahlte die pure Lebensfreude aus. Dieses

Strahlen, das diejenigen umgibt, die einfach alles haben, was sie wollen. Alles in mir sträubte sich dagegen, in meiner Kellner Uniform und den unordentlich hochgebundenen Haaren zu ihrem Tisch zu gehen. Aber ich hatte keine andere Wahl. Ich hoffte einfach, dass sie mich nicht erkennen würde.

»Deliah!«, rief Victoria jedoch erstaunt, als sie mich sah.

Mist.

»Hey, Vicky.«, grüßte ich verlegen.

»Was machst du denn hier? Hast du Semesterferien?«

Ich zögerte. Sollte ich lügen? Nein, wenn sie das bemerkt hätte, hätte ich mich noch lächerlicher gemacht.

»So ähnlich.«, stammelte ich also eine Halbwahrheit.

»Oh, was studierst du denn?«

Ihre dunkelbraunen Augen weiteten sich vor Aufregung.

»Nun... nichts. Was darf ich euch denn bringen?«, versuchte ich das Gespräch schnell in eine andere Richtung zu lenken.

Vicky zog nachdenklich die Augenbrauen zusammen. Sie schien zu begreifen, was ich so ungeschickt zu verbergen versuchte.

»Aber du hattest doch immer so große Träume! Was ist aus der Band geworden, die du gründen wolltest? Spielst du noch Volleyball? Ich dachte immer, du kommst mal ganz groß raus.«

»Das waren doch nur Träumereien. Nichts Ernstes. Ich muss jetzt weiterarbeiten. Also, was wollt ihr essen?«

Ich fürchtete der Kugelschreiber in meiner Hand könnte zerbrechen, so fest hielt ich ihn.

Zu meinem Glück betraten kurz darauf mehrere Familien die Pizzeria, sodass ich zu viel zu tun hatte, um ein weiteres Gespräch mit Vicky anzufangen. Ihre Bestellungen brachte ich ihnen wortlos mit einem erzwungenen Lächeln an den Tisch. Ich hatte beschlossen, einfach stur meine Arbeit zu erledigen. Als sie endlich bezahlten und das Lokal verließen, konnte ich aufatmen.

Dennoch verfolgten ihre Worte mich den ganzen Abend.

Was ist aus der Band geworden, die du gründen wolltest? Nun, ich habe nie gelernt, wie man ein Instrument spielt, weil … ich weiß doch auch nicht.

Spielst du noch Volleyball? Nein, weil ich keinen Sinn mehr darin gesehen habe. Ich habe es zwar geliebt, aber besonders gut war ich nie. Was hätte es also noch für einen Sinn gehabt?

Abgesehen davon waren das doch alles nur Hobbies. Nichts, womit man Geld verdienen kann. Zumindest nicht jeder.

Bei Nico hatte ich einen guten, sicheren Arbeitsplatz und dazu noch nette Kollegen. Es hätte mich deutlich schlimmer treffen können.

Warum also quälte mich das Gespräch mit Victoria so? Kellnerin ist kein schlechter Beruf. Es ist teilweise sogar sehr anstrengend, also durchaus eine Arbeit, der Respekt gebührt.

Was also bedeutete der tonnenschwere Stein, der sich seit dieser Unterhaltung in meinen Magen gelegt hatte?

Ganz einfach.

Dieses Leben entsprach in keiner Weise dem, was ich mir für mich erträumt hatte.

Ich musste da raus, sonst wäre ich für immer gefangen gewesen.

Etwa zwei Wochen später, als ich online nach meiner Zukunft suchte, stieß ich auf eine Stellenanzeige, in der eine Haushaltshilfe für eine ältere, allein lebende Dame gesucht wurde. Weg von zu Hause, neue Umgebung, neue Eindrücke, neues Leben. Vielleicht würde ich dort etwas finden, das mich wirklich erfüllt. Außerdem wäre das Gehalt um einiges höher, als ich beim Kellnern je bekommen habe und so begann ich meine Bewerbung zu tippen.

Ich, jung, arbeitswillig, ungebunden, flexibel und nach Veränderung suchend bekam genau eine Woche später eine Antwort vom Neffen der alten Frau. Ein kurzes Telefoninterview später hatte ich einen neuen Job. Dreihundert Kilometer von meiner Familie entfernt und allem, was ich kenne und liebe.

Und da fahre ich heute hin.

»Hör doch auf sie zu behandeln, als wäre sie zehn Jahre alt!«, tadelt mein Vater meine Mutter, als er über den gepflasterten Weg zu uns schlendert.

Der warme Sommerwind lässt seine kurzen grauen Haare erzittern.

»Sie ist erwachsen. Und wenn sie ihre Jacke vergisst und deshalb im Sommer erfriert, wird sie diesen Fehler kein zweites Mal machen.«

Sein Schnauzer zieht sich auseinander, als er bei seinem Vortrag stolz grinst und mir mit einem Auge zuzwinkert.

»Edgar!«, empört sich meine Mutter, die doch nur ihr Baby beschützen möchte. Beim entsetzten Aufstampfen mit ihren kurzen Beinen fällt ihr die Brille von der Nase. Sie wird jedoch von dem goldenen Kettchen gerettet, an dem sie befestigt ist.

»Ich muss los.«, unterbreche ich die in der Luft hängende Diskussion über meine Schutzbedürftigkeit.

»Oh mein Schätzchen!«, fällt mir meine Mutter um den Hals und drückt dabei meine langen, hellblonden Locken platt.

Unsere Umarmung wird verstärkt, als auch mein Vater die Arme um uns legt. Ein liebendes Trio, ein letztes Mal vereint, für eine unbestimmt lange Zeit.

Tränen glitzern in den hellblauen Augen meiner Mutter, die meinen so sehr gleichen.

»Ich wünsche dir viel Spaß und dass du findest, wonach du suchst.«, flüstert sie mir zu.

Ich lächle sie an, während ich mich vorsichtig aus der Umarmung löse.

»Ich melde mich, sobald ich angekommen bin.«, verspreche ich meinen Eltern, dann steige ich in mein Auto.

Der Rückspiegel zeigt mir nur mein lachsfarbenes Haarband, also verstelle ich ihn bis ich die beiden darin erkenne, wie sie noch immer Arm in Arm hinter dem Auto stehen.

Kurz hält die Nervosität mich gefangen, doch dann siegt die Vorfreude und ich starte den Motor.

Als ich unsere Straße entlangfahre, kann ich meine Eltern weiterhin im Rückspiegel winken sehen. Immer kleiner und kleiner, bis sie nur noch zwei Punkte auf der Straße sind und schließlich ganz verschwinden, als ich auf die Hauptstraße abbiege. Also dann, volle Kraft voraus!

Ich stehe im Stau. So viel zu dem neuen Schwung in meinem Leben. Das Schicksal lacht sich wahrscheinlich gerade schlapp, als die Dame im Radio davon singt, wie dringend sie einen Helden benötigt. Meine Jeans beginnt an meinen Beinen zu kleben, als die Temperatur im Auto steigt. Die Nervosität vor dem Unbekannten macht die Schweiß-Situation auch nicht gerade besser. Aber immerhin ist das schon spannender als alles, was in den letzten Jahren passiert ist.

Was mich wohl an meinem Ziel erwarten wird?

Alexander Griffin, der Neffe der alten Dame namens Eleonore Griffin, hat mich am Telefon schon grob über meine Aufgaben informiert. Seine Tante ist wohl eine allein lebende Frau, die laut ihm nicht unbeaufsichtigt sein sollte, da sie vieles nicht mehr selbstständig kann. Ich soll also Dinge wie den Haushalt, das Kochen und Einkaufen übernehmen. Ihr das Leben leichter machen. Krankheiten scheint sie nicht zu haben, was wohl auch der Grund dafür ist, warum ich den Job, ohne jede Ausbildung in diesem Bereich, bekommen habe. Mein neuer Chef kann leider nicht persönlich an meinem ersten Tag anwesend sein, doch er hat seine Tante wohl informiert, dass ich komme. Na, hoffentlich erinnert sie sich auch daran.

Der Verkehr beginnt wieder zu fließen, was mich aus meinen Gedanken reißt. Ein Blick auf mein Navi verrät mir, dass ich die nächste Ausfahrt nehmen muss, also setze ich den Blinker und wechsele die Spur.

Abseits der Autobahn erwartet mich sehr viel Grün. Hoch aufragende Wälder, endlos wirkende Wiesen. Es fühlt sich an, als wäre ich nur einen Katzensprung von zu Hause entfernt.

Ein hölzernes Willkommensschild ziert den Eingang des Dorfes, in dem ich die nächste Zeit leben werde.

Einzelne Häuser, umgeben von Sträuchern und bunten Holzzäunen, erscheinen nach einem hoch aufragenden Maisfeld vor mir. Es wirkt alles so friedlich in der goldenen Nachmittagssonne.

Doch die Idylle wird durch einen dunklen Fleck gestört. Ein zerfallenes Haus, schwarz durch die Spuren eines Feuers. Balken hängen schief, der Zerfall beginnt den Rest des Gebäudes an sich zu reißen. Die Haustür steht offen, als würde das Haus seinen Schmerz hinausschreien.

»Ihr Ziel befindet sich auf der linken Seite«, informiert mich die Stimme aus dem Navi.

Tatsächlich, Weidenstraße, Hausnummer sieben. Ich lenke mein Auto in die Einfahrt, weg von dem düsteren Anblick zwei Häuser zuvor.

Als ich aussteige, traue ich meinen Augen nicht. Vor mir erstreckt sich ein wunderschönes Haus, umgeben von Rosen, die sich um ein Türmchen mit großen Fenstern winden. Blumen quellen in allen Farben über die Blumenkästen am Balkon im zweiten Stock. Gekrönt durch ein spitz zulaufendes, schwarzes Dach sieht dieses Gebäude aus wie aus einem Märchen. Ein magischer Ort, der von Geheimnissen umgeben zu sein scheint.

Dann hoffen wir mal, dass da drinnen nicht die böse Hexe wohnt!

Ein Mädchen. Lange, blonde Locken, die ihr Gesicht einrahmen. Wer bist du? Was tust du hier?

So schön. Wie ein Engel!

Kann es sein? Kamst du, um mich zu erlösen? Ich will... NEIN! Ich kann nicht! Nichts überstürzen. Werde auf Abstand bleiben. Werde sie beobachten. Hinter den Rosen, so weiß und rein wie ihre Seele.

Die alte Dame

Meinen Koffer in der Hand laufe ich über den gepflasterten Hof, die drei steinernen Stufen hinauf zu einer schwer aussehenden Holztür. Ich möchte gerade klingeln, als mir auffällt, dass die Tür offensteht. Vorsichtig stoße ich sie mit meinem Fuß an, woraufhin sie zu meiner Überraschung ganz leicht aufschwingt. Langsam trete ich ein, kühle Luft streicht über meine nackten Arme.

»Hallo?«

Meine Stimme verläuft sich in den Winkeln des Flures.

»Aaaahiiiaaa! Waahaaaaiiiaaa!«, ertönt eine alte kratzige Stimme von oben.

Ich erhole mich von dem kurzen Schreckmoment und haste, ohne weiter darüber nachzudenken, die Holztreppe rechts von mir nach oben.

»Haaaa iana waaa!«, kreischt es erneut aus einem Raum dessen Tür verschlossen ist.

Um Himmels willen! Was ist geschehen? Diese Frau

muss furchtbare Schmerzen haben! Ein großer Satz lässt mich die letzten zwei Stufen auf einmal nehmen, Adrenalin rauscht durch meinen Körper, als ich die Tür aufreiße.

Vor mir steht eine ältere Dame, in bunte Tücher gewickelt und den Staubwedel schwingend.

»Anawahiaaaaaa!«, kreischt sie, als ich den Raum betrete.

Vor Schreck taumele ich zurück, stolpere über den Absatz und lande unsanft auf meinem Hintern.

»Ach du liebe Güte!«

Geschockt legt sie die Hände an die Wangen, dann eilt sie zu mir, da ich noch immer am Boden sitze und um Atem ringe. Himmel, was ist denn hier los? Habe ich mich im Haus geirrt?

»Geht es dir gut, Kindchen? Was machst du denn hier?«, fragt sie mit ihrer krächzenden Stimme und sieht mich aus, von tiefen Falten umgebenen, graublauen Augen an.

»Ich bin Deliah. Ich bin die Haushaltshilfe.«, stoße ich schmerzerfüllt hervor. Mein Steißbein fühlt sich an, als hätte es einen Hammerschlag abbekommen.

»Jetzt lass mich dir erst einmal hoch helfen und dann

mache ich dir einen Tee.«, sagt sie, während sie mir einen Arm reicht, der mich mit unerwarteter Kraft nach oben zieht.

Ungläubig sehe ich mich um. Ich hatte eine, in dicke Wolldecken gewickelte, alte Frau erwartet, die den ganzen Tag vor dem Fernseher sitzt und nicht ansprechbar ist. Diese Dame hingegen scheint vor Energie zu sprühen.

Ich folge ihr die Treppe nach unten, ihr buntes Gewand streicht bei jedem Schritt sachte über die Stufen. Wo bin ich hier nur gelandet?

Unten angekommen führt sie mich in das Esszimmer, welches durch einen großen Rundbogen vom Eingangsbereich getrennt wird. Grün gepolsterte Stühle stehen um einen hölzernen Esstisch. Auf diesem befindet sich eine Dose mit Keksen.

»Nimm dir ruhig ein Zimtplätzchen. Selbst gebacken! Möchtest du Apfelmus dazu?«, fragt die alte Dame.

»Vielen Dank. Und nein danke.«, erwidere ich.

»Sie sind Eleonore Griffin?«, erkundige ich mich.

Wie eine hilfsbedürftige alte Dame sieht sie nämlich nicht gerade aus. Vielleicht bin ich tatsächlich im falschen Haus.

»Nenn mich Elli, Kindchen. Bei meinem vollen Namen nennen mich nur Versicherungsvertreter. Außerdem fühle ich mich sonst so alt.«, erwidert sie kichernd, was bei ihr klingt wie ein Auto, welches nicht anspringen will.

»Pfefferminze?«

»Wie bitte?«

»Der Tee. Magst du Pfefferminze? Aus meinem Garten.«

»Oh, ja, sehr gerne.«

Was für eine seltsame Situation. Ich, die Haushaltshilfe, lasse mir Tee machen von der Dame, die ich betreuen soll.

»Kann ich helfen?«, frage ich deshalb.

»Oh nein, Kindchen. Setz dich ruhig. Diese alten Knochen müssen bewegt werden, solange sie noch funktionieren. Ich bin jeden Tag dankbar für jeden Schritt, den ich gehen darf.«

Ich beginne mich zu fragen, was ich eigentlich hier mache. Diese Frau scheint kerngesund zu sein.

Nachdenklich betrachte ich wieder die bunten Tücher, die sie sich umgehängt hat.

»Darf ich fragen, was sie, ähm, was du da oben getan

hast?«, will ich etwas kleinlaut wissen.

»Na, ich habe Staub gewischt.«

»Und dabei hast du… gesungen?«

»Suaheli. Das haben Theodor und ich auf unserer Afrikareise gelernt. Auch wenn ich eher den Klang, als die tatsächlichen Worte wiedergebe.«, erklärt sie kichernd.

»Wer ist Theodor?«

»Er war mein Ehemann.«

»Oh, das tut mir leid.«, entschuldige ich mich.

Super Deliah, erwähne im ersten Gespräch den toten Ehemann.

»Das muss es nicht, Kindchen. Hier.«

Sie hält mir ein in Gold gerahmtes Bild vor die Nase, welches sie eben aus einem Hängeschränkchen geholt hat. Auf dem Schnappschuss vor einem Berg strahlt sie neben einem älteren Mann mit weißem Schnauzer und Hut um die Wette. Sie wirken sehr glücklich.

»Ein Autounfall.«, erklärt sie mit belegter Stimme.

Ich bleibe stumm. Solche Situationen waren mir schon immer unangenehm. Der Anstand gebietet es, sein Beileid zu bekunden. Doch weil mir das zu sehr nach Floskel klingt, bekomme ich es nicht über die Lippen.

Eleonore atmet tief ein und mit einem lauten Seufzen wieder aus. Dann schüttelt sie sich, wie um die traurigen Erinnerungen zu vertreiben und setzt wieder ihr Lächeln auf.

»Es ist schon okay.«, sagt sie mehr zu sich selbst, »Weißt du, ich glaube er hat mich nie wirklich verlassen. Ich könnte schwören, nachts höre ich sogar noch sein gottverdammtes Schnarchen.«

Ein Lächeln stiehlt sich auf unsere Gesichter.

Ich hoffe nur, mir bleibt sein Schnarchen erspart.

Vier Stunden. Vier Stunden dauert mein neues Leben nun schon. Was ich in dieser Zeit gelernt habe?

Eleonore, lieber Elli genannt, liebte es, mit ihrem verstorbenen Mann Theodore zu verreisen. Sie war schon in mehr Ländern und Städten, als ich überhaupt kenne und kann auf fünfzehn Sprachen ein Käsebrot und ein Glas Wein bestellen.

Ihr Lieblingsessen sind Zimtkekse, die sie leidenschaftlich gerne in Apfelmus tunkt. Eine Tatsache, die sie mir nicht erzählt hat, die ich jedoch schon nach kurzer Zeit feststellen konnte. Besagtes Apfelmus füllt etwa die Hälfte ihres Kühlschrankes.

Elli hat keine Kinder, nur einen Neffen, den ihr der verstorbene Bruder ihres Mannes hinterlassen hat.

Meine Vorstellung von diesem Job hat sich verändert. Ob positiv oder negativ kann ich nicht sagen. Ich habe immer mehr das Gefühl, ich bin hier weniger als Helferin und mehr als Gesellschaft eingestellt. Aber auch das ist für mich völlig in Ordnung. Elli ist nett, lacht gerne und viel und auch wenn ich mich an ihren Gesang wohl gewöhnen muss, fühle ich mich schon sehr heimisch hier. Außerdem macht sie einen wahnsinnig leckeren Pfefferminztee.

Ein langer Tag neigt sich für mich dem Ende zu. Die Strahlen der Abendsonne tauchen den Himmel in ein sattes Orange, welches durch die Küchenfenster dringt. Elli hat sich nach oben verzogen, um ihre Regale fertig abzustauben. Helfen sollte ich ihr nicht.

Ich habe es versucht, ehrlich. Sie meinte jedoch, sie würde den Vorgang genießen, ihre Erinnerungen immer wieder zu durchleben, während sie jedes einzelne Stück anhebt und von Staub befreit.

Dagegen habe ich keine Argumente gefunden. Ich bin hier, um diese Frau glücklich zu machen und wenn dazu gehört sie die Hausarbeit soweit möglich selbst erledigen zu lassen, dann bitteschön. Putzende soll man nicht aufhalten. Oder so ähnlich.

Die Beschreibung, die Alexander Griffin mir über seine Tante gegeben hat, ist so was von daneben. Sieht er sie wirklich so? Oder spielt Elli nur die energetische Frau, um mich wieder loszuwerden? Blödsinn! Man kann zwar so tun, als sei man gebrechlich, obwohl man kerngesund ist, aber andersherum ist es dann doch schwierig. Sehr mysteriös das Ganze.

Das Wetter und die Neugier treiben mich in den Garten. Vom Hof aus führt ein mit vereinzelten Steinen gepflasterter Weg hinter das Haus, über dem ein großer Laubbaum aufragt. Warmer Wind lässt meine Haare tanzen, während ich von Stein zu Stein nach hinten in den Garten hüpfe. Mein inneres Kind lässt mich dabei breit grinsen.

Als ich meinen Weg beende, erstreckt sich vor mir ein wunderschöner Garten. Eine große Wiese, umgeben von hohen Bäumen, verschiedensten Blumen und Sträuchern. Am hinteren Ende des Grundstücks kann ich eine kleine Holzhütte erkennen. Wahrscheinlich ein Geräteschuppen.

Daneben steht ein Gewächshaus, durch dessen milchige Wände das kräftige Grün wachsender Pflanzen schimmert. Dahinter führt ein schmales Stück Rasen in die dicht bewachsene Dunkelheit. Bei meiner Hausführung habe ich eine Tür entdeckt, die direkt in den Garten führt. Es sah nicht ungepflegt, aber dennoch sehr verwachsen aus, weshalb ich den käferfreien Weg durch die Haustür gewählt habe.

Der Duft von frisch gemähtem Rasen weht mir um die Nase, als mich ein lautes Plätschern zusammenzucken lässt.

Bei all der Begeisterung über das, was vor mir liegt, habe ich doch glatt den kleinen Teich mit den Goldfischen übersehen. Drei, vier, fünf Fische in unterschiedlichen Gold- und Orangetönen tummeln sich im Wasser, während die Pflanzen unter ihnen wirken, als würden sie tanzen. Weiße Steine schimmern am Grund durch die Wasseroberfläche.

»Beruhigend nicht wahr?«, erklingt eine tiefe Männerstimme hinter mir.

Erschrocken und mit einem hörbaren Atem holen fahre ich herum und sehe in die Augen des attraktivsten Mannes, der mir je begegnet ist.

Ein eisiges Blau mustert mich, wobei es so fehl am Platz wirkt an diesem warmen Ort. Goldene Locken umrahmen ein markantes Gesicht. Er scheint etwa in meinem Alter zu sein, vielleicht auch ein wenig älter.

»Oh, tut mir leid! Ich wollte dich nicht erschrecken.«, entschuldigt er sich mit sanfter Stimme.

»Ich bin Callum.«, fährt er fort und reicht mir die Hand.

»Deliah.«, antworte ich, als ich seine Hand berühre.

Mein Herzschlag beschleunigt sich, meine Knie werden weich. Es ist als wäre ich in einem Kitschfilm gefangen.

Okay cool bleiben! Das kenne ich so überhaupt nicht von mir.

»Du bist also die neue Beschützerin von Elli?«, erkundigt er sich.

Seine Mundwinkel verziehen sich zu einem leichten Lächeln. Ich bin wie hypnotisiert von diesem Gesicht.

»Beschützerin?«, frage ich etwas verwundert nach.

Ich glaube nicht, dass diese Frau irgendwelchen Schutz nötig hat, geschweige denn eine Hilfe im Haushalt, aber das behalte ich besser für mich.

»Nun, wie ich hörte spukt der Geist ihres verstorbenen

Gatten noch durch die Wände.«, erklärt Callum mit einem breiten Grinsen im Gesicht.

»Ah ja, davon habe ich schon gehört. Ich denke, damit werde ich fertig.«, kontere ich möglichst selbstbewusst.

»Da bin ich mir ganz sicher.«, entgegnet er mit einem Augenzwinkern.

Moment mal, flirtet er mit mir? Er flirtet mit mir!

Mein Herz klopft, als hätte ich einen hundert Meter Sprint absolviert. Nach der langen Autofahrt rieche ich wohl auch so. Himmel, hoffentlich bemerkt er das nicht!

»Bist du verwandt mit Elli?«, frage ich vorsichtig nach, obwohl ich mir sicher bin, dass Alexander der einzige lebende Verwandte meiner Schutzbefohlenen ist.

»Nein. Ich bin der Gärtner.«, bestätigt er meine Vermutung.

Der Gärtner also. Das heißt, er ist für die ganze Schönheit hier verantwortlich. Ich möchte mehr über ihn erfahren, will nicht, dass diese Unterhaltung ein Ende findet.

»Elli hat bei der Hausführung gar nicht erwähnt, dass sie einen Gärtner hat.«, versuche ich das Gespräch am Laufen zu halten.

»Sie vergisst es manchmal selbst. Du weißt schon, erst

fragt sie mich, ob ich ihr die Einkäufe aus dem Auto holen kann und im nächsten Moment rennt sie mit erhobenem Besen auf mich zu und ruft ‚*haltet den Dieb*'!«

Er äfft ihre krächzende Stimme nach, was mich zum Lachen bringt.

»Apropos Garten«, fährt er fort, »genau dieser verlangt jetzt wieder nach mir. War nett, dich kennen zu lernen, Deliah.«, beendet er unser Gespräch mit einem Nicken in meine Richtung noch bevor es richtig begonnen hat.

Innerlich stampfe ich frustriert auf.

Nun gut, ich lächle ihm zur Bestätigung zu und sehe ihm anschließend verträumt hinterher, bis er hinter der Tür des Geräteschuppens verschwindet.

Ich sehe schon, das wird eine sehr interessante Zeit werden.

Der Schrei. So laut. Was ist passiert? Kann hier draußen nichts sehen, verdammt! Kleiner Engel, sag, was ist geschehen?

Doch dann, Erlösung. Deine liebliche Stimme im Garten. Die Sonne in deinen Haaren. Es geht dir gut, doch der Teufel beobachtet dich.

Wie lange kann ich mich zurückhalten?

Wie ein Engel

Bei jeder Stufe verfluche ich ein weiteres Kleidungsstück in meinem Koffer. Elli hat sich etwas hingelegt, was für mich bedeutet, ich kann in Ruhe mein neues Zimmer beziehen. Und das würde ich auch wirklich gerne, doch die Schwerkraft und mein Koffer scheinen gemeinsam gegen mich zu arbeiten.

»Verdammtes Dreckszeug!«, fluche ich, während ich rückwärts laufend am Griff des Koffers zerre.

»Sieht aus, als könntest du ein Paar starke Arme gebrauchen.«, höre ich Callums Stimme, der mit verschränkten Armen lässig gegen den Rahmen der Haustür lehnt.

Oh, wie recht er hat. Doch ich werde hier nicht die Jungfrau in Nöten spielen. Er soll nicht denken, dass ich schwach bin. Ergibt das Sinn? Und wie schafft er es bitte immer plötzlich in meiner Nähe zu erscheinen?

»Nein danke, ich komme schon zurecht.«, lehne ich sein Angebot ab und wuchte meinen metallicrosa Koffer eine Stufe weiter nach oben.

»Jetzt sei doch nicht so stur! Warte!«, fordert er und kommt zu mir.

Die starke unabhängige Frau in mir fühlt sich herausgefordert und versucht den Koffer anzuheben, um ihn wie eine federleichte Handtasche nach oben zu tragen.

Der Tollpatsch in mir stolpert jedoch über seine eigenen Füße, verliert das Gleichgewicht und landet unsanft auf dem Hintern. Die Luft wird aus meinen Lungen gestoßen, als mein Steißbein heute zum zweiten Mal Bekanntschaft mit dem Boden macht. Diesmal direkt auf die Treppenstufe.

Aus Reflex habe ich nun auch noch den Koffer losgelassen, welcher die Treppe mit voller Wucht und unter lautem Scheppern nach unten saust.

Callum, der schon fast bei mir war, rettet sich gerade noch auf das Geländer, verliert jedoch das Gleichgewicht und fällt in meine Richtung. Kurz bevor er mich unter sich begräbt, kann er sich allerdings an der Treppenstufe abstützen.

Ich höre den Aufprall meines Koffers nur ganz am Rande, da ich viel zu sehr damit beschäftigt bin, in Callums wunderschönes Gesicht zu blicken, welches direkt über meinem schwebt. Würde ich mich ein kleines Stück aufsetzen, könnten sich unsere Nasenspitzen berühren.

»Weißt du, ein einfaches ‚*ich will deine Hilfe nicht*', hätte auch gereicht.«, haucht er mir atemlos entgegen.

»So ist es doch gar nicht! Ich ähm... wollte dich nur nicht belästigen.«, ringe ich mir eine Ausrede ab.

Ein stummes Lachen gibt den Blick auf seine strahlend weißen Zähne frei. Ich bin gefesselt von seinem Anblick.

Der angenehme Geruch von Pfefferminze steigt mir in die Nase, gemischt mit dem pudrigen Duft seiner Haut.

»Dann sehen wir uns das Chaos einmal an, oder? Geht es dir gut?«, fragt er und holt mich somit aus meiner Trance.

Ich nicke und murmele ein verlegenes »Mhm.«

Daraufhin richtet er sich auf, um das untere Ende der Treppe zu sehen.

»Ohje!«, ist alles, was er sagt, als er sich umdreht und ich stelle kurz darauf fest, was der Grund für seine Reaktion ist.

Der Verschluss meines Koffers muss etwas abbekommen haben und der gesamte Inhalt liegt nun auf dem Boden verteilt. Inklusive meiner Unterwäsche.

Ungeachtet meines schmerzenden Hinterns haste ich an Callum vorbei, um alle eventuellen Peinlichkeiten einzusammeln. Er lässt mich gewähren und anstatt mir zu helfen steht er nur da und lacht, während er mich beobachtet.

Ich laufe feuerrot an vor Scham. Warum muss mir das ausgerechnet vor ihm passieren? Mit einem unattraktiven, hundertjährigen Gärtner mit Halbglatze hätte ich lieber meine Unterwäsche geteilt! Obwohl, nein, das wäre auch irgendwie schräg.

Als alles wieder verstaut ist, kommt Callum schließlich doch zu mir.

»Lass mich das diesmal machen, okay?«, bittet er, doch er wartet meine Antwort nicht ab, sondern schnappt sich den Koffer, als wäre er so leicht wie ein Kulturtäschchen und trägt ihn nach oben.

Das letzte Zimmer auf der rechten Seite, hat Elli gesagt. Vorbei an dem Zimmer, in dem sie vorhin noch abgestaubt hat.

Callum öffnet die Tür mit seinem Ellbogen und geht voraus. Ich trotte ihm wie ein Welpe hinterher.

Helles Licht scheint mir durch ein großes Fenster mit Spitzengardine entgegen. Es ist ein kleiner Raum, doch für mich völlig ausreichend. Alles ist in edlem Dunkelgrün gehalten, genau wie das Wohn- und Esszimmer unten. Rechts von mir befindet sich ein Kleiderschrank, links das Fenster und an der Wand direkt vor mir steht ein gemütlich aussehendes Bett mit vielen Kissen. Ein süßes, kleines Zuhause.

Meinen Blick weiterhin forschend durch den Raum schweifen lassend bemerke ich nicht, dass Callum stehen geblieben ist und stoße prompt mit ihm zusammen.

»Oh mein Gott, es tut mir so unheimlich leid!«, platzt es aus mir heraus.

Mein Kopf sieht wohl mittlerweile wieder aus, wie eine leuchtende Sirene.

»Mir scheint, zwischen uns gibt es eine gewisse Anziehungskraft.«, witzelt er.

Ich erstarre angesichts der Zweideutigkeit hinter dieser Aussage. Interpretiere ich da zu viel hinein?

Als ich nicht antworte lacht er nur und verabschiedet sich mit den Worten:

»Es war eine sehr interessante Erfahrung dir helfen zu dürfen, Deliah. Bis später, Kollegin.«

Ich will im Erdboden versinken und doch Luftsprünge machen.

Dafür, dass der Koffer so unheimlich schwer war, habe ich die Sachen erstaunlich schnell in meinem Schrank verstaut.

Elli schläft noch immer, also beschließe ich die freie Zeit und die letzten Sonnenstrahlen für einen Spaziergang zu nutzen. Ein wenig die Umgebung kennenlernen und dabei versuchen nicht allzu oft an diese blauen Augen und die blonden Locken zu denken. Und an diesen Duft nach Pfefferminze sowie die Wärme seines Körpers über meinem, die meinen Herzschlag beschleunigt und meine Knie weich werden lässt.

Genau. Einfach die Natur genießen.

Es ist nur ein kleines Dörfchen, ich sollte mich also leicht zurechtfinden. Nach diesem langen und aufwühlenden Tag brauche ich einfach etwas Zeit für mich allein.

Ich biege am Ender der Einfahrt nach links ab, entgegengesetzt der Richtung, aus der ich hier angekommen bin. Süße, kleine Häuser mit schönen

Gärten zieren die Straße. Hellblaue, rosafarbene und weiße Fassaden glühen im Licht der untergehenden Sonne. Wieder biege ich links ab und lande am Ende einer kurvigen Straße vor einem großen Teich, auf dem Enten ihre Bahnen schwimmen. Niedliche kleine Entenküken spielen, jagen sich gegenseitig und paddeln dann fix der Mutter wieder hinterher. Ab und an taucht ein Fisch auf, der nach Mücken schnappt.

Alles scheint so friedlich, als ob es kein Leid auf dieser Welt geben würde. Ein einsamer Baumstumpf bietet mir eine Sitzgelegenheit, von der aus ich entspannt auf das Wasser blicken kann. Es heißt immer, das Leben auf dem Land hätte nichts zu bieten, dabei sind es Momente wie diese, die einem Frieden bringen. Es ist so wichtig, in dieser schnellen Welt ab und an einmal auf Pause zu drücken.

Die Sonne ist schon fast verschwunden, nur noch ein Rest ihres Lichtes lässt die Welt glimmen. Ich mache mich auf, meinen Rundgang zu beenden. Der See erstreckt sich noch eine Weile parallel meines Weges, bis ein schmaler Feldweg mich wieder zurück zur Hauptstraße führt.

Vor dem niedergebrannten Haus nahe dem

Ortseingang halte ich kurz inne.

In dem riesigen Maisfeld direkt daneben scheinen die Blätter im Wind zu flüstern. Eine unheimliche Stille umgibt dieses Grundstück und doch ist es, als könne man die Flammen noch immer lodern hören. Ein Vogel sitzt auf einem eingestürzten Dachbalken und scheint mir von dort direkt in die Augen zu sehen. Ein Schauer läuft mir über den Rücken.

Da breitet er seine Flügel aus und saust in Richtung des Maisfeldes davon. Ich folge ihm mit meinem Blick, wodurch mir ein Loch in dem hölzernen Gartenzaun auffällt.

Ob sich Kinder dort hereinschleichen? Ein Eingang zu dem mysteriösen Geisterhaus. Was mag hier wohl geschehen sein?

Plötzlich sehe ich einen Schatten in meinem Augenwinkel vorbeihuschen. Sofort drehe ich mich um, kann jedoch niemanden erkennen.

Im Nachbarhaus ist es völlig ruhig. Ich verenge die Augen, um in die offenstehende Garage spähen zu können. Nichts regt sich.

Und doch beschleicht mich dieses seltsame Gefühl, beobachtet zu werden. Der Gedanke beschert mir eine

Gänsehaut. Ich sehe mich noch einmal um. Es scheint die Aura dieses zerstörten Hauses zu sein, die mich nervös alle Richtungen absuchen lässt. Doch weit und breit ist keine Menschenseele.

Die Kirchturmglocke reißt mich aus meinen Gedanken. Ich sollte mich wirklich auf den Heimweg machen. Schnellen Schrittes entferne ich mich von diesem unheimlichen Ort.

*

Elli wuselt wieder mit dem Staubwedel durch das Haus, als ich zurückkomme. Scheint, als wären ihre Akkus wieder geladen.

»Hat dir unser kleines, malerisches Dörfchen gefallen, Kindchen?«, fragt sie im Vorbeihuschen.

Wo hat sie nur diese ganze Energie her?

»Es ist wirklich wunderschön.«, bestätige ich ihre Aussage.

»Elli, kann ich dich etwas fragen?«, richte ich mich an sie, woraufhin sie den Kopf schief hält. Ein Zeichen, dass ich loslegen soll.

»Was ist in dem Haus am Ortseingang passiert?«,

stelle ich also die Frage, die mir unter den Nägeln brennt, seit ich das Ortsschild passiert habe.

»Oh.«, stößt Elli aus, ihr Blick verfinstert sich.

»Eine furchtbare Geschichte. Wahrscheinlich Brandstiftung. Ein junges Mädchen war allein in dem Haus, als das Feuer ausbrach. Sie hat es nur knapp überlebt. Noch heute finden viele, es sei ein Wunder, dass sie überhaupt aufgewacht ist, als das Feuer schon im Gange war.«, berichtet Elli.

Sie atmet tief ein und seufzt, dann fährt sie fort: »Lydia, so heißt das Mädchen, behauptet jemand hätte an ihr Fenster geklopft, was sie wiederum aus dem Schlaf gerissen hat. Die Tür war abgesperrt. Lydia schwört jedoch, dass sie es nicht war. Demnach hätte sie jemand eingesperrt, dann das Feuer gelegt und sie schließlich ihrem Schicksal überlassen.«

»Aber warum sollte jemand so etwas tun?«

Ich bin geschockt von dieser Grausamkeit.

»Das, Kindchen, ist nur eines der ungelösten Rätsel dieser Nacht.«

Ich kann es nicht fassen. Brandstiftung? Versuchter Mord? Direkt nebenan?

»Hat man herausgefunden, wer das war? Und warum

er das getan hat?«

»Leider nein. Die Menschen hier lebten daraufhin lange in Angst. Wie du bestimmt bemerkt hast, gibt es hier nicht allzu viele Möglichkeiten. Jeder hat jeden verdächtigt. Einige behaupten, es wäre ein missglückter Selbstmordversuch gewesen. Niemand weiß, wer damals die Feuerwehr gerufen hat. Da liegt es nahe, dass das Mädchen es sich anders überlegt haben muss.«

Meine Kehle schnürt sich zu bei dem Gedanken an das arme Mädchen.

Elli atmet tief durch, bevor sie fortfährt.

»Ein schrecklicher Gedanke, nicht wahr? Die Polizei vermutete jedoch, Jugendliche aus der Stadt hätten sich einen Streich erlaubt, der außer Kontrolle geriet. Ihr schlechtes Gewissen muss sie dann dazu veranlasst haben, die Feuerwehr zu rufen.

Allerdings bin ich mir ziemlich sicher, dass sie das nur behauptet haben, damit die Nachbarschaft sich hier nicht mehr ständig gegenseitig anzeigt. Hier war es immer äußerst harmonisch, doch seit diesem Vorfall sind alle sehr verschlossen. Ich möchte wetten, dass dich bereits das ganze Dorf beobachtet hat.«

Bei dem letzten Satz lacht sie leise.

Das erklärt wohl mein ungutes Gefühl von vorhin. Das Einzige, woran ich in diesem Moment jedoch denken kann, ist, dass hier jemand frei herumläuft, der beinahe einen Menschen getötet hätte.

»Hab keine Angst, Kindchen.«, dringt Elli wieder in mein Bewusstsein ein, als hätte sie meine Gedanken gelesen.

»Fakt ist«, erzählt sie weiter, »dieses Mädchen hat in jener Nacht einen Schutzengel gehabt.«

»Hast du eine Vermutung, wer es gewesen sein könnte?«, will ich wissen.

»Eine Vermutung? Ich vermute nicht, Kindchen. Was für mich zählt ist, was ich weiß. Der Rest ist unwichtig.«

Mit diesen Worten lässt Elli mich stehen. Ein Engel. Wohl eher eine ganze Schar an Engeln. Doch wenn wirklich jemand gekommen war, um Lydia zu warnen, warum ist er dann nicht geblieben? Warum hat er sich nicht zu erkennen gegeben? Könnte es sein, dass es am Ende doch der Täter selbst war, der seine Tat bereut hat? Vielleicht war ja doch alles nur ein schrecklicher Unfall. Zumindest möchte ich das von ganzem Herzen glauben.

Als ich eine Stunde später aus der Dusche steige, lockt mich ein köstlicher Duft in die Küche. Elli scheint meine Auszeit im Bad dazu genutzt zu haben, das Abendessen zu kochen.

Ich fühle mich immer mehr, als wäre ich nur zu Besuch bei meiner Oma.

»Kindchen! Du kommst genau richtig.«, begrüßt Elli mich, ein Lächeln im Gesicht und eine Salatschüssel in der Hand.

»Setz dich! Ich dachte mir, zur Feier des Tages koche ich uns etwas.«

Langsam trete ich näher an den Tisch heran. Sie hat ihn bereits eingedeckt und verschiedene Salate sowie je eine Schüssel mit Gemüse, Reis und Soße platziert.

Drei Teller.

»Kommt noch jemand?«, will ich wissen.

Es ist jedoch nicht Elli, die mir antwortet, sondern eine sanfte, tiefe Stimme hinter mir.

»Bin ich schon zu spät?«, fragt Callum.

Herrje, das hat mir noch gefehlt. Was hat das Schicksal vor? Will es, dass ich ihn mit Soße bekleckere? Ich habe mich doch heute wirklich schon genug vor ihm blamiert!

Auch wenn ich zugeben muss, dass ein winziger Teil

von mir sich sehr über seine Anwesenheit freut.

»Hallo Kollegin.«, begrüßt er mich mit einem breiten Grinsen und die Röte schießt mir ins Gesicht.

Mir ist, als würde mein Magen Achterbahn fahren. Dann erinnere ich mich an meine Unterwäsche, die noch vor Kurzem vor seinen Augen auf dem Boden verteilt lag.

Ein beschämtest Lächeln, gefolgt von einem knappen Nicken sind deshalb alles, was ich als Antwort zustande bringe.

Callum setzt sich auf die Seite des Tisches, auf der nur ein Teller steht. Ich möchte mich gerade zu dem freien Platz schräg gegenüber begeben, als Elli mit einer weiteren dampfenden Schüssel zum Tisch tippelt und mich wortlos einen Stuhl weiter drängt, sodass ich Callum direkt gegenübersitze.

Mein Herz hämmert in meiner Brust, als ich Platz nehme.

Das hat sie mit Absicht gemacht!

Nervös knete ich die Hände in meinem Schoß und versuche so gleichgültig wie möglich zu wirken, indem ich meinen Blick durch den Raum schweifen lasse.

Lässig überschlage ich die Beine, wobei ich leicht an das Tischbein stoße.

Erschrocken halte ich die Luft an. Der Tisch hat nicht einmal gewackelt, keiner hat es bemerkt. Gerade noch mal gut gegangen.

Am besten nicht mehr bewegen und den Fuß abgestützt lassen, an dem starken, warmen…

Moment mal!

Erschrocken sehe ich Callum an, der auf der anderen Seite des Tisches in sich hinein grinst.

»Tut mir leid!«, stoße ich hervor und nehme mein Bein weg von seinem.

Er hält seine Hand leicht vor den Mund, um sein Lächeln zu verbergen. Ich möchte am liebsten nach oben rennen und mich in meinem Zimmer einschließen.

Da stellt Elli sich an das Tischende, räuspert sich, dann beginnt sie eine kleine Rede.

»Ich bin wirklich dankbar, dass ich diesen Abend in so freundlicher Gesellschaft verbringen darf.«, sagt sie und sieht mich danach direkt an, »Kindchen ich hoffe, du findest hier ein zweites Zuhause.«

Eine einladende Handbewegung von Elli gibt uns zu verstehen, dass wir nun essen sollen.

Zwar habe ich es geschafft, mir ohne weitere Vorkommnisse den Teller zu füllen, meine Beine lasse ich jedoch vorsichtshalber eng angewinkelt unter meinem Stuhl. Um weitere Herzrasen verursachende Berührungen zu vermeiden.

Ich habe darauf bestanden, wenigstens den Abwasch zu machen, während Elli sich noch mit Callum unterhält. Schweigend lausche ich ihrem Gespräch, wobei ich immer wieder heimlich zu ihm hinüber schiele. Das Licht der Lampe über uns lässt seine Locken schimmern. Callum erzählt träumerisch von den Ideen, die er für den Garten hat und Elli stimmt ihm immer wieder mit begeistertem Nicken zu.

»Wir könnten die Blumen farblich anordnen und so einen Regenbogen schaffen. Vielleicht mit fließendem Farbverlauf.«, schlägt Callum vor.

Die Leidenschaft in seinen Worten lässt mich lächeln.

Was für eine wunderschöne Idee von ihm. Ich kann es kaum erwarten diesen Regenbogen zu sehen!

»Nein.«, erwidert Elli, »Ich mag, dass es so wild ist. Gerade das Durcheinander macht es doch erst interessant. Du kannst die Blumen stundenlang betrachten und wirst doch immer wieder etwas Neues entdecken. Außerdem ergänzen sie sich herrlich.«

Meine Hände plätschern im mit Wasser und Schaum

gefüllten Spülbecken. Der Zitronenduft des Spülmittels kitzelt in meiner Nase.

Ich fand Callums Idee wirklich toll. Warum will Elli sich nicht auf etwas Neues einlassen?

»Ich weiß nicht, ob du schon einmal das Bild gesehen hast, auf dem Theodor und ich vor dieser wunderschönen Blumenwiese in Irland stehen. Ich möchte in meinem Garten an diesen Tag erinnert werden.«, erklärt Elli.

Ihre Stimme wird dabei immer leiser.

Oh! Nun gut, das erklärt natürlich, warum sie gegen den Regenbogen ist. Ein Glück bemerkt niemand, wie ich mich dafür schäme, dass ich sie verurteilt habe, ohne ihre Geschichte zu kennen.

Sie tut mir so unendlich leid. Warum musste ihr ihr Glück so früh genommen werden?

Callum nickt knapp, um ihr zu zeigen, dass er verstanden hat.

»Dann lassen wir es so.«, versichert er ihr.

Es klingt wie der Schwur ihre Erinnerung zum Leben zu erwecken.

Ich trockne mir die Hände am Geschirrtuch ab und möchte gerade zum Tisch zurück, als Callum sich erhebt.

»Vielen Dank für den schönen Abend, Eleonore. Ich

hoffe, wir wiederholen das bald.«

Beim letzten Satz sieht er mir direkt in die Augen. Ich werde rot. Schon wieder.

Hör endlich auf damit! Himmel, ich kenne diesen Mann seit einem Tag und er macht mich wahnsinnig!

»Du kannst noch nicht gehen, Jungchen! Ich habe noch einen Likör im Kühlschrank!«, empört sich Elli und springt von ihrem Stuhl auf, um das alkoholische Getränk zu holen.

Callums Lachen klingt melodisch durch den Raum.

»Für mich bitte nicht, danke.«, lehnt er noch immer grinsend ab und hebt die Hand zum Abschied.

Bevor ich mich ebenfalls aus sicherer Entfernung verabschieden kann, dreht Elli sich zu mir.

»Nun gut. Kindchen, wärst du so nett und würdest ihn zur Tür bringen?«

Ist das ihr Ernst? Er arbeitet hier schon länger, als ich, er weiß doch wohl, wo die Tür ist.

»Natürlich.«, antworte ich und gehe voraus.

Als ich meine schweißnassen Hände fühlen kann, kippt meine Stimmung. Ich will das nicht. Ich will nicht in einem fremden Haus an meinem ersten Tag mein Herz an einen Mann verlieren, den ich überhaupt nicht kenne!

Ich bin auf der Suche nach mir selbst und nicht nach einer Beziehung. Mal abgesehen davon, dass ich keine Ahnung habe ob er mich auch auf diese Weise mag.

»Was für ein Service!«, witzelt Callum, als wir im Flur ankommen.

Ich will etwas Schlagfertiges erwidern, wie »Die Tür wirst du ja wohl allein öffnen können.«, doch als ich mich umdrehe steht er direkt vor mir. So nah, dass ich seine Körperwärme spüren kann.

Ich lege den Kopf in den Nacken, um ihm in die Augen sehen zu können.

Eine Weile stehen wir schweigend voreinander, den Blick tief in den Augen des anderen versenkt.

»Na das kann ja interessant werden.«, haucht er zu mir herunter, ein schiefes Lächeln stiehlt sich auf sein Gesicht.

»Wie meinst du das?«, frage ich verwundert.

Doch Callum antwortet mir nicht. Stattdessen greift er sanft meine Schultern, dreht uns schwungvoll herum, sodass wir Plätze tauschen und lässt mich wieder los. Ich stehe wie versteinert da, als er die Tür öffnet und nach draußen geht. Er hat sie schon fast geschlossen, als sein goldblonder Lockenkopf noch einmal im Türspalt auftaucht.

»Gute Nacht, Kollegin.«

Er zwinkert mir zu, dann verschwindet er und die Tür fällt ins Schloss.

Jetzt stehe ich hier, allein mit meinem klopfenden Herzen. Ich bin noch gefangen in seiner Berührung und erschrocken über meine Gedanken. Trotz meines Widerstandes gegen aufkommende Gefühle ihm gegenüber hofft ein verräterischer Teil von mir, dass er zurückkommt, um mein Verlangen nach einem Kuss von ihm zu stillen.

Ich sehe dich, mein Engel. Mutig von dir, allein um die Häuser zu ziehen. Es lauern Gefahren da draußen. Doch keine Angst!

Ich lege meine schützenden Hände um dich.

Du bist nie allein.

Doch was muss ich sehen? Du versuchst Dinge auszugraben, die ich so sorgfältig beerdigt habe. Reize mich nicht! Nichts wird uns entzweien! Ich habe dich gefunden und werde an deiner Seite bleiben! Und ich werde sie alle zum Schweigen bringen, wenn du mich durch deine Neugier dazu zwingst!

Neue Freunde

Am nächsten Morgen bereite ich gerade ein paar Pfannkuchen für das Frühstück vor, als Elli in ihrem violetten Morgenmantel durch die Küchentür schreitet. Ihre grauen Haare stehen in alle Himmelsrichtungen ab. Sie wirkt noch ganz verschlafen, wie sie vor sich hin schmatzend zum Esstisch tapst.

Ich beobachte sie wortlos. Sie scheint mich überhaupt nicht bemerkt zu haben.

Gerade als ich ihr einen guten Morgen wünschen will, beginnt sie sich schnüffelnd umzusehen. Ihr Blick fällt erst auf die Pfannkuchen auf dem Esstisch, dann auf mich und schließlich sieht sie an sich herunter. Mit großen Augen betrachtet sie mich, dann krächzt sie: »Entschuldige meinen Aufzug, ich… ich habe ganz vergessen, dass du… ich bin sofort wieder zurück.«

Ihr Stuhl knarzt, als sie ruckartig aufsteht, danach tippelt sie schnell aus der Küche. Ich höre die Badezimmertür zuschlagen, gefolgt vom Scheppern eines herunterfallenden Gegenstandes und einem lauten »Verflucht nochmal!«.

Grinsend decke ich weiter den Tisch. Diese Frau ist wirklich einmalig.

Die Morgensonne taucht den Raum in helles Licht, ich fühle mich wie in einem schönen Traum.

Das Geräusch eines Gartenschlauches, der gerade voll aufgedreht wird, lässt meine Füße zum Fenster laufen, noch bevor ich darüber nachdenken kann. Ich komme mir wie eine Geheimagentin vor, wie ich Callum so hinter dem Vorhang beobachte.

Seine Muskeln zeichnen sich durch sein hellgraues T-Shirt ab, als er die Blumen gießt. Noch nie war ich von einem Körper so angetan. Eigentlich ist er überhaupt nicht mein Typ, doch ich habe das Gefühl, seit ich ihn das erste Mal sah, habe ich keinen anderen Typ mehr. Ich will ihm nah sein, will wissen, wer hinter dieser attraktiven Fassade steckt. Es ist, als könnte ich noch immer seine Hände spüren, wo er gestern Abend meine Schultern berührt hat. Ich hatte noch nie so sehr diesen Wunsch nach einem Kuss verspürt. Dieses starke Verlangen, dass dein Herz höherschlagen lässt und eine wohlige Wärme durch deinen Körper schickt.

»Ein hübscher Junge, nicht wahr?«

Ellis Stimme neben meinem Ohr lässt mich erschrocken nach Luft schnappen. Wann ist sie zurückgekommen?

Die Arme auf die Küchentheke gestützt, versuche ich mein Herz zu beruhigen. Sie hat mich eiskalt erwischt.

»Oh Kindchen, ich wollte dich nicht erschrecken.«, entschuldigt sich die alte Dame, bevor sie sich zum Tisch wendet und sich mit einem breiten Grinsen über die Pfannkuchen her macht.

Ich setze mich zu ihr.

»Also, was steht heute an?«, will ich wissen.

Ich habe mich zwar damit abgefunden, dass ich hier keine gebrechliche alte Frau betreuen muss, einen Aufgabenbereich hätte ich aber trotzdem gerne. Nicht nur, weil ich für irgendetwas bezahlt werden muss, sondern aus dem ganz egoistischen Grund heraus, dass mir ohne Aufgabe langweilig wird. Außerdem möchte ich ja herausfinden, was ich im Leben möchte und das geht nun mal schlecht, wenn ich hier nur herumsitze.

»Was immer du tun möchtest, Kindchen.«, antwortet Elli mit vollem Mund. Apfelmus tropft ihr aus dem Mundwinkel auf den Teller, als sie den Bissen hinuntergeschluckt.

Als ich zögere, ergreift sie erneut das Wort.

»Ich verstehe deine Unsicherheit. Du fragst dich wahrscheinlich, was genau deine Aufgabe hier ist. Du wirst die Wahrheit noch herausfinden, wenn du aufmerksam zuhörst. Bis dahin sieh das hier einfach als eine Art bezahlten Urlaub mit gelegentlichem Haushaltsdienst.«

Nicht gerade die Antwort, die ich erwartet hatte. Das erscheint mir doch sehr seltsam, schließlich werde ich hierfür gut bezahlt. Ich hole Luft, um zu widersprechen, da klingelt das Telefon.

Elli tupft sich den Mund mit einer Serviette sauber, dann entschuldigt sie sich und verschwindet im Flur.

Wie hat sie das gemeint, ›*wenn ich genau zuhöre*‹? Sie kann mir doch nicht einfach so einen Informationsbrocken hinwerfen und mich dann sitzen lassen! In mir macht sich eine starke Unruhe breit. Hat sie vielleicht wirklich den Verstand verloren? Ich kenne sie nicht. Ihr Neffe muss einen guten Grund haben, wenn er jemanden dafür einstellt, bei ihr zu sein. Vielleicht ist sie verrückter, als sie scheint?

Ein Klopfen am Fenster reißt mich aus meinen

Gedanken. Es ist Callum. Als unsere Blicke sich treffen, hebt er die Hand zum Gruß und strahlt dabei mit der Sonne um die Wette. Ich verdränge meinen Spionageversuch von vorhin und winke verlegen zurück, was er mit einem koketten Zwinkern erwidert. Mir wird heiß.

Wie kann er mich nach so kurzer Zeit nur dermaßen um den Verstand bringen?

Hinter mir wird die Tür zum Flur aufgerissen, Elli steht im Türrahmen, ihre Wangen sind stark gerötet, sie atmet flach.

»Wir müssen in die Stadt, ich muss Besorgungen machen. Würdest du bitte fahren?«, fragt sie mich, die Augen weit aufgerissen.

»Was ist passiert?«

Sorge überkommt mich. Wer war da am Telefon? Ist jemand gestorben?

»Wir bekommen Besuch, Kindchen, wir bekommen Besuch.«, antwortet Elli, während sie einen Korb aus der Ecke holt.

Sie ist wegen Besuch so aus dem Häuschen?

»Wer kommt denn?«, will ich wissen.

Elli beginnt hektisch in einer Schublade zu wühlen.

»Bei meiner Seele, der Leibhaftige persönlich beehrt uns morgen mit seiner Anwesenheit.«

Um Himmels willen! Ist sie jetzt doch durchgedreht? Sollte ich ihren Neffen anrufen?

Sie packt ihren Geldbeutel in einen Korb, hält mir die Autoschlüssel hin und fragt: »Was ist denn nun? Kommst du?«

Ein knappes Nicken und ich springe auf. Besser ich begleite sie und sorge dafür, dass sie keinen Blödsinn anstellt. Wo bin ich hier nur gelandet?

*

Die Einkaufsstraße der Innenstadt ist wirklich wunderschön. Mit den gepflasterten Straßen, schwarzen Laternen und den Blumen überall erinnert es an Paris. Ich war erst einmal in Paris, damals mit meinen Eltern, aber ich werde diese Atmosphäre nie vergessen.

Wir befinden uns an einer Kreuzung am Stadteingang. Um uns herum reihen sich die verschiedensten Geschäfte aneinander. Weiter hinten kann ich den Eingang zu einem Park oder einem Marktplatz erkennen. Anzug tragende Männer eilen telefonierend über die Straße. Vor einem

Bekleidungsgeschäft bellen sich zwei Hunde die Seele aus dem Leib, während deren Besitzer den neuesten Tratsch austauschen. Motorengeräusche werden von lachenden Kindern übertönt, die an den Händen ihrer Mütter mit bunten Rucksäcken an den Straßenrändern warten.

Unser Weg endet vor einem kleinen Café, dessen Türschild eine Tasse ziert, deren heraus schwappender Kaffee das Wort »Kuchenstube« schreibt.

»Ach, Kindchen, würdest du mir in dem Café drei Stücke von dem Apfel-Nuss-Kuchen besorgen? Ich muss noch einmal flugs in die Apotheke.«, wendet Elli sich an mich.

Ohne meine Antwort abzuwarten, macht sie sich schon auf den Weg zur gegenüberliegenden Straßenseite.

Sie lässt mich einfach hier stehen.

Mich würde wirklich interessieren, wer oder was sie so durcheinandergebracht hat.

Ich wende mich wieder dem Café zu und steige die Steinstufen zur Eingangstür hinauf.

Das helle Bimmeln eines Glöckchens über der dunkelgrün gestrichenen Holztür verkündet meine Ankunft. Der Duft von frisch gebrühtem Kaffee steigt mir in die Nase. Links von mir erstreckt sich eine lange Theke, hinter deren Glasscheibe köstlich aussehende Kuchen und Gebäckstücke präsentiert werden. Rechts vom Eingang befinden sich einige Tische, die mit bunten Blumen dekoriert sind. Um sie herum stehen Stühle und Bänke, deren türkise Samtpolster zum Verweilen einladen.

Ganz nach alter Gewohnheit verschaffe ich mir einen Überblick über die Situation. Zehn Tische, vier davon besetzt. In der Ecke lesen zwei junge Frauen vertieft die Karte.

Hey Deliah, das ist nicht mehr deine Aufgabe!

Etwas wehmütig wende ich mich ab.

»Darf ich deine Bestellung aufnehmen, oder siehst du dich nur um?«, fragt eine helle, sanfte Männerstimme neben mir.

Ich drehe mich um und blicke in Augen, so dunkel und warm zugleich, wie heiße Schokolade. Um diese bilden sich kleine Lachfältchen, die, wie Sonnenstrahlen, das Lächeln des jungen Mannes zu verstärken scheinen.

»Oh, ja, ähm… ich hätte gern drei Stücke von dem Apfel-Nuss-Kuchen. Bitte.«, stammele ich ihm meine Bestellung entgegen.

Diese Ausstrahlung der puren Lebensfreude hat mich

doch glatt aus dem Konzept gebracht.

»Neu hier?«, fragt er mit einem schiefen Lächeln.

»Ja. Woher …?«

»… ich das weiß?«, beendet er meine Frage, »Das hier ist das beste Café dieser doch recht überschaubaren Kleinstadt. Jeder, der hier wohnt, war mindestens einmal hier und dich habe ich noch nie gesehen. Das hätte ich nämlich sicher nicht vergessen.«

Ich bin ein wenig überfordert mit diesem Kompliment und bringe nur ein verhaltenes Kichern zustande.

»Ich bin Andrew.«, stellt er sich mir vor.

»Deliah.«

»ICH WILL SCHOKOLADE, MAAAMAAA!!«, schreit ein kleiner rundlicher Junge neben mir seiner Mutter ins Ohr, als diese das Café betreten.

Die Frau ermahnt ihren Sohn peinlich berührt, dass er doch bitte ruhig sein soll. Sehr begeistert scheint er davon nicht zu sein, was er mit einem tränenreichen Wutausbruch kundtut.

Andrew ignoriert das Geschehen und wendet sich wieder mir zu.

»Also Deliah, was führt dich hierher?«, will er wissen.

»Was zum Teufel, Andy?«, flucht eine Frauenstimme

aus der Küche.

Die Person zu der diese Stimme gehört, tritt kurz darauf schwungvoll durch die Küchentür und hinter den Tresen.

Sie hat ihre langen, dunklen Haare zu einem Pferdeschwanz gebunden, aus dem sich einige Strähnen gelöst haben. An ihrer Wange klebt Mehl, die weiße Küchenschürze ist in der schlanken Taille zusammengebunden. Sie wirkt wie eine wunderschöne Kriegerin mit stechendem Blick.

Ich fürchte mein neuer Freund hier wird jetzt einen Kopf kürzer gemacht.

»Andy! Beschränke deine lächerlichen Flirtversuche gefälligst auf deine einsamen Abende vor dem PC und mach deinen verdammten Job!«, fährt sie ihn an.

»Eifersüchtig, Liv?«, kontert Andrew, die Arme vor der Brust verschränkt.

»Ja! Nämlich auf die Tatsache, dass sie«, Liv zeigt auf mich, »einfach wieder gehen kann und dich nicht den ganzen Tag ertragen muss. Jetzt kümmere dich um unsere Kundschaft!«

Oh, Schachmatt Andrew.

Schnaubend wendet er sich ab und geht zu dem noch

immer weinenden Jungen, um ihm endlich seinen sehnsüchtigen Wunsch nach Schokolade zu erfüllen. Wie schön doch das Alter war, in dem man in aller Öffentlichkeit ohne Probleme wegen einem Kuchen weinen konnte und ihn dann auch noch bekam. Ich kann dich gut verstehen, kleiner Kuchenjunge.

Ich wende mich wieder Liv zu, die mir daraufhin die mehlbestaubte Hand entgegen reicht.

»Hi, ich bin Liv, also eigentlich Olivia, aber so nennen mich nur meine Großeltern. Den Flirtversuch neben mir hast du ja schon kennengelernt. Tut mir leid, man muss ihn ständig daran erinnern, für was er hier eigentlich bezahlt wird.«, stellt sie sich mit einem netten Lächeln vor.

Wow, die Löwin kann auch ein richtiges Kätzchen sein.

»Hi, ich bin…«, beginne ich, doch sie unterbricht mich.

»Deliah. Ich weiß schon. Die Wände hier sind sehr dünn.«, erklärt sie mit einem vielsagenden Blick in Andrews Richtung.

Das Türglöckchen bimmelt erneut, als Mutter, Sohn und Schokoladen-Sahne-Torte das Café verlassen.

Andrew kommt wieder zu uns und legt Olivia den Arm um die Schultern.

»Hey Liv, soweit ich weiß, ist dein Arbeitsplatz nicht hier vorne. Wir wollen doch nicht den Kundenverkehr aufhalten.«, neckt er sie.

»Vergiss nicht, wer hier der Boss ist, Andy. Außerdem bediene ich hier nur unsere neue Freundin Deliah.«, erklärt sie ihm, während sie mir meine Bestellung in einem Karton mit dem Logo der Kuchenstube übergibt.

Ich lege ihr das Geld auf den Tresen.

Also ist Olivia hier die Chefin? Sie ist kaum älter als ich und hat ihren eigenen Laden? Ein Knoten beginnt sich in meiner Brust zusammenzuziehen. Eine Mischung aus Anerkennung und Neid.

»Jetzt erzähl doch mal«, setzt Andrew unsere Unterhaltung fort, »was verschlägt dich in dieses weltfremde und doch wunderschöne Städtchen?«

»Ich arbeite hier.«, antworte ich knapp.

Olivias Augen weiten sich.

»Oh, eine studierte Landschaftsdesignerin, die unseren ungepflegten Park auf Vordermann bringt?«

Ein kleiner Stich durchfährt mich, als ich an Callum und den wunderschönen Garten denken muss. Es wäre sicher interessant, mehr über seine Arbeit zu erfahren. Wenn ich ehrlich bin, habe ich mich nie mit anderen Dingen als der Pizzeria beschäftigt. Ich habe mich nie ausprobiert, um herauszufinden, worin meine Talente liegen.

»Nein.«, antworte ich, »Nicht studiert. Und auch keine Landschaftsdesignerin. Ich bin die Haushaltshilfe von Frau Griffin.«, erkläre ich etwas kleinlaut.

Beide reißen erstaunt die Augen auf.

»Bei der alten Griffin?«, ruft Andy fast erschrocken aus, »Nicht schlecht, die Letzte hat es genau zwei Monate ausgehalten, bevor sie schreiend das Haus verlassen hat.«, erzählt er mit einem breiten Grinsen.

Ich wusste gar nicht, dass es eine vor mir gab.

»Die Letzte?«, hake ich neugierig nach.

»Man hat sie in der ganzen Gemeinde schreien hören.«, erzählt Andy lachend.

»Das stimmt doch gar nicht!«, widerspricht Liv ihm und boxt ihm mit dem Ellenbogen in die Seite.

»Wir wollen uns nicht mit Details aufhalten. Auf jeden Fall hat sie behauptet, es würde spuken in dem alten Haus. Anscheinend der tote Ehemann.«, berichtet er weiter, hebt dabei bedeutungsvoll die Hände, um einen Geist nachzuahmen. Unheilvolle Laute inklusive.

Liv verdreht nur die Augen und ich muss lachen. Wenn auch etwas unbehaglich.

Erneut erklingt das Glöckchen der Eingangstür. Diesmal ist es Elli, die atemlos hereinstolpert.

»Kindchen, wo bleibst du denn? Oh, guten Tag Olivia!«, begrüßt sie meine neue Bekanntschaft.

Hier kennen sich wohl wirklich alle.

Liv hebt die Hand zum Gruß.

»Bin gleich fertig, Elli!«, rufe ich ihr zu, doch sie ist schon wieder nach draußen verschwunden.

Ich will mich gerade verabschieden, als Olivia mich aufhält.

»Hey, komm doch mal auf einen Kaffee vorbei. Geht aufs Haus. Ich arbeite von Montag bis Mittwoch in der Küche.«

»Und ich bin immer hier.«, wirft Andy strahlend ein.

Die Tür öffnet sich erneut.

»Kindchen, wo bleibst du denn?«

Entschuldigend lächle ich die beiden an und verabschiede mich schnell, bevor Elli mich noch an den Ohren herauszerrt.

»Ich muss los, aber ich komme auf jeden Fall einmal

vorbei.«, verspreche ich, dann verlasse ich die Kuchenstube mit drei Stückchen Apfel-Nuss-Kuchen und der Freude darüber zwei nette Menschen kennengelernt zu haben, die vielleicht zu Freunden werden.

*

Um mich herum herrscht Chaos.

Elli bereitet sich auf unseren mysteriösen Besuch vor und wuselt seit Stunden hin und her. Es kommt mir vor, als wäre sie überall gleichzeitig. Hinter mir scheppert ein Topf, vor mir brodelt es, ich zupfe mir ein Stück Kartoffelschale von den pinken Socken, das gerade in hohem Bogen durch die Luft geflogen und auf meinen Füßen gelandet ist.

»Sag mir doch bitte, wobei ich dir helfen kann.«, beschwöre ich Elli.

Sie möchte unserem Gast, von dem ich noch immer nicht weiß, wer er ist, ein Essen zubereiten. Shepherds Pie, nannte sie es. Ich habe es schon einmal gehört, doch meine Kenntnisse beschränken sich eher auf Pizza und Pasta. Die wiederum mache ich sehr gerne.

»Ich brauche keine Hilfe, Kindchen. Nicht hierfür.«,

brabbelt sie im Vorbeigehen.

Ich muss zur Seite ausweichen, da sie mich sonst über den Haufen gerannt hätte. Sie ist völlig durch den Wind und doch hoch konzentriert. Es kann kein Fremder sein, wenn sie ihn zum Mittagessen einlädt. Sie wird doch nicht etwa für den Geist kochen? Nein, Blödsinn. Jetzt werde ich selbst verrückt.

»Möchtest du mir wenigstens verraten, wer uns besuchen kommt? Ich könnte ein Tiramisu für den Nachtisch vorbereiten.«, biete ich an.

Eleonore hält abrupt inne und sieht mich aus großen, geschockten Augen an, dann flüstert sie mit ihrer Reibeisenstimme: »Kein Nachtisch! Ich hoffe doch, dass wir bis zum Nachtisch wieder Frieden in diesem Haus haben werden.«

Sie führt sich auf, als wäre sie eine Drogendealerin, deren Boss kommt, um die Schulden einzufordern. Moment, könnte es sein, dass…? Unmöglich, diese Dame hier wäre wahrscheinlich selbst die Anführerin der Gang.

KLIRR!!

Ein Glas ist von der Theke gefallen, viele kleine Glassplitter verteilen sich auf dem Boden.

»Vermaledeit noch mal!«, flucht Elli.

Ich ergreife meine Chance, für mein Geld tatsächlich etwas zu tun und schnappe mir schnell Schaufel und Besen, um den kleinen Unfall aufzukehren. Ein dankendes Lächeln aus falschen Zähnen strahlt mir entgegen.

Ich möchte gerade die Scherben wegwerfen, als ich bemerke, dass der Mülleimer voll ist, also bringe ich ihn wortlos nach draußen. Wahrscheinlich ist es da auch sicherer, als in der Küche mit der wild gewordenen Oma.

»Sieht schwer aus, kann ich dir helfen?«, höre ich Callum aus dem Garten rufen, als ich den Müllbeutel zur Tonne trage.

»Schon okay, danke!«, lehne ich ab.

Ich werde einen Teufel tun und diesem attraktiven Mann die vergammelten Essensreste der letzten Woche in die Hand drücken. Außerdem werde ich nicht noch einmal als die Schwächere hier herausgehen. Als wäre ein Müllbeutel zu schwer für mich. Lächerlich. Schnell werfe ich ihn in die Tonne. Ha! Auftrag ganz ohne fremde Hilfe ausgeführt.

Callum kommt dennoch näher, was mich innerlich einen Freudentanz aufführen lässt. Jetzt nur noch geschickt den Standort weg von den Mülltonnen und hin zu den wohlriechenden Rosen lenken. Schultern zurück, Gewicht auf ein Bein verlagern und versuchen ihn sexy anzulächeln.

Okay, lassen wir das mit dem gespielten Sex-Appeal, sonst denkt er noch, ich hätte einen Schlaganfall.

»Ist irgendetwas passiert? Von außen wirkt es, als wäre ein Tornado in der Küche zugange.«, fragt er schmunzelnd.

Er trägt ein schwarzes T-Shirt. Ich mag es lieber, wenn er helle Sachen trägt und so seine goldenen Locken noch engelhafter wirken. Wie ein himmlischer Retter. Obwohl der dunkle Dämon mit den eisblauen Augen ihm auch steht.

Wow, Deliah, wann sind wir gedanklich wieder im Teenie Alter angekommen?

Warte mal, er hat mich gerade etwas gefragt. Was war es? Was nur? Ah ja!

»Elli erwartet Besuch. Frag mich gar nicht erst wen, sie verrät es mir nämlich nicht.«

Puh, gerade noch die Kurve bekommen. Fast hätte er mich wohl als zurückgeblieben eingestuft.

Seine Augen verengen sich, mit ernster Miene sieht er zum Haus hinüber, als könnte er Elli durch die Wände beobachten. Was macht ihm solche Sorgen?

»Stimmt etwas nicht?«

»Ich frage mich nur, wer sie so durcheinanderbringt. Kein gutes Zeichen bei Eleonore.«, antwortet er.

Er ist plötzlich sehr ernst, keine Spur mehr von seiner koketten Art.

Das ist ganz und gar nicht die Stimmung, die ich heraufbeschwören wollte. So sehr ich mich auch gegen diese kleine Flamme sträube, die er in mir entfacht hat, möchte ich ihm dennoch nah sein. Ich hatte schon eine Handvoll Dates, doch keiner dieser Männer hat mich je so verzaubert wie Callum. Ich will mich nicht mehr dagegen wehren. Will der Sache eine Chance geben und meine Gefühle zulassen, auch wenn diese noch sehr frisch sind. Vielleicht gibt es ja tatsächlich so etwas wie Liebe auf den ersten Blick?

»Hey, sag mal, ich war neulich in einem Café in der Stadt. Kuchenstube. Es war wirklich sehr schön dort. Hättest du Lust, naja, dort einmal gemeinsam hinzugehen? Mit mir?«, frage ich mit dem ganzen Mut, den ich in mir zusammenkratzen kann.

Mein Magen rebelliert, ich fürchte Callum macht gleich Bekanntschaft mit meinem Frühstück. So nervös war ich zuletzt, als die Prüfungsergebnisse der Abschlussklasse verkündet wurden.

Callum sieht mich allerdings an, als hätte ihn gerade eine Biene in den Hintern gestochen.

»Nein.«, antwortet er.

Kurz, knapp, endgültig.

Mein Herz zerspringt in tausend Teile. Habe ich den Small Talk, das Lächeln, etwa falsch gedeutet? Nach all den kleinen Momenten jetzt dieses eiskalte »Nein«? Nicht einmal eine halbherzige Ausrede? Wie kann er mir nur solche Hoffnung machen und mich dann so gnadenlos fallen lassen?

»Oh. Okay. Dann nicht. Ich dachte… ich muss wieder rein.«

Den letzten Teil kann ich nur flüstern.

Ohne ein weiteres Wort stürme ich an ihm vorbei zurück ins Haus.

Er folgt mir nicht. Versucht nicht einmal mich aufzuhalten. Das gibt mir den Rest.

Da nehme ich all meinen Mut zusammen und werde doch enttäuscht. Wie konnte ich mir auch einbilden, dass es da etwas zwischen uns gäbe? Ich kenne ihn ja kaum! Er hat mich in seinen Bann gezogen, ich wollte einfach Teil seiner Welt sein. Doch er will mich nicht. Will mir nicht einmal eine Chance geben. Gut. Dann eben nicht! Dann hat er mich auch nicht verdient.

Nein! Nein! NEIN! Das war nicht gut. Du dummes Ding! So wird das nichts, mein Engel. Ein Plan, ich brauche einen Plan, sonst werde ich mich vergessen.

Wie damals.

Der Teufel

Trotz meines verletzten Stolzes habe ich diese Nacht sehr gut geschlafen. Na dann, neuer Tag, neues Glück. Keine Zeit, blöden, gutaussehenden Gärtnern hinterher zu weinen! Ich muss Elli bei den Vorbereitungen helfen. Auch wenn sie mir noch immer nicht gesagt hat, auf wen wir uns genau vorbereiten.

Noch bevor ich einen Fuß auf die erste Stufe setze, vernehme ich das Klappern von Töpfen. Natürlich hat sie schon angefangen. Warum sollte sie auch warten?

»Guten Morgen!«, rufe ich in die Küche.

Ein Schnauben gefolgt von einem »Gut ist an diesem Morgen überhaupt nichts!«, erklingt dumpf hinter der geöffneten Schranktür.

Ich lege Elli die Hand auf die Schulter, woraufhin sie erschrocken zusammenzuckt.

»Was willst du, Kindchen?«, fragt sie gehetzt.

Eine Locke hängt ihr lose ins Gesicht.

»Sag mir, wie ich dir helfen kann. Du wirst noch

umkippen.«, ermahne ich sie.

»Oh, ich komme ganz wunderbar allein zurecht.«, lehnt sie mein Angebot ab.

»Aber Elli, ich werde dafür bezahlt, dir zu helfen. Also ist es quasi mein Recht, beschäftigt zu werden.«, kläre ich sie auf.

Elli braucht definitiv keine rundum Betreuung. Ich sollte ihren Neffen darauf ansprechen. Aber dieser Job wird wirklich gut bezahlt.

Geld verdienen, bis ich meinen Weg gefunden habe. Das war der Plan. Wer weiß, wo ich lande, wenn allen klar wird, wie wenig ich hier gebraucht werde? Warum habe ich plötzlich Bilder von Schlachthöfen im Kopf? Ich schüttele mich, um die Gedanken loszuwerden.

»Nun? Eine Aufgabe bitte!«, fordere ich Elli erneut auf etwas zu delegieren.

»Na schön!«, krächzt sie, gefolgt von unverständlichem Gebrabbel.

Nach kurzem Überlegen dreht sie sich schwungvoll zu mir um und verkündet: »Blumen! Kindchen, geh in den Garten und hole mir einen Strauß gelbe Nelken. Keine Rosen! Nur viele gelbe Nelken.«

»Wird erledigt!«, bestätige ich ihren Auftrag, dann

mache ich mich auf den Weg in den Garten.

Blumen pflücken. Nicht unbedingt die Art von Hilfe, die ich im Sinn hatte, aber immerhin besser als nichts. Nur was zum Teufel sind Nelken?

Wie ein Dieb presse ich mich an die Hauswand, die Augen weit aufgerissen, die Lippen aufeinandergepresst, als ich um die Ecke spähe. Keine Spur von Callum. Sehr gut. Nach dem gestrigen Vorfall möchte ich ihn erst einmal nicht mehr sehen.

Aus ganz egoistischem, gekränktem Stolz.

Ich gehe hinüber zum Blumenbeet. Rot, lila, blau, ah! Da sind ja gelbe Blumen. Es sind die Einzigen, also werden das hoffentlich die Richtigen sein. Mehrlagige Blütenschichten strecken sich der Sonne entgegen. Sie sind wirklich wunderschön.

Direkt neben dem Beet liegt eine Schere. Ich nehme sie und beginne die Blumen zu schneiden.

»Willst du jemandem den Krieg erklären?«, erklingt eine tiefe, mir sehr bekannte Stimme hinter mir, die mich frustriert aufstöhnen lässt.

So eine Scheiße! Hat er sich im Gebüsch versteckt? Ich war mir so sicher er wäre nicht hier!

»Hi, Callum.«, begrüße ich ihn, ohne von meiner

Arbeit aufzusehen.

Ich weiß, ich wollte nur eine Nacht lang verletzt sein und diesen Vorfall vergessen. Doch anscheinend ist mein Selbstbewusstsein dafür nicht stark genug. Deshalb behandele ich ihn wie ein trotziges Kind, beachte ihn nicht weiter und lasse meine Wut an den Blumen aus, als ich ihre Stiele mit der scharfen Schere durchtrenne.

Er antwortet nicht weiter, also ist er wohl wieder gegangen. Gut so! Halte dich bloß fern von mir mit deinem bescheuerten, perfekten Grinsen!

Als ich kurz darauf mein Werk vollendet habe, stehe ich auf und muss beim Umdrehen erschrocken feststellen, dass Callum noch immer hinter mir steht. Mit geneigtem Kopf betrachtet er mich neugierig. Stalkt er mich jetzt oder was?

Gerade als ich etwas sagen möchte, nimmt er mir eine Blume aus der Hand und dreht sie begutachtend zwischen seinen Fingern. Ich bin so überrumpelt, dass ich kein Wort herausbekomme und ihn einfach gewähren lasse.

»Ich hoffe doch, die sind nicht für mich?«, fragt er mit einem schiefen Lächeln.

Wie bitte? Was bildet der sich eigentlich ein? Glaubt er nur weil er ein hübsches Gesicht hat, renne ich ihm nach, wie eine läufige Hündin? Ich wollte ihn doch nur netterweise auf einen dämlichen Kaffee einladen!

»Sicher nicht. Wir bekommen Besuch, erinnerst du dich?«, erwidere ich trotzig, wobei ich den Rest des Straußes so fest umklammere, dass ich den Saft aus den Stilen an meinen Fingern fühlen kann.

»Na da bin ich aber erleichtert.«, antwortet er, sein Lächeln wird noch breiter. Er hält mein Herz in seinen Händen und zerreißt es vor meinen Augen. Wut brodelt in mir, lässt meine Brust schmerzen.

Doch gerade als ich ihn fragen will, was er sich hier eigentlich erlaubt, beginnt er zu erklären.

»Gelbe Nelken, das Symbol der Abneigung. Schenkst du diese Blumen einer Person, sagt das so viel wie ‚*ich mag dich nicht*‘.«

»Oh.«, antworte ich kleinlaut.

Blumensprache war noch nie mein Fachgebiet. Hätte ich das gewusst, wäre das hier nur halb so peinlich. Das hätte er aber wirklich früher erklären können! Gelbe Nelken. Elli wollte unbedingt gelbe Nelken. Bestimmt weiß sie, was es bedeutet.

»Du guckst ja immer noch so grimmig.«, dringt Callum in meine Gedanken ein.

»Was?«, erwidere ich wenig geistreich.

»Du wirktest gerade so verärgert. Dachtest du, ich würde deine Blumen ablehnen?«, erkundigt er sich.

Goldene Locken umrahmen seine neugierig dreinschauenden Augen.

»Ich, nein! Nein, das dachte ich nicht.«, lüge ich ihm und mir eiskalt etwas vor.

»Oh, da bin ich aber erleichtert. Nur, wenn ich so frei sein darf, mir wäre ein Strauß roter Rosen viel lieber.«

Geschockt reiße ich die Augen auf. Was soll das? Rote Rosen? Was das bedeutet, weiß sogar ich! Warum tut er das?

»Warum tust du das?«, schreie ich ihm meine Gedanken entgegen.

Völlig überrumpelt von meiner Reaktion sieht er mich fragend an.

»Du bist so ...«, mir entweicht ein verzweifeltes Schnauben, als ich um die richtigen Worte ringe, »Ich frage dich, ob du mit mir etwas unternehmen willst und du lehnst ab. Schön. Ist in Ordnung. Jetzt willst du plötzlich rote Rosen von mir? Hast du zu viel am Dünger geschnüffelt oder was?«

Ich muss mich anstrengen, um nicht hysterisch zu

kreischen. Himmel, dieser Mann hat mich wirklich verletzt und das wollte ich ihm eigentlich nie zeigen. Tja, Mission gescheitert. Jetzt weiß er wohl, was Sache ist.

»Deliah, ich wusste nicht ... ich wollte doch nicht ...«, beginnt er, doch ich lasse ihn nicht ausreden.

Aus Furcht, er könnte mich noch einmal verletzen.

»Lass gut sein!«, kotze ich ihm entgegen und stapfe mit meinen Antipathieblumen davon.

Die eine, die er noch in der Hand hält, darf er von Herzen gerne behalten.

*

Mein Herz in Scherben decke ich den Tisch für unseren mysteriösen Gast. Warum nur habe ich zugelassen, dass er sich in mein Herz lächelt? Er wirkte wie ein Engel auf mich, der mich aus der Unsicherheit meines Lebens retten sollte. Ich habe mich auf den ersten Blick verliebt. Liebe heißt, dem Anderen Macht über dich geben. Und dennoch werfe ich mir vor, dass ich ihn vorhin hätte ausreden lassen sollen. Hätte seine Erklärung anhören sollen. Doch ich hatte Angst. Davor, dass er mich endgültig zurückweist. Und davor, dass er es nicht tut, sondern im Gegenteil, mir Hoffnung macht. Pure Macht über mich.

Elli hat währenddessen den ganzen Vormittag in der Küche hantiert. Helfen durfte ich ihr bis auf die Nelken-Sache nicht weiter. Ich habe sie noch einmal gefragt, wen wir erwarten, woraufhin sie sich theatralisch bekreuzigte und »Satan« murmelte.

So langsam bin ich mir nicht sicher, ob ich beunruhigt oder genervt sein soll. Sie verhält sich, als würde demnächst irgendein Mafiaboss die Tür eintreten. Wer kann denn bitte so wichtig sein, dass man einen solchen Aufwand betreibt?

Das laute Klingeln der Türglocke durchbricht das Klappern unserer Handgriffe. Als der Ton verklingt, erwachen wir aus unserer Starre. Kurz darauf stürmt Elli aus der Küche, streift sich den Rock glatt und bekreuzigt sich, wobei sie »Gott steh mir bei.«, murmelt.

Ich lege die letzte Serviette auf den Tisch und folge ihr nun doch beunruhigt. Durch das milchige Glas des Fensters neben der Haustür kann ich nur eine schemenhafte Gestalt erahnen. Groß und in viel Schwarz gehüllt, wippt der Schatten ungeduldig hin und her.

Dann öffnet Elli die Tür und offenbart mir unseren

Gast. Ein Mann mit blonden, kurzen Haaren und eisblauen Augen steht vor uns. Er trägt einen sportlich geschnittenen Anzug und scheint Mitte dreißig zu sein.

Wer ist das und was mag er hier wollen?

In diesem Moment zeigt er durch ein breites Lächeln, das seine Augen nicht erreicht, eine Reihe strahlend weißer Zähne. Eine spitz zulaufende Nase lässt ihn überheblich wirken. Als meine Neugier gerade unerträglich zu werden scheint, breitet er die Arme aus und sagt mit rauer Stimme: »Tante Eleonore! Wie schön dich zu sehen!«

Tante? Dann muss das Alexander Griffin sein. Mein Boss.

»Guten Tag, Alexander.«, begrüßt Elli ihn und bestätigt damit meinen Verdacht.

»Oh, du erinnerst dich an meinen Namen. Das ist toll, du scheinst einen guten Tag zu haben.«, lobt er und tritt ein.

»Gab schon bessere Tage.«, nuschelt Elli hinter ihm.

Ich habe das Ganze bis jetzt vom Ende des Flurs beobachtet, doch nun kommt Herr Griffin direkt auf mich zu.

Eine große, gepflegte Männerhand wird mir

entgegengestreckt, gefolgt von einem: »Guten Tag! Sie müssen Deliah sein. Es ist mir eine große Freude.«

Ich stimme ihm zu und begrüße ihn ebenfalls freundlich, auch wenn seine Erscheinung mich dermaßen einschüchtert, dass ich mich neben ihm wie ein kleines Mädchen fühle. Außerdem bin ich verwundert, wie jung er noch ist. Sein Händedruck ist kräftig und kurz fürchte ich, er würde mich gar nicht mehr loslassen, doch dann meldet sich Elli zu Wort.

»Setz dich. Das Essen ist bereits fertig.«

»Deck doch schon einmal den Tisch, Tantchen. Aber Vorsicht mit den Messern, okay? Ich würde mich gern noch einmal mit deiner netten neuen Freundin unterhalten.«, antwortet er mit derart liebevollem Ton, dass ich es ihm fast abgekauft hätte. Wäre da nicht diese Kälte in seinem Blick.

Eleonore schnaubt nur und drängt sich an uns vorbei Richtung Küche. Es steht doch schon alles bereit. Warum sagt sie nichts? Ist das etwa der Moment, in dem ich genau zuhören soll? Was will ihr Neffe von mir?

Wir betreten ein kleines Zimmer rechts von uns. Über dem ehemaligen Arbeitszimmer von Theodor Griffin schlängelt sich die Treppe nach oben. Es ist nur ein kleiner Raum, doch er ist mit großartigen Erinnerungen gefüllt. Die alte, mittlerweile gelbliche Tapete wird fast komplett von Bildern aus aller Herren Länder überdeckt. Aufnahmen von den vielen Reisen der Griffins. So schön sie auch sind, sie verleihen dem Raum etwas Bedrückendes, wenn man das Schicksal des lachenden Paares kennt, das hier abgebildet ist.

Rechts befindet sich ein alter Schreibtisch mit dazugehörigem Holzstuhl. Links von mir wird die Wand komplett von einem Bücherregal bedeckt. Der Geruch von Staub und altem Papier erfüllt den Raum.

Alexander Griffin schließt die Tür hinter uns und lehnt sich locker dagegen. Eine einfache Geste, die auf mich jedoch plötzlich sehr bedrohlich wirkt. Ich weiß nicht, was es ist, das den Alarm in mir auslöst, doch meine Gedanken kreisen nur noch darum, dass ich gerade wirklich nicht hier sein möchte. Elli muss einen Grund dafür haben, dass sie bei seinem Besuch derart durch den Wind ist.

Bevor meine Unruhe sich jedoch zu Panik entwickeln kann, ergreift er das Wort.

»Nun, Deliah, was halten sie von meiner Tante? Kommen sie mit ihr zurecht?«

Die Tatsache, dass er mich einfach beim Vornamen nennt, macht die Sache noch unbehaglicher. Diese eisblauen Augen, die bei Callum wie der Himmel an einem schönen Sommertag wirken, scheinen bei ihm wie eisige Gletscher den Tod zu versprechen. Dennoch versuche ich zu lächeln und antworte ihm.

»Elli ist eine wirklich sehr interessante Frau.«, formuliere ich eine vage Antwort.

Ich möchte ungern darauf hinweisen, dass Elli meiner Meinung nach keine Hilfe nötig hat.

Er lacht. Habe ich etwas Witziges gesagt?

»Interessant? Sie dürfen ruhig offen sprechen. Ich weiß, dass Tante Eleonore verrückt ist.«, antwortet er und stößt sich von der Tür ab, was mich einen Schritt rückwärts machen lässt.

Verrückt? Elli?

»Nun, ich würde es nicht verrückt nennen. Sie hat eben ihre eigene Art zu leben.«, erwidere ich unsicher.

Ist das sein Ernst oder werde ich hier gerade getestet?

»Keine falsche Bescheidenheit, meine Liebe. Meine Tante hat komplett den Verstand verloren.«, zischt er mir entgegen.

Was will er denn von mir hören? Er steht mittlerweile

unangenehm nah bei mir, sodass ich sein zugegeben gutes Parfum deutlich riechen kann.

»Ihre Tante macht auf mich einen völlig normalen Eindruck Herr Griffin. Ich finde nicht, dass sie geistig in irgendeiner Art und Weise auffällig wäre. Im Gegenteil, sie ist eine sehr weise und intelligente Frau.«, schildere ich ihm meine Sicht der Umstände und riskiere dabei meinen Job hier.

So, jetzt ist es raus.

»Ist das so?«, entgegnet er nachdenklich, wobei er die Arme verschränkt.

Eingeschüchtert nicke ich nur knapp woraufhin er sich frustriert mit der Faust auf den Oberschenkel schlägt.

Ich zucke zusammen. Was ist denn bitte sein Problem? Will er etwa von mir hören, dass Elli verrückt ist?

Er atmet hörbar ein und aus, dann wendet er sich wieder an mich.

»Gut, Deliah, ich will ganz offen sein. Meine Tante ist in einem Alter, in dem es durchaus normal ist, dass Menschen nicht mehr für sich selbst sorgen können. Eleonore mag ihnen mit ihrem ungeschulten Auge womöglich gänzlich normal erscheinen, doch sie befindet sich durchaus in einem Zustand der geistigen

Verwirrung.«

Oh wow, einer in diesem Haus ist ganz sicher geistig verwirrt und ich bin mir sicher, dass es nicht Elli ist! Da er aber mein Boss ist, schlucke ich diese Bemerkung wieder herunter.

Ich hatte mit Nico, meinem vorherigen Chef, ein sehr freundschaftliches Verhältnis und auch so einige Meinungsverschiedenheiten. Aber so etwas Bizarres wie diese Situation hier habe ich noch nie erlebt.

»Ich widerspreche ihnen nur ungern«, lüge ich ihn an, »aber ich habe keinerlei Probleme mit ihrer Tante. Das ist doch kein Grund zur Beunruhigung. Dafür bin ich doch hier.«

Wie ich es hasse, gute Miene zum bösen Spiel zu machen. Ich möchte ihm lieber ordentlich die Meinung sagen, angefangen dabei, dass er mich für meinen *ungeschulten Blick* tadelt. Dann stell dir doch eine Krankenschwester ein, du Anzug tragender Trottel!

Erneutes Durchatmen seinerseits.

»Ihre bescheidene Meinung in allen Ehren, aber ich kenne meine Tante wohl am besten.«, antwortet er mit einem schiefen Grinsen.

Bescheidene Meinung? Ich stehe kurz davor mich zu

vergessen, da spricht er weiter.

»Deliah, ich möchte sie um einen Gefallen bitten.«

Ich bin sprachlos. Erst beleidigen, dann Hilfe anfordern? Macht man das nicht allein der Höflichkeit wegen anders herum? Ich bin neugierig. Was kann meine bescheidene, ungeschulte Person für den großen Alexander Griffin tun?

»Was wollen sie?«, frage ich ohne eine Spur meiner anfänglichen Freundlichkeit.

»Sie verstehen sich anscheinend sehr gut mit meiner Tante. Seien sie weiterhin an ihrer Seite, werden sie ihr eine Freundin, wenn sie so wollen und wenn der richtige Augenblick gekommen ist, sprechen sie sie auf ihr Problem an. Ihr Problem nicht mehr bei Sinnen zu sein. Dieses große Haus ist viel zu viel für eine Dame ihres Alters. Die Welt da draußen ist zu kompliziert für eine einsame, zurückgebliebene Frau. Ich möchte nur ihr Bestes, dessen können sie sich sicher sein. Deshalb wäre ich, nun ja, um einiges weniger in Sorge um sie, wenn ich dazu, sagen wir, berechtigt wäre, ihre Angelegenheiten für sie in allen Lebensbereichen zu regeln.«, erklärt er ausweichend.

Ich brauche einen Moment, um ihm folgen zu können,

doch dann begreife ich.

»Eine Generalvollmacht?«, spreche ich meinen Verdacht aus.

Nico hatte so etwas ebenfalls für seine Mutter. Diese litt allerdings unter starker Demenz und war ständig gefährdet irgendetwas in Brand zu stecken. Davon ist Elli meilenweit entfernt.

»Betrachten sie es als ihren Job, sie davon zu überzeugen, dass dies unbedingt notwendig ist.«, redet er auf mich ein.

Wieder kommt er näher, was mich weiter nach hinten ausweichen lässt. Als ich die Lehne des Stuhls an meiner Hüfte spüren kann, fühle ich mich endgültig gefangen. Er steht nun direkt vor mir, ich kann ihn beinahe berühren. Dieser Mann hat eindeutig eine Grenze überschritten und doch hindert mich eine unerklärliche Angst davor, ihm genau das klar zu machen.

Ganz ruhig, er kann mir nichts tun. Oder?

»Deliah, es ist äußerst wichtig, dass meine Tante begreift, wie schwer krank sie ist. Verstanden?«

Das letzte Wort wirkt auf mich wie eine Drohung. Ich weiß nicht, was ich antworten soll. Mein Herz scheint mir aus der Brust zu springen. Er möchte, dass ich Elli einrede, sie sei verrückt! Das ist mein Job, deshalb bin ich hier. Aber das kann und werde ich nicht tun!

Ich versuche mich zu beruhigen und ihm genau das zu sagen, als ein lautes Poltern über uns die Anspannung zerschlägt. Kurz darauf kommt Elli herein und bittet uns zum Essen.

Ich sitze am Tisch und bekomme keinen Bissen hinunter. Wie kann dieser Mann hier so seelenruhig sitzen und essen, während er plant, die Person zu entmündigen, die für ihn gekocht hat?

»Tante Eleonore, es schmeckt wirklich wunderbar! Was für ein Glück, dass deine neue Freundin so gut kochen kann!«, lobt er mich.

Dabei wirkt er so aufrichtig fröhlich, dass ich kotzen möchte. Ich will widersprechen, doch Elli berührt mich am Arm. Fragend sehe ich sie an, sie aber hat den Blick auf Alexander geheftet, der gierig seinen Teller leer isst. Anscheinend möchte er so schnell wieder verschwinden, wie er aufgetaucht ist. Ein Sturm, der in kurzer Zeit alles vernichtet und plötzlich abklingt, als wäre er nie hier gewesen.

Ich will mich gerade dazu zwingen, auch einen Bissen

zu nehmen, da richtet Elli sich an mich.

»Ach, Kindchen, wärst du so lieb und würdest mir ein Glas Wasser aus der Küche holen?«

Heute ist ein Tag voller Überraschungen. Elli hat mich seit ich hier bin noch nie um eine solche Kleinigkeit gebeten. Naja, vielleicht will sie ihren bösartigen Neffen nicht aus den Augen lassen. Wer kann es ihr verübeln?

Wortlos gehe ich hinüber zur Küche. Als ich ein Glas aus dem Hängeschrank über der Spüle holen möchte, sehe ich ein merkwürdiges Fläschchen am Waschbecken neben dem Auflauf stehen.

Es ist geöffnet. Ich kenne mich nicht mit Medikamenten aus, doch ich bin mir sicher, so eine Flasche habe ich hier noch nie gesehen.

Skeptisch betrachte ich das Etikett: »Abführ-Tropfen«.

Moment, sie hat doch nicht?

Als ich zum Tisch zurückkehre, sehe ich, dass Elli noch immer vor ihrem gefüllten Teller sitzt. Mein Boss hingegen hat brav aufgegessen. Das kann sie nicht getan haben, oder?

»Was machen die Geschäfte, Alexander?«, fragt Elli.

»Oh, laufen gut, laufen gut.«, antwortet er kurz

angebunden.

Elli blickt zu mir, ein hämisches Grinsen auf den Lippen, dann richtet sie sich wieder an ihren Neffen.

»Das freut mich natürlich sehr. Weißt du, dass hier in der Nähe ein neues Pflegeheim entstehen soll?«, fragt sie ihn.

»Tatsächlich? Das ist doch großartig, so in deiner Heimat! Oder nicht? Ich wusste gar nichts davon.«

Er klingt wirklich begeistert.

»Ach, habe ich Pflegeheim gesagt? Ich meinte, ein neuer Supermarkt. Das andere hättest du wahrscheinlich noch vor den Architekten erfahren.«

»Wieso sollten mich solche Heime interessieren Tante Eleonore?«, fragt er anscheinend verwirrt nach.

»Nur so ein Verdacht, mein lieber Neffe.«

Dieses Puzzle aus Informationen entwickelt sich langsam zu einem großen Bild. Nur ein Teil fehlt mir. Warum ist er derart hinter Ellis Vermögen her? Es scheint ihm doch selbst an nichts zu fehlen. Soll ich wirklich glauben, dass die Aussicht auf Geld ihn derart skrupellos macht?

Im Moment gibt es jedoch ein ganz andres Rätsel zu lösen: Der Verbleib der Abführ-Tropfen. Hat Elli sie tatsächlich ins Essen gemischt?

Alexander legt sein Besteck auf den Teller, tupft sich die sauberen Mundwinkel mit einer Serviette ab, dann erhebt er sich.

»Nun denn, es war mir wirklich eine Freude, mit zwei so reizenden Damen zu essen. Jetzt ruft mich allerdings wieder die Pflicht eines viel beschäftigten Geschäftsmannes.«

Ich muss mir ein Augenrollen verkneifen. Elli hatte recht, er ist ätzend.

Wir begleiten ihn zur Tür. Auf der Schwelle dreht er sich noch einmal zu uns um und reicht mir zum Abschied die Hand.

»Es war mir eine Freude, sie kennengelernt zu haben, Deliah. Ich kann unser nächstes Treffen kaum erwarten.«

Ich bleibe stumm, doch das ist nicht weiter schlimm, denn Elli drängt sich zwischen uns, um ihm eine gute Fahrt zu wünschen.

Als er verschwunden ist, muss ich meinen Verdacht einfach loswerden.

»Elli, hast du etwa Abführmittel in das Essen gemischt?«, flüstere ich mehr, da ich es selbst nicht glauben kann.

Doch Elli lacht nur verschwörerisch, wobei sie klingt wie eine alte Hexe, dann fast sie sich in gespieltem Entsetzen an die Brust.

»Oh nein! Das muss ich wohl im Zuge meiner geistigen Verwirrung mit dem Salz verwechselt haben! Der arme Alexander. Ich hoffe inständig der Stau auf der Autobahn hält ihn nicht allzu lange auf!«

In dieser Familie sind doch alle verrückt! Wie wollte sie denn verhindern, dass ich auch davon esse?

»Nun, den guten Auflauf muss ich wohl entsorgen.«, sagt Elli enttäuscht, wobei sie übertrieben die Mundwinkel nach unten zieht.

»Oder hast du noch besondere Bekannte, die du zum Essen einladen möchtest?«, fragt sie mich, während sie mir mit dem Ellbogen neckend die Seite knufft.

Ich ziehe die Augenbrauen nach oben und schüttele nur den Kopf, woraufhin sie lachend in der Küche verschwindet und ihre Schandtat beseitigt.

Die Sprache der Blumen, mein Engel, ist eine weltbekannte.

Eine wahrlich erotische Vorstellung, die Geschlechtsorgane der Natur zu verschenken. Eines Tages werde ich dich in weißen Lilien betten. Die Blume des Todes. Deine Unschuld werde ich nehmen und sicher verwahren, mein Engel, sodass du niemandem rote Rosen schenkst, außer mir.

Die Geister, die ich rief

Es ist Samstagabend.

Die Woche verging wahnsinnig schnell seit meinem Gespräch mit Alexander Griffin. Ich sehe noch immer seinen bedrohlichen Blick vor mir. Allein die Erinnerung an den Klang seiner Stimme jagt mir eiskalte Schauer über den Rücken.

Eine Generalvollmacht. Was hat er dann mit ihr vor? Elli hat diese Pflegeheim-Bemerkung ihm gegenüber gemacht. Doch soll ich glauben, dass er wirklich so hinterhältig ist? Dass er sie in ein Heim stecken würde und… was dann? Oder ist er in Wirklichkeit einfach sehr besorgt um sie? Schließlich ist sie verrückt genug, sein Essen mit Abführtropfen zu versetzen und wer weiß, was sie mit der letzten Haushaltshilfe angestellt hat?

Ich muss Andrew und Olivia unbedingt fragen, was sie noch über den Vorfall wissen. Elli hat den Geist ihres Mannes selbst an meinem ersten Tag erwähnt. Glaubt sie daran oder ist das ihre Art, ungebetene Gäste loszuwerden? Will sie mich vielleicht überhaupt nicht hier haben?

Diese ganze Aufregung um mich herum und das Chaos in mir wecken die Sehnsucht nach der einen Person, die immer an meiner Seite war. Es ist eh schon viel zu lange her, dass wir miteinander gesprochen haben, also schnappe ich mir mein Handy und durchsuche meine Kontakte nach der Nummer meiner besten Freundin Rachel.

Ein Blick aus dem Fenster verrät mir, dass der Himmel sternenklar ist, weshalb ich beschließe, das Telefonat nach draußen zu verlegen. Da kommt mir allerdings ein Gedanke, der mich auf halbem Weg umkehren lässt.

Ob Callum wohl schon weg ist?

Ich lösche das Licht in der Küche, um mein Spiegelbild im Fenster verschwinden zu lassen. Ein prüfender Blick in den Garten. Kein Licht, ein aufgerollter Gartenschlauch und niemand, der sich bewegt. Wunderbar, also ab nach draußen!

Auch als ich um die Hausecke in den Garten spähe, kann ich keine Anzeichen von Callum entdecken. Was sollte er um diese Uhrzeit auch noch hier wollen? Also hüpfe ich wieder über die Steinfliesen bis hin zu der

Holzbank, die gegenüber vom Gartenteich an der Hauswand steht. Direkt neben dem Beet mit den gelben Nelken.

Die Sterne funkeln und kühle Spätsommerluft weht um mich herum. Die Stille wird nur von gelegentlichem Plätschern eines auftauchenden Fisches durchbrochen.

Ich genieße noch eine Weile den Frieden dieses Augenblickes, dann drücke ich auf den grünen Hörer.

Es klingelt. Einmal, zweim…

»Juicy!«, meldet Rachel sich mit freudiger, fast piepsender Stimme.

Meinen alten Spitznamen zu hören fühlt sich an, wie nach einem langen Tag endlich nach Hause zu kommen.

»Hi Rachel.«, antworte ich.

Sie bombardiert mich geradezu mit Fragen. Wie es mir gefällt, ob ich Freunde gefunden habe und wie die Arbeit läuft. Ihre Euphorie hebt meine Laune augenblicklich und so erzähle ich ihr von Elli und wie ich sie beim Abstauben kennengelernt habe.

»Suaheli? Abgefahren!«, bemerkt Rachel lachend.

»Nicht witzig! Ich habe mich zu Tode erschreckt, als ich sie schreien gehört habe!«, tadle ich meine Freundin, was einen erneuten Lachanfall ihrerseits auslöst.

Ich kann sie quasi vor mir sehen, wie sie mit ihren schwarz-weißen Dreadlocks im Schneidersitz auf dem Bett sitzt und sich den Bauch haltend hin und her wippt.

»Klingt nach einer außergewöhnlichen Frau, diese Eleonore.«

»Ist sie. Und das ist gerade einmal die Spitze des Eisbergs.«, bestätige ich ihre Vermutung und berichte ihr von dem Vorfall mit dem Abführmittel, was sie mit einem lauten »Oha!«, kommentiert.

Über meine Begegnung mit Alexander Griffin erzähle ich ihr nur die Hälfte. Ich werde dem was er von mir verlangt sowieso nicht nachkommen, also muss ich auch nicht darüber sprechen.

Das Treffen mit Liv und Andy in der Kuchenstube hingegen beschreibe ich ihr bis ins kleinste Detail.

»Also werde ich jetzt ersetzt?«, haucht sie dramatisch und mit gespieltem Schluchzen in den Hörer.

»Wer könnte dich je ersetzen? Du bist einmalig.«

»Sag mir etwas, das ich noch nicht weiß. Und dieser Andrew, ist er heiß?«

»Rachel!«

»Also ja?«

»Er ist ganz süß, ja. Aber…«

»Oh mein Gott, es gibt ein Aber! Wie heißt er?«

Sie kennt mich einfach zu gut.

»Nein, es ist nur, ach, es ist blöd. Vergiss es.«, verwerfe ich den Gedanken ihr von Callum zu erzählen, während mein Blick erneut auf die Nelken fällt.

»Na dieses Nichts scheint dich doch sehr zu beschäftigen. Komm schon, rede es dir von der Seele!«, drängt sie weiter.

»Ach, da ist dieser Mann…«

Ein entzückter Laut am anderen Ende der Leitung unterbricht mich.

»Es ist nicht so einfach, Rachel!«

»Ach, das ist es mit den Männern doch nie!«, ruft Rachel aus, was mir ein zustimmendes Schnauben entlockt.

»Ich glaube ich habe es einfach falsch gedeutet. Für mich war es, als suchte er meine Nähe und ich habe das genossen. Dann wiederum lässt er mich plötzlich eiskalt fallen. Und gerade als diese Wunde zu heilen beginnt, macht er wieder diese zweideutigen Anspielungen. Ich verstehe es einfach nicht und ich will das so auch nicht.«, gebe ich ihr die Kurzfassung.

»Heilige Scheiße.«

»Ich sage ja, es ist nicht so einfach.«

»Oh, ganz im Gegenteil, Juicy, es ist sehr einfach. Dieser Typ scheint selbst nicht zu wissen, was er will und er zieht dich in seine Scheiße mit rein. Wenn du ihn das nächste Mal siehst, läufst du am besten so schnell weg, wie du kannst.«

Mein Blick wandert wieder einmal zu den gelben Nelken, die im Mondschein ihre Farbe verloren zu haben scheinen.

»Warum gerate ich nur immer wieder an die Psychos?«, frage ich mehr mich selbst.

»Wir sind doch alle Psychos. Die Kunst liegt darin jemanden zu finden, der das gleiche Rad ab hat, wie du. Mach dir keinen Kopf. Männer kommen und gehen, wie die Jahreszeiten. Aber nach einem besonders kalten Winter kommt immer auch ein sehr heißer Sommer.«

»Wo hast du das denn gelesen?«, pruste ich ihr entgegen, woraufhin sie mit einstimmt.

Es ist seltsam, ihr diese Zusammenfassung der letzten Woche zu geben, wo sie doch über Jahre hinweg ein Teil meines Alltags war.

Doch egal wie lange wir nicht miteinander gesprochen haben, es fühlt sich immer wieder an, als wären wir nie getrennt gewesen.

Jetzt geht es mir wieder besser.

Zum Teufel mit Callum. Die Sache mit dem Davonlaufen überlege ich mir aber noch einmal.

Wir reden noch eine Weile, sie erzählt mir, dass sie neulich ihre Eltern besucht hat. Die Erkenntnis, dass ich meine beste Freundin um ein Haar verpasst habe, bricht mir das Herz. Der neueste Tratsch aus meiner Heimat lässt mich jedoch schmunzeln. Nico hat tatsächlich seine Tochter Nadja eingestellt, welche den Laden in ein ziemliches Chaos zu stürzen scheint. Genauso, wie Nico es befürchtet hatte.

Als wir auflegen, sitze ich noch einen Moment in der Stille.

Ich will nicht, dass mein Herz ein solches Drama um diesen Gärtner macht. Doch ich muss ehrlich zu mir selbst sein. Akzeptanz ist der erste Schritt zur Besserung.

»Ich habe mich in dich verliebt, du blöder Idiot!«, sage ich in die Dunkelheit, woraufhin ich ein Knacken aus dem Gebüsch höre.

Abrupt richte ich mich auf.

»Hallo?«, frage ich ängstlich.

Ein Massenmörder würde jetzt wohl kaum antworten,

also höre ich noch einmal genau hin, die Augen zu Schlitzen verengt. Nichts.

Ich stehe auf. Auf einmal wirkt jeder Baum, jeder Schatten bedrohlich. Langsam taste ich mich den Steinweg entlang Richtung Haustür, den Blick suchend auf die Büsche gerichtet.

Ein lautes Rascheln lässt mich erschrocken quieken und gibt mir den Startschuss für einen Sprint. Das Handy fest umklammert renne ich über die Steine, wobei ich versuche weder zu stolpern, noch auszurutschen. Ich muss mich an der Hauswand festhalten, um in der Kurve nicht in den Rosen zu landen. Als die Tür hinter mir ins Schloss fällt atme ich auf und versuche meinen Herzschlag wieder zu beruhigen.

Ich alter Angsthase.

*

»Deliah!«, reißt mich eine aufgekratzte Elli Sonntagmorgen aus dem Schlaf. Ich nehme die Welt noch verschwommen wahr, als ich zu meiner Uhr blinzele. Fünf Uhr morgens.

»Kindchen, wach auf!«

Elli rüttelt an mir, da erwache ich plötzlich aus meiner Schlaftrunkenheit und erinnere mich, wo ich bin.

»Was ist los? Geht es dir gut?«

»Es ist weg!«

»Was ist weg?«

»Das Geld ist weg!«

Okay, ich komme nicht mehr mit. Hat sie schlecht geträumt?

»Welches Geld, Elli?«, frage ich ruhig, während ich mir die Augen reibe, um den Schlaf endgültig abzuschütteln.

»Na das auf dem Esstisch, Kindchen. Du weißt doch, das für Hildes Geburtstag.«, erklärt sie verzweifelt.

Da erinnere ich mich wieder. Elli hatte gestern Abend ein wenig Bargeld auf den Tisch gelegt, welches sie für das Geburtstagsgeschenk ihrer Freundin Mathilde ausgeben wollte.

»Hast du es vielleicht verlegt?«, frage ich, während ich mich aus der Bettdecke befreie und mich anziehe.

Elli sieht mich empört an.

»Kindchen, diese Hirnwindungen mögen alt sein, aber sie sind noch sehr gut in Schuss. Ich weiß, wo ich meine Sachen hinlege.«

»Das hat doch nichts mit dem Alter zu tun. Jeder verlegt einmal etwas.«

»Ich nicht!«

Ich atme tief durch, dann mache ich mich auf den Weg nach unten, eine nervöse alte Frau hinter mir her tippelnd.

Unten angekommen stelle ich fest, dass das Geld tatsächlich fehlt.

»Es ist weg.«, äußere ich meine Entdeckung.

»Ach, dachtest du etwa, meine Augen sind so schlecht, dass ich es übersehen habe?«

»Irgendwo muss es ja sein.«, übergehe ich ihre Stichelei.

»Denkst du es könnte Theodor gewesen sein?«, fragt Elli mich kleinlaut.

Ihr Blick ist starr auf den Tisch gerichtet.

»Wozu sollte ein Geist denn Geld brauchen?«

Keine Ahnung, ob sie das wirklich glaubt oder ob sie es einfach glauben will. Ich vermute Letzteres, deshalb spiele ich ihr Spiel mit.

Ein Seufzen entweicht ihr.

»Wahrscheinlich habe ich es wirklich verlegt. Verzeih, dass ich dich geweckt habe, Kindchen.«

»Schon gut. Aber, was wolltest du denn um diese

Uhrzeit hier unten?«

Verlegen beginnt Elli an ihrem Morgenmantel herumzufummeln. Ich folge ihrem Blick, der zur Küchentheke wandert, auf welcher sich ein geöffnetes Glas Apfelmus und daneben ein angebissenes Zimtplätzchen befinden.

*

Es ist Montag. Ich konnte Elli dazu überreden, einen Haushaltsplan zu erstellen, in dem sie feste Aufgaben an mich abgibt. Ihre Begeisterung hielt sich zwar in Grenzen, doch sie hat eingesehen, dass ich ihr tatsächlich helfen möchte und nach der Sache mit dem verschwundenen Geld war auch sie der Meinung, dass sie eventuell ein wenig Ruhe bräuchte.

Also gehe ich meiner hart erkämpften Pflicht nach, während Elli in die Stadt gefahren ist.

Im Haus ist es totenstill und auch Callum ist nirgends zu sehen. Der perfekte Moment, um ein wenig den sonnigen Tag zu genießen.

Das Vogelgezwitscher in den Bäumen hat etwas Meditatives. Wenigstens kann ich heute genau sehen, was um mich herum passiert und muss keine Angst vor Mördern in den Büschen haben. Ein Schmunzeln stiehlt sich auf meine Lippen, als ich an meine Flucht neulich Abend denke.

Sonnenstrahlen wärmen meine Haut, ich schließe die Augen und atme tief ein. Ich darf nicht zu lange trödeln, Elli wird bald zurück sein und ich bin heute für das Mittagessen verantwortlich. Eine Aufgabe, derer ich mich von Herzen gerne annehme.

Ein Kitzeln an meiner Hand holt mich zurück ins Hier und Jetzt. Neugierig hebe ich den Arm, um sie zu betrachten und erkenne einen Marienkäfer, der quer über meinen Handrücken krabbelt. Im Stillen zähle ich die Punkte und wünsche mir etwas. Zeig mir meinen Weg, kleiner Käfer.

Kurz darauf breitet er seine Flügel aus und fliegt davon. Ist das jetzt ein gutes oder ein schlechtes Zeichen?

»Deliah?«, ruft eine Frauenstimme hinter der Hecke, die der Straße am nächsten ist.

Ich erkenne sie.

»Liv?«

Da erscheint sie auch schon auf dem Weg.

»Was machst du denn hier?«, will ich wissen.

»Ich habe in der Nähe eine Bestellung abgeliefert und dachte, ich besuche dich.«, erklärt Liv.

Was für eine wundervolle Überraschung.

Anmutig wie eine Katze kommt Liv zu mir in den Garten. Das Grün ihrer Augen wird von dicken, schwarzen Linien umrandet. Die Haare hat sie wie bei unserer letzten Begegnung zu einem Zopf gebunden.

Als sie bei mir steht, begrüßen wir uns mit einer herzlichen Umarmung.

»Hier arbeitest du also.«, stellt Liv staunend fest, wobei sie den Blick über das Grundstück schweifen lässt.

Ich nicke.

»Bist du allein?«, will sie wissen.

»Elli ist bei einer Freundin. Kann ich dir etwas anbieten?«

»Lieb von dir, aber ich muss gleich wieder weiter.«, schlägt sie mein Angebot mit einem entschuldigenden Schulterzucken ab.

»Aber was hältst du davon, wenn du morgen Abend nach Ladenschluss im Café vorbeikommst? Andy ist auch da. Wir sperren die Tür ab und können uns in Ruhe richtig kennenlernen.«

Liv sieht mich aus großen Augen erwartungsvoll an.

Wir wollten uns sowieso einmal verabreden, also warum eigentlich nicht? Zumal Elli morgen auch nicht hier sein wird.

»Das klingt wunderbar!«, stimme ich also zu.

»Sehr schön. Dann...«, beginnt Liv, wird jedoch durch ein Poltern hinterm Haus unterbrochen.

»Ich dachte, du bist allein.«, richtet sie sich an mich.

»Das dachte ich auch. Ist bestimmt Callum.«

»Wer ist Callum?«, fragt Liv mit finsterer Miene.

»Der Gärtner.«, antworte ich knapp.

»Aha. Also, ich muss los. Bis morgen dann?«

Bei der Frage setzt sie ein breites Lächeln auf.

»Ja, bis morgen, Liv.«, bestätige ich ihre Einladung, dann verschwindet sie auch schon wieder so plötzlich, wie sie gekommen ist.

Ich warte nicht lange und beeile mich ebenfalls wieder nach drinnen zu kommen. Mein Bedürfnis, auf Callum zu treffen, ist nämlich gleich null.

Ein kurzer Schauer durchfährt mich, als ich die Auflaufform für das Mittagessen aus dem Schrank hole und die Erinnerung an den Shepherds Pie sich in mein Bewusstsein drängt. Ich schüttele mich, um den

Gedanken loszuwerden und beginne mit den Vorbereitungen.

Die Lasagne nach dem Geheimrezept des »A Tavola« ist meine leichteste Übung. Damals habe ich Nico so lange genervt, bis er mir endlich die berühmte geheime Soße beigebracht hat. Beim Gedanken an meinen alten Chef wird mir schwer ums Herz. Wer hätte gedacht, dass ich diesen Laden je so vermissen werde?

Ein Blick auf die Uhr verrät mir, dass Elli jeden Moment wieder hier auftauchen müsste. Ich sollte mich ranhalten.

Durch das gekippte Fenster kann ich das Geräusch einer Hacke hören, die sich durch das Unkraut im Blumenbeet zu arbeiten scheint. Also war das vorhin tatsächlich Callum.

Ein Vorteil des Putzplans ist, dass ich die ganze restliche letzte Woche in den hintersten Ecken des Hauses unterwegs war und meinem Herzensbrecher somit nicht über den Weg gelaufen bin. Das darf gerne noch eine Weile so bleiben.

Ich beginne die vorbereiteten Bestandteile der Lasagne zu schichten und schiebe sie anschließend in den Ofen.

Und während meine Gedanken so umherschwirren,

quält mich mein Gewissen, da ich die Sache mit der Generalvollmacht noch immer nicht angesprochen habe. Vielleicht weiß Elli sogar davon und hat Angst, dass ich dem Ganzen zustimmen könnte. Ein guter Grund, sie so schnell wie möglich zu beruhigen. Mal abgesehen davon, dass dieser Plan sowieso nicht funktionieren wird. Elli wird ihre Freiheit niemals kampflos aufgeben.

Gedankenverloren räume ich die Küche auf. Etwa zwanzig Minuten später meldet sich der Timer meines Handys und ich hole das Essen aus dem Ofen. Heißer Dampf wirbelt durch den Raum, es riecht nach Tomatensoße und Oregano. Genau wie an meinem letzten Arbeitstag in der Pizzeria.

»Das duftet köstlich, Kindchen.«, lobt Elli, als sie die Küche betritt.

Auch ich bin sehr stolz auf mein Werk. Kochen war schon immer eine große Leidenschaft von mir, der ich in Nicos Küche nach Feierabend gerne nachgehen durfte. Das waren die Momente, in denen ich den Stress des Arbeitstages vergessen konnte. Oh, wie sehr es mir gefehlt hat, den Kochlöffel zu schwingen!

Langsam, fast schon wie eine Katze schleichend, nähert Elli sich der Theke, wo die Lasagne dampfend abkühlt. Leise schmatzend dreht sie sich zu mir.

»Ich habe einen Gast zum Essen eingeladen. Ich hoffe, das ist in Ordnung für dich, Kindchen.«, fragt Elli.

Allein, dass sie mir diese Frage stellt lässt mich verwirrt die Stirn runzeln.

»Es ist dein Haus, Elli. Du darfst einladen wen immer du möchtest.«, erinnere ich sie.

Ich hoffe nur es ist ein freundlicher Gast! Vielleicht ihre beste Freundin Hilde, von der sie mir hin und wieder berichtet. Sie scheint ein sehr fröhlicher Mensch zu sein.

»Wunderbar.«, klatscht Elli in die Hände und verschwindet wieder.

Was hat sie nun wieder ausgeheckt? Zumindest scheint es jemand zu sein, über den sie sich freut. Wie schlimm kann es schon werden?

»Komm nur herein!«, höre ich ihre Stimme nebenan.

Der Besuch ist schon hier? Ich habe gar keine Klingel gehört. Hat dieser jemand etwa die ganze Zeit vor der Tür gewartet?

Ich trage die Auflaufform zum Esstisch, als Elli unseren Gast hereinführt und bleibe geschockt stehen.

»Sieh, wer uns heute Gesellschaft leisten wird, Kindchen. Ich dachte mir, dass Callum nach all der harten

Arbeit durchaus einmal eine kleine Pause verdient hat.«

Warum?

Das ist das Einzige, was mir gerade im Kopf herumschwirrt. Warum muss das heute sein? Was soll ich tun? Wie soll ich mich verhalten? Cool und reserviert? Offen und als wäre nichts gewesen?

»Hallo, Deliah.«, begrüßt Callum mich.

Ein Stich durchfährt mich und ich bringe nur ein Nicken zur Begrüßung zustande. Eine Mischung aus Scham und zerstörten Tagträumen ballt sich in meinem Magen zusammen. Vor meinem inneren Auge sehe ich rote Rosen und gelbe Nelken.

Mir ist der Appetit vergangen. Die Spannung zwischen uns ist schon fast spürbar und wird nur durch Elli unterbrochen, die ein Lied vor sich hin summt. Schweigend widme ich mich wieder dem Decken des Tisches und ignoriere die unausgesprochene Frage, die zwischen Callum und mir im Raum steht. Ich wende mich der Schublade hinter mir zu, während Elli unseren Gast drängt, sich an den Tisch zu setzen. Meine Hand greift nach dem Besteck. Für mich, für Elli und für… ihn. Kurz zögere ich über der dritten Gabel, doch dann atme ich durch und ergreife sie.

Mach es wie im Restaurant. Du musst die Gäste nur bedienen, du musst sie nicht mögen. Stures, sachliches abarbeiten.

Als jedoch der Platz gegenüber meinem an der Reihe ist, gedeckt zu werden, verlassen mich meine guten Vorsätze.

Auf keinen Fall möchte ich ihm zu nah kommen, aus Angst, er könnte mein Herz hören, das noch immer für ihn schlägt.

Ich kann nicht über meinen Schatten springen, ich will nicht. Also recke ich mich über den Tisch, um ihm sein Besteck an den Teller zu legen, doch ich bin zu kurz und komme nicht mal in die Nähe seines Tellers. Super.

»Warte, ich helfe dir.«, sagt Callum und streckt mir seinen Arm entgegen.

Da passiert es.

Seine Hand an meiner. Nur eine kurze, sanfte Berührung, doch es reicht aus, um mich erstarren zu lassen.

Das war Absicht! Er hätte mich nicht berühren müssen, er wäre ohne jede Anstrengung an seine dämliche Gabel gekommen! Er wollte es.

»Alles in Ordnung, Kindchen? Lass uns essen, bevor

es kalt wird!«, fordert Elli, da bemerke ich, dass ich Callum noch immer anstarre.

Mit knallrotem Kopf setze ich mich. Diese Situation ist so dermaßen unangenehm. Ich möchte verschwinden und doch bleiben. Möchte in seiner Nähe bleiben. Alles an ihm verzaubert mich. Sein Lächeln, sein Geruch, der Klang seiner Stimme. Nie fühlte ich mich mehr zu einem Menschen hingezogen. Ich möchte ihm sagen, dass ich mehr über ihn erfahren möchte, dass ich es genieße bei ihm zu sein. Doch die Angst vor erneuter Ablehnung und die Vermutung, dass er sich über mich lustig macht, lässt mich schweigen und ich schlinge nur stumm die heiße Lasagne hinunter.

Warum nur bin ich diesem Idioten, der nicht weiß, was er will, so verfallen? Vielleicht sollte ich Rachels Rat folgen und einfach davonlaufen. Ich war mir so sicher, dass ich ihm widerstehen könnte, doch diese kleine Berührung ließ meine Mauer bröckeln. Verdammt!

Es ist totenstill am Tisch. Das ist überhaupt nicht meine Art, doch das Wort an Callum zu richten, wage ich nicht. Er hingegen, das sehe ich im Augenwinkel, sieht mich die ganze Zeit über an. Betrachtet mich wie ein Kunstwerk in einem Museum. Als würde er mich erforschen. Diese Sehnsucht in seinem Blick, als würde er mich bewundern. Lächerlich.

Nach einer gefühlten Ewigkeit ist es Ellis Räuspern, welches die Stille vertreibt.

»Nun, das war nicht gerade das, was ich ein *fröhliches Beisammensein* nenne. Lasst uns doch bei einer Tasse Tee und Zimtplätzchen etwas plaudern.«, schlägt sie vor.

»Ich muss noch die Wäsche fertigmachen.«, verkünde ich, springe auf, räume meinen Teller weg und verlasse ohne ein Wort die Küche.

Das hat bestimmt überhaupt nicht kindisch oder seltsam gewirkt. Herrje.

*

»Was war das, Kindchen?«, fragt Elli mich, als sie etwa eine halbe Stunde später zu mir in die Waschküche kommt.

»Was war was?«, stelle ich mich unwissend.

Bitte sprich mich nicht darauf an, Elli!

»Können wir uns darauf einigen, dass du nicht versuchst mich für dumm zu verkaufen? Die Luft da beim Essen eben war dicker als ein afrikanischer

Buschelefant!«, rügt sie mich.

»Ich möchte nicht darüber sprechen.«, antworte ich, während ich die Wäsche in den Trockner stopfe.

»Was auch immer es war, du verletzt den Jungen damit, Kindchen.«

Wie bitte? Ich verletze ihn? Das soll wohl ein Witz sein! Diese Frau ist wahrlich verrückt.

»Es ist deutlich zu erkennen«, fährt Elli fort, »dass er deine Nähe sucht und du kränkst ihn mit einer Kälte die ich so nicht von dir kenne.«

»Hör auf! Er will meine Nähe nicht! *Er* weist mich einsilbig ab, warum also muss *ich* mich erklären?«, entgegne ich ihr lauter, als ich es wollte.

Jetzt steigen mir auch noch Tränen in die Augen. Klasse.

Sie kennt diese Kälte nicht von mir? Na, weil sie mich überhaupt nicht kennt!

»Du musst dich nicht erklären, Kindchen. Ich kenne diesen Jungen schon sehr lange und ich weiß, dass er nicht leicht zu durchschauen ist. Ich möchte dir nur den Rat geben, genau hinzuhören, bevor du vorschnell urteilst, denn für mich war es sehr eindeutig. Und vielleicht ist das für ihn genauso verwirrend wie für dich.«, sagt sie und lässt mich mit diesen Worten zurück.

Genau hinhören. Was will sie nur immer damit? Oh, da fällt mir ein...

»Elli!«, rufe ich, während ich ihr nacheile.

Sie ist schon oben an der Treppe, als ich sie erreiche. Ist sie gerannt?

»Hast du etwas vergessen, Kindchen?«, wendet sie sich mir zu.

Ich weiß nicht, wie ich beginnen soll, also erzähle ich ihr einfach die schonungslose Wahrheit über mein Gespräch mit Alexander Griffin.

»Und du stimmst seinem Plan zu?«

Ihr Blick verfinstert sich, als sie mir diese Frage stellt.

»Nein! Natürlich nicht! Sonst hätte ich es wohl kaum erzählt.«

Elli sieht an mir vorbei nach unten in die Dunkelheit, dann sagt sie: »Na, das freut mich zu hören. Mich glauben lassen, ich sei verrückt... was für ein durchtriebener Bengel er doch ist.«

Also ich hätte ganz andere Bezeichnungen für diesen Mann!

»Aber dieser Plan ist doch total bescheuert. Man kann doch niemandem einreden, dass er verrückt ist!«

»Oh, täusche dich nicht, Kindchen. Wenn du etwas nur oft genug hörst, glaubst du es auch irgendwann. Sieh doch nur all die unglücklichen Menschen, denen immer wieder gesagt wurde, sie seien nicht gut genug oder sie könnten etwas nicht.«

Da ist etwas dran.

»Ich würde so etwas nie tun.«, versichere ich ihr.

»Und ich danke dir dafür, Kindchen. Nicht alle sind so ehrenhaft wie du.«, antwortet Elli, wobei ihr Blick auf der Dunkelheit hinter mir haftet.

Ein eiskalter Schauer läuft mir über den Rücken. Ich drehe mich um und sehe… nichts.

Verwirrt wende ich mich wieder Elli zu, doch die ist verschwunden. Nur ihre immer leiser werdenden Schritte sind zu hören. Obwohl niemand hier ist, fühle ich mich, als würde ich von allen Seiten aus beobachtet.

Also war ich nicht die Erste, die Alexander zu seiner Komplizin machen wollte? War es bei meiner Vorgängerin etwa genauso? Elli hat damals bereits geahnt, dass ihr Neffe einen Plan verfolgt. Was hat sie getan, dass diese Frau die Flucht ergriffen hat? Ich muss unbedingt mit Andrew und Olivia sprechen, um mehr darüber herauszufinden.

Ich sehe mich noch einmal um, da ich das Gefühl, beobachtet zu werden, einfach nicht loswerde. Doch als ich erneut nichts Verdächtiges erkennen kann, widme ich mich wieder der Hausarbeit.

*

Die Nacht ist sehr unruhig. Wilde Träume von Rosen, gelben Nelken und Geistern reißen mich immer wieder aus dem Schlaf. Mein Herz rast noch immer, als ich die Augen wieder schließe und erneut in einen Traum wegdämmere.

Ich sehe mein Zimmer von meinem Bett aus, wo eine große, von der Nacht geschwärzte Person direkt über mir steht. Der Schatten betrachtet mich. Ich versuche zu erkennen, wer es ist, doch es ist zu dunkel. Der Mond wird von dicken Wolken verdeckt, es ist stockfinster. Auf einmal richtet sich der gebeugte Schatten auf, als hätte ihn etwas erschreckt.

Ein Hund bellt draußen, ich sehe zum Fenster und da erkenne ich plötzlich, dass ich nicht träume.

Ich schreie, reiße die Augen auf, doch kann nur noch erkennen, wie die Gestalt aus meinem Zimmer heraus um die Ecke verschwindet.

Oh Gott, oh Gott, oh Gott, da ist jemand im Haus! Wie gelähmt umklammere ich meine Bettdecke. Mit einem Schlag bin ich hellwach. Was soll ich nur tun? Ich bleibe einfach hier und verstecke mich. Nein! Elli! Ich bin für sie verantwortlich, hinterhältiger Neffe hin oder her.

Meinen ganzen Mut zusammennehmend schleiche ich aus dem Zimmer. Meine Knie fühlen sich an wie Pudding, als ich die kühle Wölbung des Lichtschalters erreiche. Nach und nach knipse ich die Lichter im Flur und den restlichen Zimmern an.

Ich lausche angestrengt. Alles ruhig. Niemand ist hier.

Am Treppengeländer lehnt ein Besen, mit dem ich mich vorsichtshalber bewaffne. Danach gehe ich langsam die Stufen hinunter, die hin und wieder unter meinem Gewicht knarzen. Jedes Geräusch lässt mich zusammenzucken. Mein Kiefer schmerzt, da ich die Zähne unter Anspannung so fest zusammenbeiße.

Unten angekommen laufe ich Raum für Raum ab. Als das ganze Haus schließlich leuchtet wie ein Weihnachtsbaum, beende ich meine Suche. Der Keller ist von oben verschlossen, ebenso sämtliche Türen, die nach draußen führen. Hier ist absolut niemand. War es doch nur das Trugbild eines Traumes? Oder habe ich etwa gerade den berühmten Geist von Theodor Griffin gesehen?

Ich brauche dich, mein Engel!

Ich bin mir jetzt ganz sicher! Du bist es! Deine Stimme im nächtlichen Garten wie das Lied der Nachtigall.

Wenn du doch nur zu mir sprächest, du heiliges Geschöpf! Erlöse mich von meinem Leid, berühre mich und werde eins mit mir!

Neues und Altes

Dieser seltsame Vorfall von letzter Nacht steckt mir noch immer in den Knochen, als ich mich auf den Weg in die Kuchenstube mache. Ich habe die ganze Nacht kein Auge mehr zugetan, doch keine Spur von einem Eindringling.

Aber es war so real! Ich hätte schwören können, dass mich jemand angestarrt hat. Vielleicht war es jedoch nur ein sehr realistischer Traum.

Warmer Sommerwind lässt meinen hellblauen Rock tanzen, die Sonne strahlt am Himmel.

»Bist du fertig, Kindchen?«

Ich nicke und eile zu dem grauen Mercedes.

Heute ist die Geburtstagsfeier von Ellis Freundin Mathilde, weshalb sie mich auf dem Weg dorthin in der Stadt absetzt.

Das verschwundene Geburtstagsgeld ist bis heute noch ein Mysterium. Wahrscheinlich finden wir es irgendwann in einem Glas Apfelmus.

Doch genug von seltsamen Vorfällen! Jetzt freue ich mich erst einmal auf eine entspannte Autofahrt.

*

»Da war ein Stoppschild!«, rufe ich entsetzt.

»Es war frei!«, kontert Elli gelassen und brettert geradeaus über die Pflastersteine eines angedeuteten Kreisverkehrs.

Diese Frau fährt wie ein Henker!

»Elli, würdest du bitte langsamer fahren?«

»Dafür habe ich keine Zeit! Außerdem kenne ich diese Straße, Kindchen. In all den Jahren ist hier noch nie etwas passiert, wenn ich gefahren bin.«

»Ja, weil sie sich alle vor dir verstecken!«

Daraufhin lacht Elli nur ihr Hexenlachen und gibt Gas.

Sie hat alles unter Kontrolle, das muss man ihr lassen. Das ist jedoch keine Entschuldigung dafür, derart auf die Regeln zu pfeifen.

Nervös umklammere ich den Blumenstrauß für Mathilde. Bunte Wiesenblumen aus Ellis Garten. Inmitten der Blüten steckt eine Geburtstagskarte mit dem Bild eines Apfels und der Aufschrift »Du bist immer noch knackig«.

Als ich weiter vorne endlich das Schild der Kuchenstube erkennen kann, fällt mir ein Stein vom Herzen.

Ich habe überlebt!

Erleichtert steige ich aus dem Auto.

»Fahr vorsichtig, Elli.«, rufe ich ihr durch die halb geöffnete Scheibe zu, was diese nur mit einem Lachen beantwortet, bevor sie mit quietschenden Reifen davonbraust.

»Deliah!«, begrüßt Andy mich freudestrahlend, als ich das Café betrete.

»Setz dich doch schon einmal, ich mache noch schnell die Kasse fertig. Möchtest du etwas trinken?«, fragt er mich.

»Kaffee. Bitte.«, antworte ich knapp.

Die türkisgepolsterten Bänke schmiegen sich angenehm an meinen Körper, als ich mich setze. Die letzten Gäste verlassen unter lauten Gesprächen das Café, da kommt Andy schon mit meinem Kaffee. Dankend nehme ich das dampfend heiße, wohlriechende Getränk entgegen.

»Kann ich dich sonst noch irgendwie glücklich machen?«, fragt Andy, seine Wangen röten sich leicht.

Ich schüttele nur den Kopf.

»Alles bestens, vielen Dank!«

»Da ist ja unser Ehrengast!«, ruft Liv, als sie aus der Küche tritt.

Liv schließt die Tür ab und die beiden holen sich ebenfalls etwas zu trinken, ehe sie mir an meinem Tisch Gesellschaft leisten.

»Also, neue Dorfschönheit, wie zum Teufel kommt man auf die Idee, für die alte Griffin zu arbeiten?«, will Liv wissen, die sich lässig auf den Stuhl lümmelt.

»Was habt ihr denn nur immer mit Elli?«, frage ich.

Hat ihr Neffe etwa in der Stadt Gerüchte gestreut?

Andy und Liv sehen sich fragend an, dann klärt Andy mich auf.

»Ich will dir nicht zu nahetreten, Deliah, du scheinst die Griffin, ähm, ich meine Elli, zu mögen, aber…«

»Was der unbeholfene Trottel hier versucht zu sagen ist, dass die Alte verrückt ist!«, unterbricht Liv ihn, wobei sie wild mit den Armen fuchtelt.

»Sie behauptet ihr toter Mann würde durch das Haus spuken!«, erklärt sie.

»Liv!«, ermahnt Andy sie, dem die Situation sichtlich unangenehm ist.

»Was denn?«, empört diese sich,» Hast du etwa jemals diesen Geist gesehen?«, wendet sie sich nun an mich.

»Ich ... ähm ...«, stammele ich.

Ich möchte nicht unbedingt über meine eventuelle Begegnung von letzter Nacht sprechen, doch Andy versteht meine Zurückhaltung falsch und übernimmt das Wort.

»Natürlich hat sie das nicht, Liv! Verschrecke sie doch nicht so!«, fährt er seine Freundin an.

Ich nutze die Stille, die daraufhin entsteht, um selbst die Führung des Gespräches zu übernehmen.

»Die letzte Haushaltshilfe wurde immerhin von dem Geist verjagt. Irgendwas muss also dran sein, oder?«

»Das war sehr seltsam.«, beginnt Liv, »Sie war etwa zwei Monate hier. Es schien alles gut zu sein. Hat der Griffin alles abgenommen, nicht einmal einkaufen war sie mehr selbst. Ein Mann, scheinbar ihr Neffe, kam immer öfter zu Besuch. Anscheinend soll man sie mit ihm gesehen haben. Du weißt schon. Zusammen.«

Liv sieht mich vielsagend an.

»Oh!«, stoße ich aus, als ich begreife.

Ich möchte niemandem etwas unterstellen, aber ich zweifle sehr stark an guten Absichten hinter dieser Verbindung.

»Was ist passiert?«, frage ich neugierig nach.

»Sie ist durchgedreht. Eines Tages hat sie unter lautem Gezeter die Koffer gepackt und panisch das Haus verlassen. Es wird erzählt, sie hätte einen Geist gesehen. Keiner weiß, wo sie nach ihrem filmreifen Abgang gelandet ist.«, endet Liv mit ihrer Erzählung.

»Das ist wirklich merkwürdig.«, stelle ich fest.

Hat Elli ihr vielleicht einen bösen Streich gespielt? Sie scheint meiner Meinung nach vor nichts zurückzuschrecken. Wenn diese Frau tatsächlich alle Aufgaben an sich gerissen hat, könnte es sein, dass Elli sich eingesperrt gefühlt hat. War sie es, die letzte Nacht in meinem Zimmer stand? Will sie mich loswerden? Glaubt sie mir etwa nicht, dass ich auf ihrer Seite stehe?

»Wie dem auch sei!«, unterbricht Andy meine Gedanken, »Hüte dich vor der Alten, die ist nicht einmal halb so unschuldig, wie sie tut. Wahrscheinlich hat sie auch das Feuer…«

»Andrew!«, mischt Liv sich ein. »Wir wollten darüber

nicht mehr sprechen!«

»Du! Du wolltest darüber nicht mehr sprechen!«, entgegnet er scharf. »Ich bin gleich zurück«, fügt er an, dann verlässt er den Tisch Richtung Toiletten.

Was ist denn hier los? Habe ich was verpasst?

»Was hat er denn?«, frage ich nach.

»Ach er kann es einfach nicht gut sein lassen. Das Haus, es müsste ganz in deiner Nähe sein. Ein Feuer hat es zerstört. Andy versucht jeden davon zu überzeugen, dass die Griffin es gelegt hat. Aber das ist Blödsinn, sie war in jener Nacht überhaupt nicht hier.«, klärt Liv mich auf.

Dieses Feuer also.

»Warum hat er es denn so auf Elli abgesehen?«, will ich weiter wissen, doch Liv schnaubt nur und setzt ein schiefes Lächeln auf. Da kommt Andrew wieder zu uns zurück.

»Tut mir leid. Ich wollte nicht die Beherrschung verlieren. Diese Geschichte... ich werde einfach emotional, wenn es um diese Nacht geht.«, erklärt er sein Verhalten.

Ich würde zu gern mehr darüber erfahren, doch ich halte mich zurück.

Wir wechseln das Thema.

Liv erzählt mir, dass die »Kuchenstube« ihren Eltern gehört, die gerade verreist sind. Andrew ist der Sohn der besten Freundin von Livs Mutter. Er beginnt nächstes Jahr sein Raumfahrttechnikstudium und sollte bis dahin einen Job annehmen, da seine Mutter sonst seine Spielkonsole verkauft hätte.

Sie sind beide unheimlich nette Menschen, die sich wie Geschwister zanken. Ich kann mir gut vorstellen, dass wir Freunde werden. Seit meine beste Freundin Rachel für ihr Studium weggezogen ist, fühle ich mich sehr allein. Auch wenn wir ab und zu Kontakt haben, hat sich eben alles stark verändert.

Entspannt lasse ich den Blick durch den Raum schweifen und stelle erschrocken fest, dass es bereits beginnt, dunkel zu werden.

»Ohje!«, rufe ich aus und unterbreche damit Andy bei einer lustigen Geschichte.

»Was ist?«

Verwirrt sehen die beiden mich an.

»Elli wollte mich schon vor…«, ich sehe auf die Uhr, »zwei Stunden hier abholen.«, stelle ich beunruhigt fest.

Okay, keine Panik. Wenn etwas passiert wäre, hätte

man mich benachrichtigt. Ich stehe bei ihren Notfallkontakten. Das heißt, sie hat mich einfach vergessen!

»Ich kann dich mitnehmen. Ich weiß ja, wo du wohnst.«, bietet Andy mit einem breiten Lächeln an.

»Das wäre großartig!«, bedanke ich mich bei ihm.

»Super, ich mache dir schon einmal den Sitz frei.«

Andy springt auf und hastet nach draußen.

Liv und ich spülen noch unsere Tassen, bevor ich gehe.

»Andy ist einfach zu gut für diese Welt.«, bemerkt Liv.

»Er ist wirklich sehr nett. Ihr beide seid sehr nett.«, antworte ich.

Liv zieht einen Mundwinkel zu einem schiefen Lächeln nach oben.

»Eine Schande, dass sein Herz derart gebrochen wurde.«, sagt Liv mehr zu sich selbst.

Ich will fragen, was sie damit meint, doch eine Hupe beendet unser Gespräch.

*

Kurze Zeit später sitze ich in Andys Auto.

Es ist eine ruhige Fahrt, doch nicht unangenehm ruhig.

Außerdem fährt er sehr entspannt, was ich nach meiner aufregenden Herfahrt sehr begrüße.

»Das ist wirklich nett von dir.«, unterbreche ich die Stille.

»Ach, keine große Sache. Es liegt auf meinem Weg und ist ja auch nicht weit.«, tut er meinen Dank mit einer wegwerfenden Handbewegung ab.

»Außerdem«, fährt er fort, »könnten wir das doch wiederholen.«

»Die Heimfahrt?«, entgegne ich lachend.

»Die auch, aber ich meine das Treffen. Nur ohne Liv.«, beantwortet er meine Frage und ich stocke.

»Ein Date?«

»Wenn du es so nennen möchtest.«, stimmt er mir vorsichtig zu.

Mir ist, als hätte sich ein Stein auf meine Brust gelegt. Möchte ich das? Ich kenne ihn doch kaum! Aber das ist ja auch der Sinn von einem Date. Sich kennenlernen. Ich bin mir unsicher, das kommt so plötzlich. Andy ist total nett, doch reicht es für mehr? Will ich überhaupt mehr? Letzte Woche noch habe ich mich derart gegen irgendwelche Gefühle gesträubt.

Zugegeben, derartige Gefühle habe ich bei Andy nicht.

Doch das muss ja nichts Schlechtes sein. Wahrscheinlich ist diese Freundschaft, die ich Andrew gegenüber verspüre, genau das, was es braucht, um nicht verletzt zu werden. Wir sind Freunde. Wir mögen uns. Wir testen es einfach. Keiner wird verletzt.

»Also, du musst nicht, wenn du nicht möchtest.«, korrigiert Andy fast flüsternd seine Einladung.

»Doch! Sehr gern! Ich würde mich sehr freuen, wenn wir uns verabreden.«, antworte ich schnell.

Puh, gerade noch gerettet.

Andy scheint meine Antwort zu gefallen, denn er strahlt über das ganze Gesicht.

»Abgemacht! Dann hole ich dich am Wochenende ab und entführe dich an einen schönen Ort.«, schlägt er vor.

»Klingt super.«, nehme ich seine Einladung an.

Wir erreichen Ellis Haus. Ich bin noch ganz aufgewühlt, als ich aussteige.

»Also, bis dann.«, verabschiede ich mich ein wenig unbeholfen.

»Gute Nacht, Deliah.«

Andy startet den Motor, wendet sein Auto und fährt in die Richtung davon, aus der wir gekommen sind.

Aha. Meine Unterkunft liegt also auf seinem

Heimweg? Ist klar. Er ist wirklich zu gut für diese Welt.

Und mit seiner Einladung hat er meine Welt erschüttert. Ob positiv oder negativ kann ich noch nicht sagen, dafür lässt die Aufregung die Schmetterlinge in meinem Bauch noch zu sehr flattern.

»Schönen Abend gehabt?«, fragt Callum, der gerade um die Ecke neben der Haustür kommt.

Oh, bitte nicht er. Nicht jetzt.

»Was machst du denn noch hier?«, wundere ich mich.

Es ist bestimmt schon halb zwölf.

»Ich habe noch die Geräte sauber gemacht.«

»Aha«, antworte ich knapp, denn eigentlich interessiert es mich überhaupt nicht.

Schweigend setze ich meinen Weg fort, doch Callum läuft mir nach.

»Hey, Deliah. Ich weiß nicht, was ich sagen soll, aber wenn ich dich irgendwie verletzt habe, dann tut es mir wahnsinnig leid!«

»Hast du nicht.«, lüge ich.

Ich habe jetzt keine Nerven für diese Art von Gespräch.

»Bitte! Lass. Mich. Ausreden.«, fordert er und greift meine Schulter, um mich zum Stehen zu bringen.

Es ist, als müsste er jedes einzelne Wort erzwingen. So habe ich ihn noch nie erlebt. Er wirkt... verzweifelt? Gut, dann höre ich ihn eben an. Nichts, was er sagen könnte, würde mich davon abbringen ihn auf Abstand zu halten. Ich verschränke die Arme und nicke ihm auffordernd zu.

»Die Wahrheit ist«, beginnt er, »ich würde sehr gerne mit dir einen Kaffee trinken gehen. Ich gehe nur nicht gerne in die Stadt. Ich mag die Menschen hier nicht besonders und halte mich außerhalb. Ich wollte es dir ja erklären. Es war dumm von mir, dich so stehen zu lassen. Also, wenn du mir noch einmal verzeihen kannst, dass ich dir nicht annähernd die Erklärung gegeben habe, die du verdient hast, dann würde ich dich sehr gerne einmal einladen, um mein dämliches Verhalten zu entschuldigen.«

Das ist jetzt nicht sein Ernst, oder? Oh Elli! Sie hat mich bestimmt verraten. Meine Reaktion im Keller war so offensichtlich. Doch was, wenn er das jetzt nur wieder sagt, um mich dann erneut unter dem Deckmantel der Freundschaft fallen zu lassen? Nein, nein. Diesmal nicht, diesmal drehe ich den Spieß um. Leide!

»Tut mir leid, ich habe schon eine Verabredung.«, entgegne ich ihm cool, woraufhin er noch verzweifelter wird.

Meine Mauer beginnt zu bröckeln, als ich in seine traurigen Augen sehe. Wie sehr ich mir doch wünsche, dass ich ihm glauben könnte!

»Bitte, lass es mich wieder gut machen!«, fleht er.

Warum schlägt mein Herz schon wieder schneller? Hör auf damit, du dummes Organ! Ich wollte ihm keine Chance mehr geben, mich zu verletzen! Keine Macht mehr über mich!

»Gut, aber nur als Freunde.«, nehme ich sein Angebot an, noch bevor mein Kopf versteht, was mein Mund da gerade gesagt hat.

Höre ich mir eigentlich selbst zu? Ich will es zurücknehmen. Sein Spiel spielen und so etwas wie »obwohl, wenn ich es mir recht überlege«, sagen, doch Callums breites Lächeln und die zum Sieg geballten Fäuste machen mich sprachlos. Er scheint sich wahrhaftig zu freuen. Fein! Dann unternehmen wir eben etwas gemeinsam. Ich habe ja nie gesagt, wann. Und rein freundschaftlich, jawohl!

Ohne ein weiteres Wort nicke ich Callum zum Abschied zu und begebe mich Richtung Haustür.

Dieses dämliche Gefühl, Andy zu hintergehen, lässt

mich nicht los. Was ich ja irgendwie auch tue. Warum hat Callum nicht schon früher erklärt, was das an jenem Abend sollte? Ach ja, weil ich ihm aus dem Weg gegangen bin. Ich habe mich wie ein Feigling vor ihm versteckt.

Aber ich werde Andy jetzt nicht hängen lassen! Schließlich ist er derjenige, der von Anfang an ehrlich zu mir war. Und wer weiß, vielleicht entwickelt sich ja noch mehr zwischen uns. Er sieht gut aus, ist nett und wird einmal einen tollen Job haben. Ein absoluter Traummann.

Und doch lehne ich gerade mit dem Rücken innen an der Haustür und denke an einen anderen.

»Wer s da?«, lallt es aus dem Wohnzimmer.

Elli? Die hatte ich ja total vergessen! Toll Deliah, du machst deinen Job wirklich großartig!

Schnell begebe ich mich in das Zimmer links von mir. Was ich dort vorfinde, ist eine betrunkene, Zimtplätzchen mampfende Eleonore Griffin, die aus glasigen Augen zu mir hinüber schielt.

»Kindchn, wo wahsdu?«, will Elli wissen, als sie sich vom Sofa aufrichtet.

»Bist du betrunken Auto gefahren?«

Ich stemme die Hände in die Hüften, wie eine Mutter,

die ihr besoffenes Kind zusammenstaucht.

»Nee. Henri.«

Aha. Nun gut, ihr Auto stand nicht im Hof, weshalb ich daraus schließe, dass Henri, wer immer das sein mag, sie nach Hause gefahren hat.

»Komm schon du alte Schnapsnase, wir bringen dich ins Bett.«

Vorsichtig nehme ich ihr die Dose mit den Zimtplätzchen aus der Hand und bringe auch das Apfelmus in Sicherheit. Dann lege ich ihren Arm um meine Schulter und stütze sie. Schön vorsichtig, damit keine von uns beiden stolpert, torkeln wir gemeinsam zur Treppe.

Wir haben gerade den Flur erreicht, als ein Schlüssel in der Haustür gedreht wird und ein blonder Lockenkopf erscheint.

»Theodor?«, fragt Elli in seine Richtung.

»Nein, Elli. Das ist nur Callum.«, erkläre ich ihr schweren Herzens.

Dann wende ich mich an ihn.

»Du hast einen Schlüssel?«, spreche ich das Offensichtliche an, weil ich nicht weiß, was ich sagen soll.

Er arbeitet schon Jahre hier und Elli hat sonst

niemanden, natürlich hat er einen Schlüssel!

»Ja. Für Notfälle. Und nach ebendiesem hat es durch das Fenster eben ausgesehen, deshalb wollte ich euch helfen.«, erklärt er und kommt herein.

Stimmt. Draußen ist es dunkel, er muss uns vom Garten aus durch das Fenster gesehen haben.

»Gut, dann übernimm die andere Seite.«, weise ich ihn an und er tut, was ich sage.

Wenn es nur immer so leicht wäre!

»Du bis schon n Schnuckelchen, Jungchn.«, lallt Elli ihm entgegen.

Ich muss kichern.

»Wasn?«, empört sie sich, während wir gemeinsam die Treppe hoch wanken.

»Wenn du ihn nich nimms, nehm ich ihn.«, verkündet Elli mit breitem Grinsen und stolz erhobenem Kinn.

Ich stocke.

Wir müssen diese tickende Informationsbombe unbedingt ins Bett bringen, bevor sie noch etwas über meine Gefühle zu Callum ausplaudert. Wenn sie das nicht ohnehin schon getan hat. Das ist alles so dermaßen unangenehm und ich kann nicht einmal weglaufen. Gefesselt an eine betrunkene alte Frau neben dem Mann, der mich wahnsinnig macht. Super.

Heimlich schiele ich zu Callum hinüber, um seine Reaktion zu erkennen. Doch etwas stimmt nicht. Er wirkt so ernst. Irgendwie traurig. Ich hatte erwartet, er strahlt wieder sein Gewinnerlächeln und lacht mich innerlich aus oder macht mich wieder mit irgendeinem blöden Spruch verlegen. Aber nichts dergleichen geschieht.

Mit vereinten Kräften hieven wir Elli ins Bett, wo sie sofort weg döst. Wortlos verlassen wir das Zimmer.

»Theodor, bleib hier!«, ruft Elli Callum im Halbschlaf zu, dann dreht sie sich um und schläft weiter.

Es zerreißt mir das Herz.

Leise schließe ich die Tür hinter mir.

»Danke.«, richte ich mich flüsternd an Callum.

»Nicht dafür.«, winkt er ab und wendet sich zum Gehen.

»Sie bedeutet dir viel, oder?«, frage ich beim verzweifelten Versuch ihn aufzuhalten.

Ich will nicht, dass er schon geht. Vielleicht ist es naiv von mir, ihn bei mir haben zu wollen, aber es ist mir egal.

Callum bleibt am Treppenabsatz stehen.

»Sie ist... wie eine Mutter für mich.«, sagt er, ohne sich zu mir umzudrehen.

»Was hast du gegen die Leute hier? Warum willst du nichts mit ihnen zu tun haben?«, stelle ich die Frage, die mir schon seit seiner Einladung unter den Nägeln brennt.

Noch immer sieht Callum mich nicht an, sondern starrt stur die Treppe hinunter.

»Sie sind zu neugierig.«, murmelt er, dann nimmt er die erste Stufe und verschwindet.

Schon wieder. Er hat mich schon wieder einfach stehen lassen.

Ich bin wie versteinert. Zu neugierig? War das ein Wink für mich, weil ich mehr über ihn erfahren möchte? Ist es das, was ihn immer wieder so kalt mir gegenüber werden lässt?

Welches Geheimnis versteckst du, Callum?

Deine Stimme am Abend versüßt mir die Nacht, mein Engel. Ich muss dich nicht stehlen, du kommst freiwillig zu mir. Wie ein Reh, das sich vor das Gewehr des Jägers wirft. Sei meine Beute, mein Engel, ich werde ein Fest daraus machen, dich zu verzehren.

Ratschläge

Eine fast schon unheimliche Stille hat sich die letzten Tage über das Haus gelegt. Jeder ging seiner Arbeit nach, keine seltsamen Vorfälle mit Geistern oder Gärtnern. Keine ungebetenen Gäste, ja nicht einmal Ellis Suaheli Gesang. Diese hatte übrigens einen drei Tage andauernden Kater, mit dem sie sich im Schlafzimmer verkroch.

Ich hingegen habe mich damit abgefunden, dass ich mich wohl mit zwei Männern verabredet habe, obwohl mein Herz nur für einen schlägt. Wenn auch für den Falschen. Vielleicht muss ich mir nur genug Mühe geben, damit ich den Richtigen auf die gleiche Weise lieben kann.

Callum ist nicht gut für mich! Er ist so undurchsichtig. Ich weiß absolut nichts über ihn. Er ist so ein verdammter Idiot mit seinem dämlichen, strahlenden Lächeln!

Andy mag mich und ich mag ihn. Er könnte mir die Sicherheit geben, nach der ich mich so sehr in meinem

Leben sehne. Vielleicht ist es genau das, was mir all die Jahre gefehlt hat.

Als Victoria damals die Pizzeria mit ihrer Begleitung betrat, wirkte sie vielleicht nur deshalb so glückselig, weil sie jemanden hatte, der sie durchs Leben führte.

Mein Handy gibt ein leises *Bing* von sich und reißt mich somit aus meinen Gedanken. Eine Nachricht. Ich werfe mir den Putzlappen über die Schulter, mit dem ich gerade den Schrank von Staub befreit habe und lese.

Liv.

Hey du! Lebst du noch?

Herrje, Liv habe ich bei all dem Chaos ganz vergessen! Ich habe mich seit unserem Treffen nicht mehr gemeldet. Schnell tippe ich eine Antwort.

Hi! Tut mir leid, hatte viel zu tun. Natürlich lebe ich noch. Wie läuft es bei dir?

Prompt kommt eine Antwort.

Du hast dich mit Andy verabredet.

Wow. Das war... auf den Punkt. Ob es sie wohl stört? Schließlich sind sie seit Ewigkeiten befreundet. Was, wenn ich ihr Andy wegschnappe? Ich lehne mich an das Sofa, welches in dem zweiten Wohnzimmer im oberen Stock steht und beginne zu tippen.

Stört es dich?

Ich warte. Keine Antwort. Da erklingt plötzlich mein Klingelton. Olivia ruft mich an.

»Ja?«, melde ich mich.

»Damit das klar ist, mir ist völlig egal, mit wem der Typ sich trifft.«

Sie klingt dabei so kühl, dass ich fürchte, der Hörer könnte einfrieren.

»Aber?«, frage ich vorsichtig nach.

Irgendetwas scheint sie ja doch zu stören, wenn sie deshalb gleich anruft.

Ein lautes Knacken hinter mir lässt mich herumfahren, doch ich kann nichts erkennen. Dann folgt Stille, die jedoch sogleich von Livs Antwort durchbrochen wird.

»Meinst du es ernst mit ihm?«, fragt sie unverblümt.

Ich will antworten, doch es bleibt mir im Hals stecken. Ich wage es nicht auszusprechen, was ich fühle. Schon gar nicht vor Andys bester Freundin. Muss ich auch gar nicht, denn Liv deutet mein Schweigen.

»Deliah. Du darfst Andy nicht verletzen! Du darfst nicht mit ihm spielen!«, antwortet sie nun viel energischer.

»Ich spiele nicht mit ihm! Ich mag ihn!«, nun werde

auch ich forscher.

Freund hin oder her, das gibt ihr nicht das Recht so mit mir zu sprechen.

Da knackt es erneut hinter mir. Ich will gerade nachsehen, als Liv etwas erwidert.

»Bist du dir sicher, dass du ihn auf diese Weise magst?«

»Naja…«, antwortet mein Mund mal wieder schneller, als mein Kopf denken kann.

»Ich wusste es! Gibt es einen anderen?«, fragt Liv schon wieder gerade heraus.

»Wie kommst du denn darauf?«, will ich wissen.

Sie kennt Callum nicht, wie kann sie dennoch etwas ahnen?

»Kann doch sein, oder? Hör zu, ich möchte mich nicht mit dir streiten. Ich mag euch beide und unklare Gefühle haben schon so manche Freundschaft zerstört.«, erklärt sie.

Ihr Tonfall hat sich gänzlich geändert und ist nun fast ängstlich. Daher weht also der Wind.

»Mach dir keine Sorgen, Liv. Ich werde einen wunderschönen Abend voll glasklarer Gefühle mit Andy haben. Welcher Art auch immer diese sein mögen. Wenn wir am Ende doch nur Freunde bleiben, ist das doch auch gut.«

Meine Antwort ist ehrlicher, als ich es wollte. Zumindest Liv gegenüber.

»Aha. Also liebst du ihn nicht. Dann sag ihm das! Hör auf ihm Hoffnungen zu machen, wenn du für jemand anderen bestimmt bist!«, fordert sie.

Ich verstehe ihre Angst, dass ich Andy verletzen könnte. Doch ich werde mir nicht vorschreiben lassen, mit wem ich mich treffe!

»Ich…«

Da werde ich durch ein erneutes Poltern hinter mir unterbrochen, gefolgt von einem erstickten Schrei. Es kam eindeutig von unten. Aus dem Garten? Callum? Elli?

»Liv, ich muss los, wir hören uns und… mach dir keine Sorgen.«, beende ich unsere Diskussion noch bevor sie richtig angefangen hat, dann lege ich auf und sprinte nach draußen.

»Elli?«

Vor meinem inneren Auge sehe ich die alte Frau mit gebrochenen Beinen auf dem Boden liegen. Mein Job hier wäre erledigt, Alexander Griffin hätte seine Bestätigung, dass Elli nicht einmal mit Betreuung sicher in diesem

Haus ist und Elli würde in einem Heim landen.

Wie der Wind tragen meine Beine mich hinters Haus in die Richtung, aus der das Geräusch kam.

Dort versucht jedoch nicht Elli, sondern ein schmerzverzerrter Callum gerade auf die Beine zu kommen. Was zum Teufel? Ich eile zu ihm.

»Was ist denn passiert?«, frage ich mit noch immer hämmerndem Herzen, während ich ihn stütze.

Seine Hose ist vom Rasen grün gefärbt. Ich kann jedoch nichts erkennen, worüber er gestolpert sein könnte.

»Ist schon gut, vielen Dank.«, ächzt er, wobei er etwas beschämt wirkt.

Wird er etwa rot? Ungeschickt versucht er meinen Arm abzuschütteln.

»Was hast du denn gemacht?«, will ich wissen.

Ich lasse mich nicht abwimmeln. Diesmal nicht.

»Ich… ähm… da hing etwas im Baum und ich wollte es herunterholen. Hat nicht so gut geklappt.«, stammelt er.

Im Baum? Skeptisch richte ich den Blick auf das saftige, grüne Laub.

Ich kann nichts erkennen, folge den Ästen mit meinen Blicken bis zu… dem Fenster. Der Baum ist nicht hoch, doch hoch genug, um durch das gekippte Fenster zu sehen, hinter dessen Raum ich gerade eben noch geputzt habe. In welchem ich gerade noch mit Liv gesprochen habe. Kleinere Äste liegen am Boden, als wären sie abgebrochen. Das Knacken!

»Du hast gelauscht!«

Callum wirkt verlegen, antwortet nicht.

»Tatsächlich! Du hast mich belauscht!«, werfe ich ihm vor.

Was denkt er sich dabei? Sein Schweigen macht mich nur noch fassungsloser und in einem Impuls aus Frust, stoße ich ihn mit der Hand gegen die Brust. Callum ist größer und stärker, als ich, doch ich habe ihn so unvorbereitet getroffen, dass die Überraschung und sein unstabiler Stand ihn zu Fall bringen. Direkt in den Gartenteich.

Vor Schreck schlage ich die Hände vor den Mund und starre ihn mit weit aufgerissenen Augen an. Das wollte ich nicht! Prustend setzt Callum sich in dem, zum Glück nicht besonders tiefen, Teich auf. Wasser tropft seine Locken entlang.

»Naja, ich schätze, das habe ich verdient.«, sagt er mehr zu sich selbst.

Ich habe mich von dem Schock erholt und muss nun

über den völlig durchnässten Mann lachen.

»Haha.«, äfft er mich nach, lächelt jedoch dabei.

Ich strecke ihm die Hand entgegen.

»Komm schon, ich hole dich wieder raus. Genug gebadet.«

Callum reicht mir seinen Arm.

Doch gerade als ich ihn herausziehen möchte, spüre ich einen starken Gegenzug.

Danach geht alles ganz schnell. Ich verliere den Halt, sehe den Teich und einen breit grinsenden Callum immer näherkommen und lande im Wasser.

Schnell richte ich mich auf. Meine langen Haare hängen mir ins Gesicht, ich kann nichts sehen. Das Wasser ist kalt und ich schwöre ich habe einen Fisch an meiner Hand gespürt, der daraufhin in den tiefen Teil des Teichs geflohen ist. Hektisch versuche ich wieder freie Sicht zu bekommen, während meine Kleidung sich immer mehr vollsaugt, was mir kalte Schauer über den Rücken jagt.

Das Erste, was ich erkennen kann, ist Callum, der sich neben mir nicht mehr einzukriegen scheint vor Lachen.

»Du!«, rufe ich.

Ohne nachzudenken stürze ich mich auf ihn und

spritze ihm Wasser ins Gesicht.

Mein ganzer Frust der letzten Wochen entlädt sich in diesem Moment.

Callum hingegen hebt nur die Arme zum Schutz und lacht lauthals.

»Was ist denn daran so witzig?«, will ich atemlos wissen.

Er steht auf, kommt zu mir und hilft auch mir auf die Beine.

»Du bist einfach niedlich, wenn du dich aufregst.«, sagt er ganz ruhig, während er mir tief in die Augen sieht.

»Also machst du dich über mich lustig?«, erwidere ich gereizt.

»Das würde ich nie wagen. Du bist der einzige Mensch, der mir seit so langer Zeit ein Lächeln ins Gesicht und Wärme in mein Herz zaubert.«

Es ist um mich geschehen. Das waren die schönsten Worte, die je jemand an mich gerichtet hat. Ungeachtet meiner weichen Knie, stelle ich mich auf Zehenspitzen, schlinge die Arme um seinen Hals und küsse ihn.

Er legt seine Arme um meine Hüfte und erwidert meinen Kuss. Erst zaghaft, dann deutlich fordernder, als wäre die kleine Flamme der Sehnsucht zwischen uns zu einem lodernden Feuer herangewachsen. Plötzlich scheint die Welt sich schneller zu drehen und wir sind der Mittelpunkt. Das ist der schönste Augenblick meines Lebens!

Als hätte mir jemand ins Gesicht geschlagen, trifft mich die Erkenntnis. Ich stehe hier knutschend mit Callum im Gartenteich und bin mit Andy verabredet. Das ist absolut nicht in Ordnung!

Erschrocken löse ich mich von Callum. Seine friedlichen Gesichtszüge verhärten sich, als er mich ansieht.

»Was ist?«, fragt er besorgt.

»Das ist falsch! Was bin ich nur für eine…«, rüge ich mich, dann stapfe ich aus dem Wasser.

Callum hält meine Hand fest.

»Deliah! Was ist denn los?«, ich kann seine Verzweiflung nahezu spüren.

»Ich kann nicht.«, flüstere ich, dann verschwinde ich tropfnass ins Haus und lasse ihn und mein Herz zurück.

Ich schäle mich aus den nassen Klamotten. Wasser sammelt sich auf den Fliesen des Badezimmers. Tränen rinnen mir über die Wangen.

Was mache ich hier eigentlich? Ich wollte mein Leben in eine andere, eine bessere Richtung lenken und jetzt habe ich nichts Besseres zu tun, als eine Dreiecksbeziehung zu beginnen, die ich überhaupt nicht möchte! Ich sollte verschwinden. Irgendwo anders beginnen. Neustart.

»Was ist denn hier los, Kindchen?«, krächzt Elli, die mit großen Augen im Türrahmen steht, während sie ein Zimtplätzchen isst.

Ein verzweifeltes Schluchzen ist alles, was ich zustande bringe. Ich stehe hier in klatschnasser Unterwäsche weinend vor der Dame für deren Betreuung ich zuständig bin. Wie nutzlos kann man sich eigentlich fühlen?

Wortlos reicht Elli mir ein Handtuch, welches ich mir dankend umwickele.

»Schieß los, Kindchen. Ich höre dir zu.«, sagt sie, während wir uns auf den Rand der weißen Badewanne setzen.

Sie schiebt sich den Rest des Plätzchens in den Mund und kaut genüsslich, während sie geduldig meinen Worten lauscht.

»Ich bin fertig, Elli. Ich weiß nicht einmal mehr, was

ich hier mache. Ich wollte raus aus meinem Leben. Wollte einfach weg. Ich dachte, woanders würde ich einfach das finden, was ich suche. Habe das erste Angebot angenommen, das ich bekommen habe, ohne mir Gedanken darüber zu machen, was mich hier erwartet und wohin das führen sollte. Ich habe es versaut! Ich mache mein Leben kaputt!«, schluchze ich.

»Aber du lebst doch.«, stellt Elli verwirrt fest und schluckt.

Ich verstehe nicht, was sie damit sagen möchte und sehe sie nur fragend an.

»Du lebst.«, wiederholt sie, »Und solange du lebst, machst du doch alles richtig. Was hattest du denn geglaubt, was passiert, wenn du von zu Hause fortgehst? Dass du plötzlich den Sinn deines Lebens erkennst?«

»Naja…«, meine Stimme ist dünn und kratzig.

»Hör mal Kindchen, der Sinn des Lebens ist das Leben selbst. Sei du selbst, hör nicht auf das, was andere von dir erwarten und lebe einfach.«

Sie klingt wie ein gutmütiger Lebenscoach.

»Aber Elli, ich habe das Gefühl alle wissen genau, was sie wollen und ich habe keine Ahnung, was in zehn Jahren ist.«, erkläre ich niedergeschlagen.

»Na hör mal! Niemand weiß, was in zehn Jahren ist. Könnte man so weit in die Zukunft sehen, hätte man sicher so manchen schon bei der Taufe ertränkt.«

»Elli!«, rufe ich erschrocken aus.

Diese Behauptung ist ziemlich makaber, dennoch muss ich grinsen.

»Entschuldige. Was ich sagen möchte ist, als Theodor und ich den Autounfall hatten, da habe ich nicht innerlich meine Abschlüsse aufgezählt, oder an meinen Kontostand gedacht. Ich habe an ihn gedacht. Und an mich. An das, was wir erlebt haben. An Zeiten, in denen wir im Chaos lebten und lachten. Und bereut habe ich nur jede sinnlos verschwendete, schlaflose Nacht, in der ich mich über Kleinigkeiten aufgeregt und gesorgt habe, die so unwichtig waren, dass ich sie jetzt nicht einmal mehr weiß. Deliah, das Leben wird dir nicht einfach einen Plan vor die Füße werfen, dem du dann bis zu deinem Ableben folgen kannst. Das Leben bietet eine unendliche Zahl an Wegen und Abzweigungen. Du kannst natürlich geradeaus gehen, aber eben auch links, rechts, dich im Kreis drehen und sogar mehrmals wieder umkehren. Du weißt nie, wo du am Ende hingelangst. Nur eines ist gewiss: Solange du immer du selbst bist, kannst du dich nicht verlaufen. Denn du bist dein eigener Kompass.«

Ich bin sprachlos. Sie hat recht. Ich habe tatsächlich erwartet, dass ich hier ankomme und einfach weiß, wo ich hingehöre. Dass ich einer Anleitung folgen kann. Ich war so beschäftigt damit, den Sinn zu suchen, dass ich mich selbst verloren habe.

Ich bin hier und betreue eine alte Dame, dabei vermisse ich die Pizzeria so sehr. Ich vermisse das Kochen mit Nico. Ich vermisse sogar den gestressten Geschäftsmann, der jeden Tag seine Mittagspause bei uns verbracht hat. Ich war immer so genervt von ihm, dabei hat er wahrscheinlich einfach einen furchtbaren Job, wenn er stets so schlecht gelaunt ist. Ich wünschte, ich hätte ihn besser behandelt. Mehr versucht ihm ein Lächeln ins Gesicht zu zaubern. Ich hätte ich selbst sein und Nico darum bitten sollen, mich in die Küche zu holen, anstatt im Service zu arbeiten.

Ich hätte Andy ehrlich sagen sollen, dass ich kein Interesse habe, anstatt mich in dem Gedanken zu verlieren, dass ein netter Mann an meiner Seite schon einmal der Anfang eines guten Lebens ist.

Ich hätte Callum nach unserem Kuss nie wieder loslassen sollen!

Diese Erkenntnis lässt mich aufspringen.

»Danke, Elli.«, verabschiede ich mich schnell, dann eile ich in mein Zimmer und werfe mir ein leichtes, weißes Sommerkleid über.

Ich haste die Treppe hinunter, durch die Haustür und nach hinten in den Garten. Ich werde es ihm sagen! Werde ihm sagen, dass ich in ihn verliebt bin und dass ich an seiner Seite sein möchte.

»Callum?«, rufe ich mit pochendem Herzen.

Doch Callum ist weg.

Ich habe es nicht ausgehalten, habe versagt! Doch ich musste dich noch einmal sehen. Dein Fenster stand offen, es war schon fast zu leicht. Ich weiß, ich weiß, das letzte Mal endete es nicht gut.

Der falsche Engel. Bin fast erwischt worden, wegen ihrem Gekreische!

Das Gesicht nun für immer entstellt, aber was hätte ich tun sollen?

Halb so schlimm, ein neuer Engel wurde mir geschickt.

Vorsichtig, ganz vorsichtig näherte ich mich. Oh, wie lieblich du aussahst, als du schliefst. Wie lieblich dein Seufzen, als ich dich berührte. An den Armen, der Brust, zwischen deinen Beinen. Ich musste gehen, bevor die Lust mich überkam und ich mich nicht mehr zu bremsen vermochte. Langsam, ganz langsam mein Engel. Bald wirst du im Rausch der Lust meinen Namen hauchen.

Sommernachtstänze

Nun scheint Callum es zu sein, der mir aus dem Weg geht. Ich habe ihn die ganze Woche nicht einmal gesehen. Meine Laune ist im Keller.

Ausgerechnet heute ist auch noch das Date mit Andy.

Nein, ich habe es nicht abgesagt. Ich habe versucht, mir einzureden, dass ich einfach persönlich mit ihm sprechen möchte. Dass er heute Abend vielleicht sogar selbst merkt, dass wir nicht füreinander geschaffen sind.

In Wahrheit war es wohl eher mein altes Verhaltensmuster, das fürchtete, irgendjemand könnte es mir übelnehmen, wenn ich diesen netten Mann gehen ließe.

Jetzt stehe ich vor dem Spiegel und versuche mein gebrochenes Herz unter einer schimmernden Fassade zu verstecken. Ich trage meine Haare offen. Große Locken winden sich bis in meine Taille. Ein weißes, mit Spitze verziertes Oberteil wird durch einen lachsfarbenen, knielangen Rock ergänzt, der bei jeder Drehung weit aufschwingt. Ich liebe diesen Rock. Ich hatte ihn nur nie oft an, da er durch seine knallige Farbe sehr auffällig ist. Nicht so schlicht und still, wie Schwarz, sondern leuchtend und laut, als ob er rufen würde »Ich will tanzen!«.

Damit beginnen, ich selbst zu sein. Das hat Elli gesagt und das werde ich tun! So gut es mir eben gelingt.

Die Sonne nähert sich bereits dem Horizont, als Andy vor dem Haus parkt. Ein Lächeln stiehlt sich auf mein Gesicht. Ich freue mich ehrlich, ihn zu sehen.

Wir umarmen uns fest zur Begrüßung, dann öffnet Andy mir die Autotür und wir fahren los.

»Also, ähm, wie geht es dir?«, versuche ich das Schweigen zwischen uns zu brechen.

»Gut. Gut.«, antwortet Andy.

»Um ehrlich zu sein, ich freue mich schon seit Tagen auf dieses Treffen. Geht es dir auch so?«, will Andy wissen.

Wundervoll. Er hat sich auf heute gefreut. Er erwartet mehr von diesem Date, als ich. Ich hätte einfach vorher mit ihm sprechen sollen. Was habe ich mir dabei gedacht? Dass ich ihm beim Essen zwischen Hauptgang und Nachspeise verkünde, dass ich zwar dankbar für die

Einladung bin, aber dass wir bitte nur Freunde sein sollen? Wo war mein Gehirn, als ich diese Idee ausgetüftelt habe?

»Wo fahren wir denn hin?«, frage ich nach.

Irgendwie muss ich das Thema auf unsere Freundschaft lenken.

»Deliah, bitte. Das ist doch der Sinn von einer Überraschung.«, neckt er mich.

»Überraschungen von Freunden sind einfach immer so spannend.«, antworte ich und trete mir innerlich in den Hintern.

Überraschungen von Freunden? Deliah du Trottel. Doch zu meiner Erleichterung scheint Andy diese dämliche Formulierung überhört zu haben.

Wir parken vor einem edel aussehenden Restaurant. Außen rekeln sich weiße Statuen von leicht bekleideten Frauen und Männern um steinerne Säulen. Warmweißes Licht lässt die rund geschnittenen Büsche vor der Tür sanft leuchten. Ein roter Teppich führt in das Innere des Lokals.

»Ich hoffe, du magst griechisch.«, sagt Andy, als er mir die Tür öffnet.

Herrje, das hier sieht viel zu teuer aus für eine rein freundschaftliche Einladung. Wie komme ich hier nur unbeschadet wieder raus?

Gar nicht. Ich komme hier nicht heil raus.

Ein großer, schlaksiger Kellner mit schwarz gefärbten Haaren und müden Augen führt uns schnellen Schrittes an unseren Tisch.

Eine gemütliche kleine Ecke, ein Tisch mit zwei bequem aussehenden Stühlen und eine sacht vor sich hin flackernde Kerze. Das ist alles so romantisch. Mir schmerzt es in der Brust, dass Andy sich so viel Mühe gegeben hat und diese doch umsonst ist. Ich sollte gehen. Sollte es beenden, bevor alles nur noch schlimmer wird. Doch ein Blick in sein Gesicht und ich werde weich. Er sieht so überglücklich aus.

»Und? Was sagst du?«, fragt er mich deutlich nervös.

»Es ist nett.«, untertreibe ich völlig.

Andy sieht aus, als hätte ich ihm ins Gesicht geschlagen.

Toll gemacht, Deliah. Spuck ihm doch direkt auf den Tisch. Ich muss das Ruder wieder herumreißen, bevor er mich für immer hasst.

»Mir ist aufgefallen, dass ich eigentlich kaum etwas über dich weiß.«, versuche ich ein Gespräch zu beginnen, als ich mich setze.

Jeder redet doch am liebsten über sich selbst. Ich tue ihm den Gefallen und höre zu, dann kann ich mich schon nicht in die nächste dumme Aussage verstricken.

»Was willst du denn wissen?«, stellt Andy mir eine Gegenfrage.

Super, damit hatte ich natürlich nicht gerechnet. Ich will überhaupt nichts wissen. Nein, das ist nicht richtig. Ich möchte gerne etwas über ihn wissen. Alles, was man über seine Freunde eben weiß. Nicht diese Informationen mit denen man versucht den anderen zu beeindrucken.

»Hattest du schon einmal eine Beziehung?«, ist die erste Frage, die mir in den Kopf kommt und wieder habe ich schneller gesprochen, als nachgedacht.

Was soll er denn jetzt von mir und meinen Absichten denken, nachdem ich das gefragt habe?

Ich sehe ihn an und stelle fest, dass sein Gesicht sich verfinstert hat.

»Ist alles in Ordnung?«, hake ich vorsichtig nach.

Da scheine ich wohl einen wunden Punkt getroffen zu haben.

Er schüttelt den Kopf, wie um einen Gedanken loszuwerden.

»Schon gut, ich… spreche nicht so gern darüber.«,

erklärt er mir.

»Oh. Das tut mir leid. Ich wollte dich nicht traurig machen.«, entschuldige ich mich aufrichtig.

»Schon gut. Du kannst nichts dafür. Es ist einfach eine sehr unschöne Geschichte.«

Gerade als ich denke, er hätte das Thema hiermit beendet, beginnt er zu erzählen.

»Wir waren nie wirklich zusammen. Ihr Name war Lydia. Das klang immer wie ein Lied für mich.«

Er lächelt beschämt bei diesem Geständnis.

»Ich habe sie wirklich geliebt, hätte alles für sie gegeben. Wir haben uns häufig getroffen. Bin gern heimlich bei ihr durchs Fenster geklettert.«

Andy lacht bei der Erinnerung daran.

»Kitschig, ich weiß. Aber so bin ich eben. Ich habe es kaum ausgehalten ohne sie. Dann eines Tages… wir haben uns gestritten. Ich wollte es endlich offiziell machen zwischen uns, doch sie hat sich so dermaßen dagegen gewehrt. Ich habe es einfach nicht verstanden. Ich meine, was konnte denn so schlimm daran sein?

Das war unser letzter gemeinsamer Abend. Sie hatte einen… Unfall. Sie wollte mich danach nie wieder sehen.«

Andy endet mit einem hörbaren Atemzug. Ich bin wie versteinert, so gebannt habe ich dieser tragischen Geschichte gelauscht.

Nie hätte ich erwartet, dass er meine Frage so aufrichtig und detailliert beantwortet. Vielleicht wird ihm jetzt klar, dass er überhaupt nicht bereit ist für eine neue Beziehung?

Was denke ich da bloß? Er legt mir sein Herz offen und ich sehe nur meinen Vorteil darin! Wie furchtbar er gelitten haben muss! Und wie schrecklich das Schicksal manchmal sein kann. Noch mehr wird mir klar, dass ich diesen Abend nicht im Streit beenden möchte.

Und doch beruhigt mich die Tatsache, dass er immer noch sehr an seiner Ex-Liebe hängt. Das könnte unsere Freundschaft nach diesem Date retten.

»Wie sieht es bei dir aus? Irgendwelche Verehrer?«, richtet Andy nun die Frage an mich.

»Ach, da gibt es nicht viel Spannendes zu berichten. Hier und da mal eine nette Bekanntschaft, doch für mehr hat es einfach nie gereicht.«, antworte ich ehrlich.

»Ist das so? Niemand, auf den du ein Auge geworfen hast? Das kann ich fast nicht glauben.«, kontert er mit einem schiefen Lächeln.

Ich zucke nur verschwörerisch mit den Schultern. Was soll ich darauf antworten? Ich kann nicht »Nein« sagen, ohne ihn zu verletzen, kann aber auch nicht »Ja« sagen, ohne ihm Hoffnung zu machen. Dieser Abend gehört definitiv in die Top Ten der unangenehmsten Situationen meines Lebens.

Zu meinem Glück unterbricht der unmotivierte Kellner unsere Unterhaltung und nimmt die Bestellungen auf. Auch wenn mir gerade überhaupt nicht nach Essen zumute ist. Aber wenn ich den Mund voll habe, kann ich schon nichts Dummes sagen.

Im Laufe des Abends stelle ich immer mehr fest, dass Andy und ich absolut keine Gemeinsamkeiten haben. Er ist begeistert von allem, was mit Technik zu tun hat. Ich hingegen verstehe nur Bahnhof und habe auch kein Interesse daran, meinen eigenen PC zu bauen.

Als Andy auf die Toilette verschwindet, habe ich endlich einen Moment, um durchzuatmen.

Er muss doch selbst gemerkt haben, dass uns nichts verbindet.

Ich werfe einen Blick auf mein Handy. Es ist halb zehn. Somit können wir beruhigt den Abend als beendet betrachten.

Erleichtert versinke ich in dem gepolsterten Stuhl.

»Also ziehen wir weiter?«

Andy legt mir von hinten die Hand auf die Schulter, was mich zusammenzucken lässt.

»Weiter?«, frage ich verunsichert.

»Natürlich! Glaubst du, ich lade dich nur zum Essen ein? Das wäre doch langweilig.«, eröffnet Andy mir mit stolz geschwellter Brust.

Mir schwant Übles. Die romantische Atmosphäre dieses Restaurants erschlägt mich fast und er möchte noch eine Schippe draufsetzen? Ich muss das einfach beenden!

»Keine Sorge, du musst mich nicht heiraten.«, witzelt Andy.

Anscheinend kann er den leisen Anflug von Panik in meinem Gesicht ablesen. Ich lächle verlegen und folge ihm gespannt zu unserem nächsten Ziel.

*

Ich kann die Musik schon hören, bevor ich die Lichter der Innenstadt sehe. Anscheinend findet in der malerischen Altstadt heute Abend eine Art Sommerfest statt.

Livemusik, Verkaufsstände mit Süßigkeiten und Alkohol. Männer, Frauen und Kinder Tanzen wild umher, erleuchtet vom orangenen Licht der Laternen.

Ich bin überwältigt von der ausgelassenen, fröhlichen Stimmung und von den verschiedenen Gerüchen, die von den Ständen zu mir herüberwehen. Es war eine ganz wundervolle Idee, hier her zu kommen.

»Möchtest du tanzen?«, fragt Andy, der mir auffordernd die Hand entgegenstreckt.

Ich erschrecke, denn bei all der Begeisterung habe ich ihn völlig vergessen. Moment, was wollte er von mir? Tanzen?

»Ich kann doch überhaupt nicht tanzen!«, protestiere ich.

Da packt Andy einfach meine Hand, wirbelt mich herum und flüstert mir ins Ohr: »Du wurdest eben noch nie richtig geführt.«

Es klingt wie Drohung und Versprechen zugleich und ich bekomme eine Gänsehaut. Andrew sieht plötzlich so entschlossen aus, als wollte er mich in seinen Bann ziehen und er wüsste genau, dass er die Macht dazu hat.

Ich darf ziemlich schnell feststellen, dass ich mit meiner Vermutung gar nicht allzu falsch lag. Sein fester und doch sanfter Griff hält mich gefangen. Meine Hand in seiner tanzt er wortlos mit mir durch die Menge, dreht mich, fängt mich und kommt mir verführerisch nahe.

Ich weiß nicht, wie ich es mache, aber mit ihm an meiner Seite scheinen die Tanzschritte einfach zu passieren, ohne dass ich darüber nachdenken muss. Wenn ich das Gefühl habe, über meine Füße zu stolpern, ist Andy schon an meiner Seite, leitet meine Schritte um und lässt mich elegant in seine Arme fallen.

Die Menschen um mich herum verschwinden. Ich höre die Musik nicht mehr, ich fühle sie. Ich bin wie verzaubert und möchte, dass es nie wieder endet.

Doch da es bekanntlich aufhört, wenn es am schönsten ist, verklingt just in diesem Moment die Musik. Andy dreht mich erneut und zu den letzten Noten des Liedes werde ich in seine starken Arme gelegt.

Sein Gesicht schwebt mit einem gewinnenden Lächeln direkt über meinem. Schwer atmend starre ich Andy fassungslos an.

»Wow.«, ist das Erste, was ich imstande bin zu sagen, nachdem er mich wieder aufgerichtet hat.

»Was denn?«, fragt er gespielt unschuldig.

Er tanzt wie ein Gott und er weiß es.

»Ich hatte ja keine Ahnung, was in dir steckt!«, schwärme ich begeistert.

»Meine Mum hat mich gezwungen, tanzen zu lernen. Zehn Jahre hat es gedauert, bis mein Protest dagegen erhört wurde und ich aufhören durfte. Versteh mich nicht falsch, ich habe es nicht gehasst, ich hatte nur nicht die Art Leidenschaft, die ich eben für andere Dinge habe. Scheinbar war es schließlich doch für etwas gut.«, stellt er, mir zuzwinkernd, fest.

Ich kichere. Ich kichere? Was soll das werden? Nein, nein, nein! Ich darf ihm keine Hoffnung machen! Der Tanz war wundervoll, ja, aber ich darf mich nicht darin verlieren!

Apropos.

In diesem Moment fällt mir auf, dass wir noch immer Händchen halten.

Ich möchte mich lösen, doch Andrews Griff verstärkt sich. Mein Blick klebt regelrecht an unseren Händen.

Da löst er seine rechte Hand und streicht mir damit über die Wange. Seine Finger wandern an meiner Haut entlang, bis er mein Kinn erreicht und es sanft, aber fordernd nach oben drückt.

»Sieh mich an, Deliah.«, haucht er.

Mein Herz klopft mir bis zum Hals. Ich kann das nicht!

Andy tritt näher an mich heran. Seine Hand berührt zärtlich meinen Arm, sein Blick ruht auf meinen Lippen.

Zitternd hole ich Luft und schließe die Augen.

»Ist alles in Ordnung?«, fragt Andy besorgt.

»Ich fühle mich nicht besonders gut.«, erkläre ich.

Zumindest ist es nicht gelogen.

»Möchtest du etwas trinken?«, will Andy wissen.

Ich nicke hastig, bin noch immer in der Situation gefangen.

Andy vergewissert sich noch schnell, dass ich alleine stehen kann, dann steuert er einen der Stände in unserer Nähe an.

Er scheint den Verkäufer zu kennen, der da in seiner hölzernen Verkaufshütte steht und wird von diesem direkt in ein Gespräch verwickelt. Besorgt sieht er zu mir, doch ich halte nur den Daumen hoch, als Zeichen, dass es in Ordnung ist, wenn er sich kurz unterhält.

Das Date habe ich wohl erfolgreich beendet.

Eine warme Hand legt sich von hinten auf meine Schulter.

»Deliah?«, sagt eine Männerstimme, die wohl zu der Hand gehört.

Ich bekomme Gänsehaut, denn ich kenne diese Stimme.

Mit einem Ruck drehe ich mich um. Vor mir, im schwachen Schein einer Lampe und wie ein gefallener Engel, steht Callum.

Vorbei! Es ist vorbei mit meiner Geduld!
Ich kann mich nicht mehr bremsen, brauche dich.
Jetzt!

Fronten

»Callum?«

»Verfolgst du mich etwa?«, neckt er mich.

»Das Gleiche wollte ich dich gerade fragen.«, erwidere ich.

Hatte er nicht gesagt, er geht nicht gern in die Stadt?

»Ich wohne in der Nähe und wollte mir das Fest ansehen.«, erklärt er.

Da fällt mir auf, dass ich in all der Zeit, die wir uns nun kennen, nicht einmal gefragt habe, wo er lebt.

Aber wir haben uns geküsst!

»Wo warst du die ganze Zeit?«, frage ich ihn, als mir der Kuss wieder einfällt und die Woche danach, in der ich verzweifelt versucht hatte, mit ihm zu reden.

»Ich war zu Hause.«, antwortet er knapp.

Keine Erklärungen, keine Gegenfrage und doch genug Inhalt um es dabei belassen zu können.

»Willst du mich weiter mit Fragen löchern, oder wollen wir etwas Spaß haben?«, fragt Callum.

Ich bin, wie so oft an diesem Abend, völlig überrumpelt und bringe nur ein wenig geistreiches »Was?«, zustande.

»Tanzen, Deliah, lass uns tanzen!«, fordert Callum und wieder einmal wird meine Hand geschnappt und ich hinterhergezogen.

Es gelingt mir jedoch mich seinem Bann zu entziehen und ihn zur Rede zu stellen. So leicht kommt er mir diesmal nicht davon!

»Was spielst du hier?«, frage ich ihn mit verschränkten Armen.

Callum sieht mich nur verdutzt an, doch ich lasse nicht locker.

»Du kannst nicht einfach eine Woche lang verschwinden und dann plötzlich auftauchen und mich zum Tanzen auffordern, als wäre nichts gewesen!«

»So wie du mich geküsst hast und dann ohne ein Wort der Erklärung davongerannt bist?«

»Ich bin zurückgekommen! Du warst einfach weg!«, verteidige ich mich verzweifelt.

Ich spüre, wie meine Augen heiß von Tränen werden.

»Hätte ich einfach in dem Teich bleiben und auf dich warten sollen? Warum konntest du es nicht einfach geschehen lassen?«, entgegnet Callum ruhig.

Um uns herum die tanzende Menge, die mit ihren Farben und der Fröhlichkeit so gar nicht zu unserem Gespräch passt.

»Es war zu spät! Warum hast du mich immer wieder weggestoßen, wenn ich dir doch anscheinend etwas bedeute?«

»Weil ich nicht wusste, ob ich dir vertrauen kann!«

Seine Stimme ist ein tiefes Grollen.

Ich schrecke zurück und auch die Pärchen in unmittelbarer Nähe bemerken, dass etwas nicht stimmt und starren uns an.

Die Tränen, die ich vorhin bereits gespürt hatte, drohen nun auszubrechen.

Die Leute sind zu neugierig. Das hat er gesagt. Welches Geheimnis darf niemand wissen? Was fürchtest du, könnte ich verraten?

Ich drehe mich um, will einfach nur weg, doch Callum ergreift meine Hand.

»Deliah, bitte, geh nicht! Lass mich nicht noch einmal stehen!«, fleht er und ich erstarre, das Gesicht von ihm abgewandt.

»Bitte verlass mich nicht.«

Seine leisen Worte werden von der lauten Menschenmenge um uns herum verschluckt, sodass nur ich sie wahrnehmen kann. Und sie zerreißen mir das Herz. Aber ich kann das einfach nicht.

Da taucht Andy neben uns auf.

»Hey, Kumpel, dürfte ich wohl mein Date zurückhaben?«, spricht er Callum gespielt freundlich an.

Seine geballte Faust ergänzt sein verbissenes Lächeln.

Callum hingegen hält meine Hand weiterhin fest, sieht nur kurz zu Andy und danach wieder zu mir.

Eine stille Frage.

Darf er mich zurückhaben? Ich müsste es nur sagen und schon wäre ich an Callums Seite. So wie ich es wollte. Doch will ich es immer noch? Noch dazu befinde ich mich auf einem Date und kann doch nicht einfach mit einem anderen Mann verschwinden!

Ich muss mich entscheiden. Jetzt. Hier. Bleibe ich bei Andy oder gehe ich mit Callum?

Herz und Kopf streiten sich und ich stehe dazwischen. Zu viel ist ungeklärt, also tue ich das Einzige, was mir in diesem Moment richtig erscheint und löse meine Hand von seiner.

»Andy, du bist schon fertig mit deiner Unterhaltung?

Wir haben uns zufällig hier getroffen und ein wenig geredet.«, erkläre ich gespielt fröhlich auch wenn ich einen Stein in meiner Brust fühlen kann.

Eine ziemlich lausige Erklärung. Callum sieht aus, als hätte ich ihm ein Messer in die Brust gerammt. Ein knappes Nicken, dann verschwindet er wortlos in der Menge. Mein Herz zerspringt, ich möchte ihm nachlaufen, doch ich halte mich zurück.

»Was sollte das?«, richtet Andy nun das Wort an mich.

»Ich lasse dich fünf Minuten allein und du schmeißt dich irgendeinem Typen an den Hals?«

Er wird lauter.

»Das stimmt doch gar nicht!«, protestiere ich, doch die Lüge in dieser Aussage lässt mir die Stimme versagen.

»Verschone mich damit, Deliah! Ich Idiot habe mir wirklich eingebildet du würdest mich mögen! Warum sagst du mir nicht, die Wahrheit? Warum gibst du nicht zu, dass es einen anderen gibt? Ist *er* es?«

Die letzte Frage zischt er mir zu wie eine giftige Schlange. Wie kommt er denn darauf? Er hat recht, doch das kann er nicht wissen. Wie kann er sich dennoch so sicher sein?

Liv.

»Was hat Liv dir gesagt?«, will ich wissen.

»Halt Liv da raus!«, schreit Andy mich an.

Einige Menschen um uns herum tuscheln und starren uns vermeintlich unauffällig an. Was sie wohl über das Mädchen denken mögen, dass sich mit zwei Männern nacheinander streitet?

»Ich hatte keine Wahl, Andy.«

Meine Stimme zittert. Genau das wollte ich doch nicht.

»Man hat immer eine Wahl! Nur wenn man sich zwischen der unangenehmen Wahrheit und der angenehmen Lüge entscheiden muss, redet man sich gern ein, keine Wahl zu haben.«.

Mit diesen Worten geht er. Lässt mich einfach allein. Die tanzende, lachende Menge um mich herum bietet einen starken Kontrast zu der tiefen Schwärze die mich gerade von innen heraus zu zerfressen droht. Die neugierigen Blicke verflüchtigen sich, es gibt hier nichts mehr zu sehen, der Kampf ist verloren.

*

Ich laufe. Ich habe kein Ziel, ich möchte einfach nur weg. Davonlaufen. Was habe ich nur getan? Ich hätte zu mir selbst und meinen Gefühlen stehen sollen. Mein Herz schlägt vom ersten Moment an für Callum. Wie naiv von mir zu glauben, Andy könnte mit viel Mühe und genug Zeit seinen Platz einnehmen! Ich belüge mich selbst. Erzähle mir die Geschichte meines Lebens und sehe mich in der Rolle der tragischen Heldin. Dabei habe ich so sehr das Gefühl, die Böse zu sein.

Nach kurzer Zeit erreiche ich einen Park. Ein breiter Weg führt um einen See herum, der von Bäumen und Büschen geschmückt wird. Auch hier leuchten die Laternen in einem magischen Orange.

»Bitte erschrick nicht.«, flüstert eine zarte Stimme hinter mir.

Alles in mir zieht sich zusammen und ich mache einen Satz nach vorne, begleitet von einem, deutlich hörbaren, Luft holen. Ich habe mich fast zu Tode erschreckt!

In dem schwachen Licht kann ich eine kleine Gestalt erkennen. Eine Frau, ihr Gesicht liegt unter der Kapuze ihrer schwarzen Jacke verborgen.

»Wer bist du?«, frage ich mit noch immer pochendem Herzen.

»Du solltest vorsichtig sein, mit wem du deine Zeit verbringst. Glaub mir.«, warnt sie mich.

»Was meinst du damit?«

Wer ist sie und wen meint sie mit ihrer unheilvollen Warnung? Und warum sollte ich ihr glauben? Das Mädchen antwortet mir nicht, kommt nur mit einem Satz auf mich zu und schubst mich in das Licht der Laterne. Ich will gerade einen Gegenangriff starten, da nimmt sie ihre Kapuze ab und offenbart mir ihr Gesicht, welches auf einer Seite gänzlich von Narben entstellt ist.

»Oh Gott…«, stoße ich bei ihrem Anblick hervor.

Nicht gerade nett von mir. Ich möchte mich entschuldigen, möchte sie fragen, was ihr passiert ist.

Plötzlich reißt sie erschrocken die Augen auf, zieht sich die Kapuze wieder über, tritt aus dem Schein der Lampe und rennt davon.

Panisch sehe ich mich um. Was hat sie gesehen, dass sie so plötzlich die Flucht ergreift?

Mit zu Schlitzen verengten Augen versuche ich in der Dunkelheit etwas zu erkennen.

Ich höre die Schritte, noch bevor ich die Gruppe Männer sehen kann, die geradewegs auf mich zukommt. Alles in mir zieht sich zusammen, Panik ergreift mich. Wenn das Mädchen vor ihnen geflohen ist, sollte ich besser auch sehen, dass ich hier wegkomme.

Mit klopfendem Herzen eile ich zurück zum Stadttor. Bloß nicht rennen, sie dürfen nicht wissen, dass ich sie bemerkt habe.

Das habe ich zumindest einmal gehört.

Doch auch ihre Schritte werden schneller und lauter. Die Gruppe kommt immer näher und näher an mich heran und obwohl ich das Stadttor bereits sehen kann, werden sie mich erreicht haben, bevor ich um die Ecke biegen kann. Ich werde es nicht rechtzeitig zurückschaffen, ich brauche Hilfe!

Ich hole tief Luft, meine Muskeln spannen sich an, bereit los zu sprinten. Als ich gerade den ersten Schritt machen will, springt mir jemand in den Weg und hält mich fest. Ich schreie.

»Deliah! Hier bist du, wir haben dich schon überall gesucht! Komm schon, die Gruppe wartet da vorne.«

Ich brauche einen Moment, bis ich Liv erkenne.

»Na komm schon!«, drängt Liv und zieht mich weg von meinen Verfolgern, die ein kleines Stück entfernt stehen geblieben sind und leise tuscheln.

»Wir müssen die Polizei rufen!«

»Die Typen sind über alle Berge, bis die Polizei hier ankommt. Was machst du auch nachts allein im Park?«, fragt Liv, während sie mich weiter in Richtung des Festes zieht.

Als der Schock sich gelegt hat, fällt mir mein Streit mit Andy wieder ein und ich bleibe abrupt stehen. Liv sieht mich aus großen Augen an.

»Was hast du zu Andy nach unserem Telefonat gesagt?«

Liv erstarrt.

»Ich habe gar nichts erzählt!«, beteuert sie, doch ich glaube ihr kein Wort.

»Ich habe nur mit dir über Andy gesprochen. Woher kommt sein Verdacht, ich könnte einen anderen haben? Wieso wusste er, dass er für mich nur ein Freund ist?«

»Keine Ahnung, wahrscheinlich hat er es dir angemerkt!«, kontert Liv.

»Wenn du die Verantwortung für dein Leben in die Hand nehmen würdest, dann müsstest du die Schuld jetzt nicht bei mir suchen!«, keift sie mir ihre Antwort entgegen.

Das tat weh. Sie hat in gewisser Weise ja recht. Dennoch war es nicht in Ordnung, mich zu verraten. Auf der anderen Seite, sie ist seine beste Freundin. Was habe ich erwartet? Moment kann es sein…

»Du bist in Andy verliebt!«, äußere ich meinen Verdacht.

Liv beginnt laut zu lachen.

»Ernsthaft? Du willst die Eifersuchtsschiene fahren?«

Diese Reaktion macht mich nur noch wütender. Es hat keinen Sinn. Ich habe an diesem Abend schon genug Streit hinter mir und hierfür keine Kraft mehr, deshalb wende ich mich von ihr ab. Ich weiß nicht mehr, was ich glauben soll. Suche ich nur einen Schuldigen für meine Lage?

»Oh nein, du wirst mich jetzt nicht einfach stehen lassen!«, ermahnt Liv mich und hält meinen Arm fest.

»Was willst du noch von mir?«, kotze ich ihr entgegen.

Ich habe keine Lust mehr mit ihr zu reden. Ich möchte nach Hause, wo immer das ist.

Liv schreckt zurück.

»Nichts, ich möchte gar nichts mehr von dir.«, mit diesen Worten lässt sie mich los und ich verschwinde.

Pech! So viel Pech! Du hast mir das Herz gebrochen, mein Engel, hast mich allein in die Dunkelheit geschickt.

Doch hast du vergessen, dass dies mein Reich ist. Ich bin die Nacht und werde dich mit mir in die Schwärze ziehen.

Erwischt! Fast erwischt! Beim Tanz hieltest du die falsche Hand, mein hübscher Engel. Fast hätte ich dich gehabt. Nah so nah.

Ein Feind schleicht sich in unsere Mitte. Doch ich gebe dich nicht auf. Du wirst mir gehören! Mir allein! Dieses Mal werde ich erfolgreich sein, werde dir das Herz aus der Brust schneiden und es bei seinen letzten Schlägen fest an mich drücken. Und so vereint sich unser beider Herzen Pochen zur Melodie deines ewigen Schweigens.

Geister

Andys verletzten Stolz in allen Ehren aber hätte er mich nicht wenigstens wieder nach Hause fahren können? Es hat eine gefühlte Ewigkeit gedauert, bis mich das Taxi endlich eingesammelt hatte.

Aber wahrscheinlich ist das meine Strafe vom Universum dafür, dass ich so verdammten Mist gebaut habe. Andy hasst mich, ich habe Callum verletzt und mich mit Liv gestritten und das alles an nur einem Abend. Wie soll ich das denn je wieder geradebiegen?

Als Erstes sollte ich wohl mit Callum sprechen. Wenn er nicht wieder vom Erdboden verschluckt wird. Ich will das einfach alles klären, reinen Tisch machen. So viel Drama macht mich fertig.

Der Taxifahrer setzt mich vor Ellis Haus ab.

Alles ist dunkel, es ist ja auch schon sehr spät. In der Finsternis schleiche ich durch das Haus. Ich möchte Elli nicht wecken und vor allem jetzt nicht gesehen werden, also verstecke ich mich in den Schatten. In meinem

Zimmer angekommen, werfe ich meine Kleidung nur achtlos in die Ecke, streife mir mein Schlafshirt über und lege mich hin, um den Abend einfach im Schlaf zu vergessen.

Seit zwei Stunden starre ich an die Decke. Meine Gedanken wandern immer wieder zu Callum und Andy. Der Abend mit Andy hätte so schön sein können. Er hat mich in ein schickes Restaurant ausgeführt und der Tanz mit ihm war der Wahnsinn. Er ist nett und er würde bestimmt alles für mich tun.

Doch Callum ist es, der mein Herz schneller schlagen lässt. Als ich seine Hand losließ, zerbrach etwas in mir und von diesem Moment an war ich mir endgültig sicher, dass ich Andy einfach nicht lieben kann. Dennoch fürchte ich dieses unausgesprochene Geheimnis, welches zwischen Callum und mir steht.

Der Gedanke, in Andy einen guten Freund verloren zu haben, schmerzt unheimlich. Und trotzdem darf ich auf Liv nicht sauer sein. Ja, sie hat Andy erzählt, was ich ihr eher unfreiwillig anvertraut habe, allerdings kennt sie ihn länger als mich. Warum sollte sie mir treu sein? Wer weiß? Vielleicht war es sogar Andrew selbst, der sie zu diesem Anruf aus dem Nichts aufgefordert hat. Eventuell hat er mir tatsächlich schon früher etwas angemerkt.

Ich möchte nicht mehr grübeln, doch einschlafen kann ich auch nicht, also stehe ich auf.

Ich habe kein Ziel, ich kann nur einfach nicht mehr hier liegen. Leise öffne ich meine Tür, damit Elli nicht aufwacht.

Sie ist so nett zu mir. Ich hoffe wirklich, ihr Neffe lässt sie einfach in Frieden. Schon allein, weil ich ihr immer mehr anmerke, wie sehr sie ihren Mann vermisst. Oft beobachte ich sie dabei, wie sie sehnsüchtig sein Foto ansieht. Ich kann mir nicht vorstellen, wie zerrissen sie sich fühlen muss, wenn sie sich sogar sein Schnarchen einbildet. Moment...

Ich lausche. Da! Tatsächlich! Ein leises Ächzen, tiefes Luftholen... da schnarcht tatsächlich jemand!

Langsam laufe ich zu Ellis Schlafzimmer und presse mein rechtes Ohr gegen die Tür. Ich höre es. Jedoch mit dem linken Ohr. Das Geräusch scheint seinen Ursprung am Ende des Flures zu haben. Je näher ich ihm komme, desto deutlicher kann ich die harten Atemzüge erkennen.

Meine Ohren führen mich in das Zimmer, welches Elli an meinem ersten Tag geputzt hat. Ich stehe mitten im

Raum, kann das Schnarchen nun dumpf, aber klar hören. Doch hier ist niemand. Reglos stehe ich in der Dunkelheit und lausche. Ja! Es sind eindeutig Atemzüge. Woher kann das kommen? Machen alte Leitungen solche Geräusche?

Nervös sehe ich mich in allen Winkeln des Raumes um.

Meine Suche bleibt jedoch erfolglos. Keine Spur von schlafenden Geistern. Frustriert möchte ich gerade aufgeben, als mir ein Gedanke kommt. Lächerlich. Ich möchte gerade kopfschüttelnd über meine Idee den Raum verlassen, doch da meldet sich meine Intuition energischer und schließlich lausche ich doch an der Wand.

Tatsächlich! Ich kann es hören! Ein mittlerweile leiseres, doch stetiges Schnarchen kommt direkt durch die Wand. Doch das hier ist der letzte Raum im Flur. Nach dieser Wand kommt nur die Treppe nach unten. Andererseits ist es eine recht dicke Wand.

Wäre es möglich?

Vorsichtig klopfe ich dagegen. Ich weiß nicht, was ich mir davon erhoffe, doch als ich ein drittes Mal anklopfe, ist es plötzlich still. Ich könnte schwören, einen kurzen, erschrockenen Atemzug gehört zu haben. Angespannt bleibe ich noch eine Weile stehen und lausche.

Dann klopfe ich erneut gegen die Wand.

Ein dumpfes Poltern folgt als Antwort.

Ich hole erschrocken Luft und renne aus dem Raum heraus.

»Elli!«, rufe ich, als ich den Flur zurückrenne.

Mein Herz rast und fast verliere ich den Halt, als ich vor ihrer Tür zum Stehen komme. Ich rüttele an ihrem Türgriff, doch es ist abgeschlossen.

»Elli! Elli, mach auf!«

Ich hämmere gegen ihre Tür.

Kurz darauf wird mir von einer völlig zerknitterten Eleonore Griffin die Tür geöffnet.

»Du liebe Güte, Kindchen, hast du einen Geist gesehen?«, fragt Elli schlaftrunken schmatzend im fliederfarbenen Nachthemd.

»Elli, hier ist jemand im Haus!«

»So?«, fragt sie skeptisch.

Sie scheint überhaupt keine Angst zu haben, tritt aus dem Zimmer und knipst das Licht an, dann wirft sie stirnrunzelnd einen Blick nach rechts und links.

»Wo hast du jemanden gesehen, Kindchen?«, will sie wissen.

»Naja, nirgendwo, aber ich habe ihn gehört! Da vorne. Wir müssen hier raus, müssen die Polizei rufen!«

Ich zeige zu dem Zimmer, in dem ich meine Entdeckung gemacht habe.

Elli beginnt zu lachen und ich verstehe die Welt nicht mehr.

»Das ist doch nur Theodor.«, klärt sie mich auf.

Hat sie nun völlig den Verstand verloren? Ist sie dement? Muss ich ihr nun erklären, dass ihr Mann tot ist?

»Elli...«, beginne ich, doch ich weiß nicht weiter und stocke.

Beunruhigt werfe ich immer wieder einen Blick über die Schulter. Während ich dieser Frau versuche, die Gefahr begreiflich zu machen, könnte, wer auch immer hier im Haus ist, seinen Mordplan in die Tat umsetzen.

»Keine Sorge, Kindchen. Dieses seltsame Geräusch, ich weiß nicht, woher es kommt, doch in all den Jahren ist es mir nie gefährlich geworden. Ich möchte einfach glauben, dass es mein Theodor ist, verstehst du?«

Ihre Stimme ist am Ende nur noch ein Flüstern.

Plötzlich tut sie mir unendlich leid. Ich nicke als Antwort auf ihre Frage. Es muss furchtbar sein, einen Menschen so sehr zu vermissen, dass man sich einreden will, man würde seinen Geist hören.

Und trotzdem, ich habe etwas gehört und es scheint auf mich reagiert zu haben! Aber Elli hat gesagt, sie hört das schon seit Jahren. Es kann also kein Serienmörder sein, der hier eingestiegen ist. Dazu kommt, dass das Geräusch aus der Wand zu kommen scheint. Vielleicht Mäuse? Doch ich bin mir sicher, es war kein Nagen, sondern ich habe jemanden atmen gehört!

»Geh wieder ins Bett, Kindchen.«

Elli tätschelt mir die Schulter, dann dreht sie sich um, schlägt mir die Tür vor der Nase zu und lässt mich allein auf dem Flur zurück.

Unglaublich. Jetzt stehe ich hier, der Körper voll Adrenalin und kann nur den Kopf schütteln. Ich bin doch nicht bescheuert!

Da kommt mir erneut ein schockierender Gedanke: Habe ich mir doch nicht eingebildet, dass mich jemand im Schlaf beobachtet hat?

Wieder einmal verbringe ich eine Nacht damit, das Haus abzusuchen. Elli, die von dieser Sache absolut nicht beunruhigt ist, hat sich schon lange wieder schlafen gelegt und schnarcht nun selbst laut genug, um Tote aufzuwecken.

Ich hingegen kann jetzt erst recht kein Auge mehr zu tun. Angenommen, ich habe mir die Gestalt neulich in meinem Zimmer nicht eingebildet und die Geräusche in der Wand waren menschlichen Ursprungs, dann würde das bedeuten, dass hier noch jemand mit uns im Haus lebt. Dagegen spricht nur die Tatsache, dass es hinter dieser Wand kein weiteres Zimmer gibt, in welchem sich jemand verstecken könnte.

Ich bekomme eine Gänsehaut von der Vorstellung, beobachtet zu werden.

Stunden vergehen, doch wie beim letzten Mal kann ich nichts Außergewöhnliches entdecken. Total erschöpft setze ich mich auf das grüne Sofa im unteren Wohnzimmer.

Was geht hier nur vor sich?

*

Völlig verwirrt erwache ich am nächsten Morgen. Ich muss eingeschlafen sein. Und niemand hat mich ermordet oder entführt, das ist doch ein gutes Zeichen, oder?

»Oh, du bist wach, Kindchen. Wie schön.«, begrüßt Elli mich, die gerade mit einem Teller Zimtplätzchen und einem Schälchen Apfelmus auf dem gegenüberliegenden Sessel Platz nimmt.

»Willft bu auf eimem?«, fragt sie mit vollem Mund und hebt den Teller in meine Richtung.

»Nein, danke.«, lehne ich lächelnd ab.

Mein Körper fühlt sich an, als wäre ich mit dem Nudelholz bearbeitet worden. Mein Schlafplatz war nicht die beste Wahl.

»Elli, wegen gestern Abend…«, beginne ich, doch sie unterbricht mich.

»Mach dir deswegen keine Gedanken. Du bist nicht die Erste, die von meinem kleinen Hausgeist verjagt wird.«, erzählt sie leise lachend.

Ich kann mir vorstellen, an wen sie da gerade denkt.

»Was war mit der letzten, mit meiner Vorgängerin?«, will ich wissen.

Erneut lacht Elli.

»Widerwärtiges Weib! Hat für meinen Neffen die Beine breitgemacht und gehofft er würde das Geld mit ihr teilen, das beim Verkauf meines Hauses und meiner Habseligkeiten herausspringen würde. Ganz zu schweigen von meinem Bankkonto, für welches mein fürsorglicher Neffe aus rein großherzigen Gründen eine

Vollmacht haben möchte. Sie versuchten wirklich mit allen Mitteln mich wahnsinnig zu machen. Mir alles abzunehmen, mir einzureden, ich könnte nicht mehr allein leben. Ich hörte sie eines Tages mit Alexander über Medikamente sprechen. Sie wollten mich ruhigstellen! Die ganze Nachbarschaft hatte gesehen, dass sie alles für mich übernahm, jeder hätte sofort geglaubt, es ginge bergab mit mir. Niemand hätte ein abgekartetes Spiel vermutet.«

Ich schlucke schwer. Wie können Menschen nur so grausam sein, einzig und allein des Geldes wegen?

»Doch dann«, fährt sie mit erhobenem Zeigefinger fort, »dann kam ein Engel, mein Theodor, zu mir. Maren, so hieß sie, konnte von da an keine Nacht mehr schlafen. Sie redete immer wieder davon, dass sie beobachtet würde. Dass sie nachts Geräusche hörte und sich plötzlich Dinge nicht mehr da befanden, wo sie sie abgestellt hatte. Vielleicht wurde sie verrückt, vielleicht war es real. Fakt ist, mir selbst sind derartige Dinge ferngeblieben. Eines Tages, sie war gerade dort drüben in Theodors Zimmer, da schien sie Stimmen zu hören, die zu ihr sprachen. Ich habe nie erfahren, was sie gehört hat, aber es war wohl schrecklich genug, um fluchtartig mein Haus zu verlassen.«, endet Elli mit einem herzhaften Lachen.

Ich bin schockiert darüber, dass sie sich absolut keine Sorgen zu machen scheint. Oder hat sie etwa selbst etwas damit zu tun? Ist am Ende sie selbst der Geist? Will sie mich auch loswerden? Aber… letzte Nacht, das konnte sie gar nicht gewesen sein.

»Und das Beste«, ergänzt Elli, »mein lieber Alexander hat sie nach ihrer überstürzten Flucht fallen lassen, wie eine heiße Kartoffel!«

Jetzt brüllt sie vor Lachen, kleine Tränen kullern ihr aus den Augenwinkeln.

»Hat sich sogar eine neue Nummer besorgt, dieser Scheißkerl!«, presst sie hervor, während ihr ganzer Körper bebt.

Das nenne ich mal die personifizierte Schadenfreude.

Es wird Zeit, mein Engel. Meine Erlösung wartet auf mich. Ich werde dich in Flammen hüllen und deine Asche in mir aufnehmen.

Gespräche

Die Nacht auf der Couch steckt mir auch nach der ausgiebigen Dusche noch in den Gliedern. Völlig steif tapse ich die Treppe hinunter zur Küche, in der Elli schon wieder am Herumwerkeln ist.

»Vergiss den Sekt nicht!«, krächzt sie in den Telefonhörer, den sie zwischen Schulter und Ohr geklemmt hat.

Sie hat die Küchenmaschine auf die Küchentheke gestellt, wo diese kontinuierlich einen Teig zu rühren scheint.

»Ich werde Henri in den Gartenteich verfrachten, wenn er nicht aufhört zu meckern!«, prophezeit Elli mit erhobenem Kochlöffel.

Was ist denn hier schon wieder los?

Vorsichtig schlängele ich an Elli vorbei, um mir ein Glas Wasser zu holen. Dabei fällt mein Blick auf die Koch- und Backbücher, die kreuz und quer in der Küche verteilt liegen.

»Sag ihm, er kann mich mal an meinem faltigen... Oh! Wärt ihr so lieb und würdet wieder ein paar Gläser Apfelmus mitbringen? Sehr schön. Also gut, bis morgen dann.«, verabschiedet Elli sich.

»Kindchen!«, begrüßt sie mich freudestrahlend, nachdem sie aufgelegt hat.

»Was ist denn hier los?«, frage ich, immer noch schockiert über dieses Chaos.

Elli hält inne, dreht sich dramatisch zu mir um und zieht einen Schmollmund.

»Jetzt sag bloß, du hast meinen Geburtstag morgen vergessen!«

Ach herrje! Das habe ich tatsächlich!

Nun, nicht wirklich vergessen. Um ehrlich zu sein, habe ich nie wirklich nachgesehen, wann er überhaupt ist.

»Ich fürchte doch.«, gestehe ich und umklammere schuldbewusst mein Wasserglas.

Elli schüttelt in gespielter Enttäuschung den Kopf.

»Mit wem hast du telefoniert?«, versuche ich von der unangenehmen Situation abzulenken.

Sofort beginnt Elli zu strahlen.

»Mathilde. Sie und ihr Mann sind auch zu der Feier morgen eingeladen.«

»Feier?«

»Natürlich! Glaubst du ich begnüge mich mit Kaffee und Kuchen?«, erwidert Elli, die Hände in die Hüften gestemmt.

Und das sagt sie einen Tag vorher?

»Was für eine Art Feier hast du denn im Sinn?«, frage ich nach und fürchte mich ein wenig vor der Antwort.

Ellis Augen funkeln.

»Ein Gartenfest! Alles soll voll von Lichtern und Blumen sein. Eine große Geburtstagstorte und ein karibisches Buffet.«

Ich starre Elli mit großen Augen an. Das will sie alles allein in einem einzigen Tag schaffen? Sie ist also doch verrückt!

*

Ich werfe alle Zutaten für die Sauce chien in den Mixer, deren Rezept Elli mir zwischen Reis abwaschen und Curry umrühren beigebracht hat. Anders als meine Französischkenntnisse mich befürchten ließen, wird hierfür zum Glück kein Hund benötigt. Die hauptsächlich aus Gemüse bestehende scharfe Soße benutzt Elli als

Dressing für ihren Salat.

»Höllisches Zeug! Theodor hat fast eine ganze Kuh ausgetrunken, nachdem er sich zu viel davon genehmigt hatte. Sei also vorsichtig mit den Chilis, Kindchen«, erzählt Elli lachend, als sie die Kidneybohnen aus der Dose in ein Sieb kippt.

Gebannt lausche ich den Geschichten von ihrem Karibikurlaub, während Elli mir alles beibringt, was sie über die dort einheimische Küche weiß.

Ich staune immer wieder über ihre Geschichten von früher. Die Abenteuer, die sie mit ihrem Mann erlebt hat. Auch wenn mir der Gedanke, dass ich ihren Theodor nie kennenlernen werde, das Herz schwer macht.

Nach einem langen und anstrengenden Tag in der Küche verstauen wir schließlich alles säuberlich verpackt im Kühlschrank. Wir haben es tatsächlich geschafft, eine Vielzahl von Speisen herzustellen und sogar noch eine Torte zu backen und zu verzieren.

Zwischendurch kam ich sogar in den Genuss von Reis, der langsam in Kokosnussmilch gekocht und anschließend mit Bohnen vermischt wird. Es war einfach köstlich, was meine Vorfreude auf die morgige Feier ins Unermessliche steigen lässt.

Todmüde und überglücklich falle ich abends ins Bett. Es tat gut, einmal einen Tag ohne Drama einfach nur meiner Arbeit nachzugehen. Morgen wird bestimmt ein toller Tag. Mit dem Gedanken an das leckere Essen versinke ich schließlich in einen traumlosen Schlaf.

Am nächsten Morgen springe ich sofort gut gelaunt aus dem Bett. Es gibt viel zu tun und ich möchte, dass es für Elli ein ganz besonderer Tag wird.

Unten angekommen muss ich feststellen, dass ich mal wieder nicht die Erste auf den Beinen bin.

Elli saust durch das Haus und erledigt hundert Dinge gleichzeitig. Als sie an mir vorbeiflitzen will, schnappe ich sie jedoch bei den Schultern.

»Stehen geblieben! Lass dich doch mal drücken, Elli.«, fordere ich, dann ziehe ich sie in eine herzliche Geburtstagsumarmung.

»Kindchen, wärst du so nett und würdest Callum draußen helfen?«, fragt Elli, wartet jedoch meine Antwort nicht ab, sondern verschwindet schon wieder durch die nächste Tür.

Helfen. Callum. Den hatte ich bis jetzt doch so wunderbar verdrängt.

Ich fühle mich, als hätte ich sein Haustier getötet, als ich den Garten betrete. Was mich dort erwartet, lässt mich jedoch stocken. Ein großer Tisch mit weißer Tischdecke steht umringt von Stühlen inmitten des Gartens. Darauf befinden sich große Vasen mit wunderschönen Blumensträußen. Es sieht aus wie in einem Märchen.

»Wie findest du es?«, fragt der Baum neben mir.

Verwundert sehe ich nach oben in die Baumkrone. Dort entdecke ich einen mir sehr vertrauten, blonden Lockenkopf.

»Es sieht einfach wunderschön aus.«, gestehe ich.

Er spricht mit mir. Das ist doch schon mal ein gutes Zeichen, oder?

Ein dumpfer Aufprall ist zu hören, als Callum vom Baum zu mir herunterspringt. Er bückt sich, hebt einen Stecker auf, der mit der Steckdose an der Wand verbunden ist und legt einen Schalter um. Auch wenn es noch hell ist, kann ich die vielen kleinen Papierlaternen im Baum erkennen, die sanft leuchten. Das wird heute Abend bestimmt wunderschön aussehen!

»Ich habe nachgedacht.«, beginnt Callum, der noch immer neben mir steht.

Ich betrachte ihn mit großen Augen, unruhig, was nun

wohl kommen mag.

»Ich war nicht fair zu dir.«, sagt er und lässt mich dann stehen, um die Blumenvasen erneut auszurichten.

Ungläubig stolpere ich ihm hinterher.

»Und was willst du mir jetzt damit sagen?«, frage ich vorsichtig nach.

Da ist es wieder, dieses Flattern im Magen. Doch ich darf nicht zu viel Hoffnung in diese Worte legen. Ich habe den Abend in der Stadt nicht vergessen.

»Ich will damit sagen, dass ich dich nicht einfach bei deinem Date hätte entführen sollen und dann erwarten, dass du den Typen für mich stehen lässt. Auch wenn ich das gehofft hatte.«, gibt er zu und grinst mich durch einen Strauß lilafarbener Blumen an.

Aha, wir sind also wieder an dem Punkt, an dem er flirtet. Doch dieses Spiel kenne ich nun schon zu gut. Ich traue diesem Lächeln kein Stück!

»Was meintest du damit, dass du mir nicht vertrauen kannst?«

»Das habe ich nie gesagt!«, widerspricht er und wendet sich dem Tisch neben dem Gartenteich zu, der später als Buffet dienen soll.

Es macht mich wahnsinnig, wie er hier steht und so tut,

als wäre das hier eine ganz einfache, beiläufige Unterhaltung, obwohl ich genau merke, dass er mir nicht in die Augen sehen kann! Ich will das jetzt ein für alle Mal geklärt haben!

Also stapfe ich zu ihm, packe ihn an der Schulter und drehe ihn schwungvoll zu mir herum.

»Entweder, du redest jetzt anständig mit mir oder wir gehen getrennte Wege. Dieses hin und her macht mich fertig!«

Den letzten Satz wollte ich eigentlich gar nicht sagen.

»Worüber möchtest du denn sprechen?«

Sein aufgesetztes Grinsen ist verschwunden.

Ich möchte über alles sprechen. Darüber, was er in mir auslöst und wie er mich durcheinanderbringt. Möchte sein Geheimnis erfahren, denn die Angst davor, was er verbergen könnte, bringt mich um den Verstand. Doch die Worte bleiben mir im Hals stecken. Ich fühle mich wie ein Teenie, der nicht wagt seinen Schwarm zu fragen, ob er mit ihr gehen will.

»Du bist mir nicht egal.«, umschreibe ich meine Gefühle für ihn und hoffe, er versteht, was ich ihm damit sagen möchte.

»Was ist mit dem anderen? Deinem Date.«, fragt

Callum ruhig, jedoch ohne mich anzusehen.

»Nichts. Ich hätte nie hingehen sollen.«, gebe ich zu.

»Warum denkst du, du könntest mir nicht trauen?«, frage ich erneut nach und hoffe ihn damit nicht zu verschrecken.

Callum atmet tief durch und ich fürchte schon fast, dass er mich einfach hier stehen lässt, doch dann sieht er mir endlich in die Augen.

»Es gibt Dinge in meiner Vergangenheit, über die ich nicht sprechen möchte. Nicht sprechen kann. Und auch jetzt, wo du vor mir stehst und mich so traurig ansiehst, dass es mir das Herz bricht, kann ich nichts weiter tun, als dich darum zu bitten, nicht weiter nachzufragen.«

Ich erstarre. Seine Worte jagen mir einen eiskalten Schauer über den Rücken.

»Was hast du getan?«, will ich wissen.

Callum atmet hörbar aus.

»Nichts. Ich habe rein gar nichts getan.«, antwortet er und wendet sich zum Gehen.

Plötzlich hält er jedoch in der Bewegung inne und dreht sich erneut zu mir um.

»Du musst keine Angst vor mir haben, Deliah. Aber vermutlich wäre es klüger Abstand zu halten. Ich hätte mich dir nicht auf diese Weise nähern sollen. Es ist meine Schuld. Aber ich bereue keine Sekunde. Ich will nur, dass du das weißt.«

Daraufhin verschwindet er hinterm Haus und lässt mich inmitten des Gartens mit tausend Fragen zurück.

Dank einer gigantischen Liste an Aufgaben, die Elli mir zugeteilt hat, hatte ich keine Zeit mehr, mir den Kopf über Callum zu zerbrechen. Doch jetzt ist alles erledigt und wie ich hier stehe und auf die Gäste warte, überfallen mich meine Gedanken.

Was verbirgt Callum? Will ich es überhaupt wissen? Er möchte es mir nicht erzählen, doch ich weiß, ich werde nicht lockerlassen. Ich wünschte, ich könnte ihn einfach aus meinem Kopf und meinem Herzen verbannen. Alles wäre dann so viel einfacher.

Es klingelt.

Elli eilt zur Haustür, ich folge ihr.

Durch das Milchglas der Tür erkenne ich einen riesigen Umriss. Elli drückt die Türklinke nach unten und eine zwei Meter hohe Frau mit dunkler Haut und ausladenden Hüften betritt das Haus. Ein knallrotes Kleid mit vielen weißen Blüten schmiegt sich um ihren kurvigen

Körper. Hellgraue, fast weiße Haare treten in kurzen Locken unter einem Strohhut hervor, der ebenfalls großzügig mit künstlichen Blumen geschmückt ist.

»Lass dich umarmen, du alte Schachtel!«, begrüßt die Frau Elli mit kräftiger Stimme und zieht sie in eine Umarmung.

»Du bist fünf Jahre älter, als ich!«, protestiert Elli in gespieltem Entsetzen.

Ich ahne, wer unser Gast ist. Ellis beste Freundin Mathilde.

Da wandert ihr Blick auch schon zu mir.

»Du bist bestimmt Deliah! Ach, Nörchen hat so viel von dir erzählt, du Gute!«

Daraufhin schließt sie auch mich in eine feste Umarmung und saust dann weiter durchs Haus und zur hinteren Tür hinaus, die in den Garten führt. Was für ein Wirbelwind!

»Nörchen?«, wiederhole ich kichernd den Spitznamen, den sie Elli gegeben hat.

»Ach das sieht ja wirklich wundervoll aus!«, ertönt Hildes Stimme, aus dem Garten.

»Diese Frau ist unmöglich.«, grummelt eine tiefe Männerstimme hinter uns.

Ich drehe mich zur Haustür, wo gerade ein klein gewachsener Mann mit Glatze und Schnauzbart einen Geschenkkorb hereinträgt.

»Henri!«, heißt Elli den zweiten Gast willkommen.

Steht er schon die ganze Zeit da? Ich war so erschlagen von Ellis Freundin, dass ich ihn überhaupt nicht bemerkt habe. Das muss dann der Ehemann von Mathilde sein.

Seine Wangen sind von einem leichten Sonnenbrand gerötet. Er wirkt viel ruhiger und ernster als seine Frau.

Wir begleiten Henri nach draußen, wo Hilde schon mit einer Flasche Sekt bereitsteht.

»Nörchen, wo hast du denn die Gläser? Oder willst du wieder aus der Flasche trinken, wie neulich?«

Ich sehe Elli mit großen Augen an, doch die zuckt nur entschuldigend mit den Schultern.

»So schnell, wie ich bei dir nachschenken muss, lohnen sich Gläser doch überhaupt nicht.«, antwortet sie ihrer Freundin.

Währenddessen hat Henri die Gläser vom Buffettisch geholt, stellt sie demonstrativ vor seiner Frau ab und setzt sich.

Mathilde öffnet die erste Flasche und schenkt ein.

»Hoffen wir, dass dein alter Magen das verkraftet.«,

sagt sie, als sie Elli ihr Getränk reicht.

»Keine Sorge, sollte mir übel werden, schnappe ich mir einfach deinen scheußlichen Hut!«, kontert Elli.

Die Freundinnen brechen in schallendes Gelächter aus, da klingelt es erneut an der Tür.

Ich eile nach drinnen, von wo aus ich die beiden noch immer hören kann. Das wird bestimmt ein sehr schöner Tag.

Doch als ich die Tür öffne und unserem neuen Gast in die Augen sehe, erstarre ich.

»Guten Tag, Deliah.«, begrüßt Alexander Griffin mich kühl.

Nah. So nah.

Ich bin bei dir, mein Engel. Kein Schritt mehr ohne mich. Ich beobachte dich.

Mach keine Dummheiten, mein Engel! Füge dich deinem Schicksal!

Bekenntnis

»Hallo.«, murmele ich eine Antwort.

Er kommt auf den Geburtstag seiner Tante? Warum? Was hat er vor?

»Kindchen, wer … oh! Alexander?«, fragt Elli überrascht, als sie ihren Neffen erkennt.

»Tante Eleonore.«, antwortet dieser ohne einen Funken Sympathie und drückt Elli einen winzigen Blumenstrauß in die Hand, der dringend Wasser zu benötigen scheint.

Wir folgen Alexander schweigend in den Garten, wo Hilde auf Ellis Neffen aufmerksam wird.

»Na was sagt man dazu? Der große Alexander Griffin beehrt uns mit seiner Anwesenheit!«

»Mathilde, Henri.«, grüßt er das Ehepaar mit einem Nicken, dann nimmt er am Ende des Tisches Platz.

Elli und ich sehen uns beunruhigt an.

»Möchtest du ein Stück Kuchen, Alexander?«, fragt Elli.

»Nein danke. Für mich heute nichts zu essen.«, lehnt dieser mürrisch ab.

Ich ahne warum.

Mathilde lässt sich von diesem Grießkram jedoch nicht den Tag verderben und stellt ihm ein Glas mit rotem Inhalt hin.

»Stoß wenigstens mit uns auf deine Tante an!«, fordert sie.

Alexander betrachtet das Getränk ungläubig.

»Kirschsaft. Du alter Spießer, jetzt hab dich nicht so!«

Ich beobachte die Szene von dem geschmückten Baum aus.

Alexander, der vorsichtig an seinem Glas nippt, es für gut befindet und einen großen Schluck nimmt. Hilde, die zufrieden lächelt, sich umdreht und eine Flasche zuschraubt, die eindeutig kein Saft ist. Als sie bemerkt, dass ich sie erwischt habe, hält sie verschwörerisch grinsend ihren Zeigefinger an die vollen Lippen.

Sie hat ihm Schnaps in das Glas gemischt? Ich mag Alexander Griffin nicht besonders, doch das ist nicht in Ordnung!

Hilde, die meinen entsetzten Gesichtsausdruck sieht, kommt zu mir herüber. Als Henri sich mit Alexander zu unterhalten beginnt, nutzt sie seine Unaufmerksamkeit, um mir zu erklären, was ich gerade beobachtet habe.

»Teuflisches Zeug.«, flüstert sie, »Du bemerkst es erst, wenn es zu spät ist.«

»Ich finde das nicht gut.«, entgegne ich.

»Das ist es auch nicht. Aber glaub mir, dieser Mann hat weitaus mehr verdient, als einen kleinen Schuss in seinem Kirschsaft. Außerdem werde ich nicht zulassen, dass er Nörchen mit seiner schlechten Laune die Feier vermiest. Und so, wie du ihn ansiehst, weißt du, wovon ich spreche.«

Und wie ich das weiß! Trotzdem geht es mir nicht gut mit diesem Geheimnis.

Etwa zwei Stunden sind vergangen, in denen freudig gefeiert wurde. Auch das kleine Buffet, welches ich mit Elli vorbereitet habe, kam wunderbar bei unseren Gästen an. Zumindest bei denen, die dem Essen trauten.

Eine Sache jedoch lässt mir keine Ruhe. Obwohl Elli ihm so wichtig ist und er immer an ihrer Seite zu stehen scheint, hat Callum sich seit unserem Gespräch vorhin hier nicht mehr blicken lassen.

Ist es wegen mir? Wir hatten uns doch mehr oder

weniger versöhnt, wenn auch nicht so, wie ich es mir vorgestellt hatte.

Warum sollte er Ellis Feier verpassen wollen? Er hat doch selbst gesagt, dass sie für ihn wie eine Mutter ist.

Ich mache mir schon wieder viel zu viele Gedanken! Ich sollte lernen, ihn loszulassen. Er scheint ein Problem zu haben und ich bin mir nicht sicher, ob ich etwas damit zu tun haben will.

Elli und Mathilde lachen und scherzen angetrunken, während Henri kopfschüttelnd daneben sitzt. Mein Blick wandert den Tisch entlang zu Alexander. Doch sein Platz ist leer.

Ist er etwa gegangen? Meine Hände werden schweißnass. Mathilde hat ihm ungefähr drei Gläser von ihrem Spezialsaft gemixt. Er wird doch nicht nach Hause gefahren sein! Vielleicht ist er auch einfach nur auf der Toilette?

Keiner hier scheint ihn zu vermissen, nicht einmal Henri, der sich die ganze Zeit mit ihm unterhalten hat. Und doch lässt es mir keine Ruhe, ich muss einfach nachsehen.

Unruhig stehe ich auf und laufe um das Haus herum in den Hof.

Sein Auto steht noch da.

KRACH

Ein lautes Poltern lässt mich zusammenzucken. Es kam von drinnen! Ich sprinte zur Haustür, fische meinen Schlüssel aus der Hosentasche und eile hinein.

»Verdammt!«

Alexander Griffins Stimme hallt durch den Flur. Ich folge ihr in das kleine Arbeitszimmer von Theodor Griffin. Unschöne Erinnerungen erwachen, als ich eintrete.

Was ich dort vorfinde, ist ein absolutes Chaos. Bücher sind aus dem Regal gezerrt und achtlos auf den Boden geworfen worden, ebenso eine kleine Lampe, die auf dem Schreibtisch stand. Davor sitzt Alexander auf dem hölzernen Bürostuhl, das Gesicht in den Händen vergraben, die Ellbogen auf die Oberschenkel gestützt.

Vorsichtig nähere ich mich ihm wie einem wilden Tier.

»Ist alles in Ordnung?«

Sein Körper bebt, dann beginnt er hysterisch zu lachen. Ich bin wie versteinert. Was ist hier los?

»Ob alles in Ordnung ist, will sie wissen!«, äfft er mich nach.

Er ist betrunken, seine Maske fällt. Ich verfluche Mathilde für das, was sie getan hat. Das hier ist weitaus gruseliger, als ein grimmig dreinschauender Alexander.

»Nein! Nein, es ist nicht alles in Ordnung!«, brüllt er mich an und sieht mich aus weit aufgerissenen Augen an.

Ich bin überfordert mit der Situation, weiß nicht, wie ich mit ihm umgehen soll. Am besten ich hole Elli. Oder Henri.

Ich wende mich ab und gehe zur Tür.

»Nein!«, schreit er erneut und springt auf.

Erschrocken drehe ich mich um, da ist er auch schon bei mir und knallt die Tür zu. Ich taumele, stoße mit meinem Rücken an die geschlossene Tür und bin zwischen seinen Armen gefangen, die er an das kühle Holz drückt. Er ist mir ganz nah. Zu nah. Seine eisblauen Augen starren auf mich herab.

»Wolltest du zu ihr?«, haucht er in mein Ohr.

Der Geruch von Alkohol und Kirsche brennt in meiner Nase. Mein Körper bebt vor Anspannung. Ich suche die richtigen Worte, um ihn zu beruhigen, doch diese unangenehme Nähe zu ihm lässt mich nicht klar denken.

»Bitte, ich möchte gehen.«, stammele ich.

Ein selbstgefälliges Grinsen, begleitet von einem

Schnauben, ist seine Antwort darauf. Ich fürchte, ich habe etwas Falsches gesagt, ihn noch angestachelt, doch da stößt er sich von der Tür ab und gibt mich frei.

»Bitteschön! Die Welt steht dir offen, kleine Deliah.«, sagt er, gefolgt von einer ausladenden Handbewegung.

Blitzschnell drehe ich mich um und greife nach dem Türgriff.

»Es ist nicht fair.«, wendet er sich erneut an mich.

Ich bleibe stehen, höre ihm zu.

»Sie hat alles. Einfach alles. Und trotzdem verlangt er von mir, dass ich mich um sie kümmere!«

»Wer verlangt das?«, frage ich und drehe mich zu ihm um.

»Mein Vater! Er hatte nichts! Sein Bruder, mein Onkel, er hatte alles. Und jetzt hat sie es!«, erklärt Alexander, wobei seine Augen feucht werden.

Soweit ich weiß, sind die Eltern von Alexander Griffin bereits verstorben. Seine Mutter verlor er sehr früh, sie war krank. Sein Vater verstarb kurz nach Theodor an einem Herzinfarkt.

»Nachdem Onkel Theodor gestorben ist, hat er zu mir gesagt, ich soll auf Tante Eleonore aufpassen. Ich habe sie nicht einmal richtig gekannt! Die beiden waren nie hier!

Und als ich nach dem Tod meines Vaters erkannt habe, in welchem Reichtum diese Frau lebt und wie arm meine Familie dagegen war... Es ist nicht fair!«

Er schlägt mit der Faust gegen die Wand und ich zucke zusammen. Jetzt ergibt alles Sinn. Deshalb will er sie aus dem Haus haben. Er denkt, er hätte einen Anspruch auf Ellis Geld.

Ich kann mir jedoch nicht vorstellen, dass Elli und Theodor ihre eigene Familie derart im Stich gelassen haben sollen.

»Hast du mit Elli darüber gesprochen?«, will ich wissen.

Ich begebe mich auf seine Ebene, spreche nicht mehr mit meinem Boss, sondern einem angetrunkenen, gebrochenen Mann.

»Damit ich nicht nur meine Familie, sondern auch meine Würde verliere? Ich werde nicht betteln, falls du das meinst. Ich werde mir nehmen, was mir zusteht!«

Alexander beginnt in dem kleinen Räumchen auf und ab zu tigern, während er sich immer wieder mit den Händen das Gesicht reibt. Ich beobachte ihn still.

»Ich habe ihm den Gefallen getan. Habe sie besucht. Doch ich konnte diesen goldenen Käfig einfach nicht mehr ertragen! Das alles zu sehen!«, er öffnet seine Arme weit, um das Haus zu beschreiben, »Diesem Schatz ausgesetzt zu sein, während meine Eltern nie etwas hatten und elendig krepiert sind! Und mir soll es jetzt genauso gehen, wie ihnen?«, richtet er seine Frage an mich.

»Aber du bist doch nicht arm.«, ist alles, was mir als Antwort einfällt.

Ich kann einfach nicht glauben, dass Elli ihn derart im Stich lassen würde.

»Ich habe nichts! Ich bin ganz allein auf dieser Welt! Ich habe nichts. Und niemanden.«, antwortet er, dann bricht seine Stimme.

»Du hast sie. Du musst es nur zulassen.«, spreche ich meine Gedanken mit zitternder Stimme aus.

Mein Herz bricht, als ich den kleinen Jungen in dem Mann vor mir erkenne, der seine Eltern vermisst und sich von der Welt verlassen fühlt. Eine einzelne Träne rinnt über seine Wange. Schnell wendet er sich ab.

»Geh.«, befiehlt er und ich gehorche.

Als ich die Tür hinter mir schließe, kann ich ein leises Schluchzen hören, welches sich mit meinem eigenen vermischt.

Ich ließ dich allein, mein Engel. Doch sei unbesorgt, meine Vorbereitungen sind abgeschlossen. Ich bin zurück und ich bin bereit, dich zu verzehren.

Entdeckungen

Der Tag nach Ellis Geburtstagsfeier beginnt mit einer lauten Diskussion, die mich aus dem Keller nach oben lockt. Schnell werfe ich die Wäsche beiseite, die ich gerade in die Maschine stopfen wollte und haste die Treppe hinauf in die Küche, aus der das Stimmengewirr zu kommen scheint.

»Sprich nicht so über ihn, du altes Weib!«, ertönt Alexander Griffins Stimme. Nachdem er mit Henris Hilfe das Chaos im Arbeitszimmer beseitigt hatte, hat er die Nacht hier verbracht. Anscheinend hat er sich nüchtern geschlafen und jetzt gibt es Streit zum Frühstück.

»Du musst der Wahrheit ins Auge sehen, Alexander! Jeder Versuch, ihm zu helfen, war zwecklos!«, kontert Elli energisch.

»Mein Vater war nicht süchtig!«

»Fein! Verschließe dich. Das wird dir aber nie den Frieden bringen, nach dem du suchst!«

Ich betrete die Küche, sofort sind alle Augen auf mich

gerichtet. Alexander betrachtet mich finster, dann kommt er auf mich zu.

»Mit ihr sprechen? Pah!«, raunt er mir zu, dann schiebt er sich an mir vorbei in den Flur.

Das Klappern eines Schlüssels und das Knallen der Haustür folgen, dann hören wir einen Motor und Alexander Griffin ist verschwunden.

Seufzend lässt Elli sich auf einen Stuhl fallen.

»Was war denn hier los?«, will ich wissen.

Ein weiteres Seufzen folgt.

Ich setze mich zu ihr.

»Elli?«

»All die Jahre.«, murmelt sie, »All die Jahre der Geheimhaltung, nur um ihn zu schützen. Und am Ende hat ihn genau das gebrochen.«

»Was meinst du damit?«

Sie sieht aus, als wäre sie unter einer Last zusammengebrochen. Tiefe Sorgenfalten zeichnen ihre Stirn.

»Er war spielsüchtig. Alexanders Vater. Theodor wollte ihm helfen, doch er nahm keine Hilfe an. Dann hat er ihm immer wieder Geld gegeben. Für den kleinen Alexander, der als ungeplantes Kind erst sehr spät in diese

Familie kam. Für seine kranke Frau. Doch das Geld kam nie an. Auch nachdem seine Frau gestorben ist, hat er nicht aufgehört. Er konnte es nicht.«

»Alexander wusste nichts davon?«

»Nein. Wir wollten ihn schützen. Wollten, dass er seinen Vater als den Helden sieht, den Kinder brauchen. Vor allem, nachdem er keine Mutter mehr hatte.« Elli kämpft mit jedem Wort, als sie mir die Geschichte dieser kaputten Familie erzählt.

»Wie wolltet ihr das denn für immer geheim halten?«, frage ich nach.

»Oh, wir hatten sehr wohl vor, es Alexander zu sagen. Du musst wissen, Theodor und ich haben viele Jahre Organisationen unterstützt, die Kindern und Jugendlichen aus ärmeren Verhältnissen halfen. Wir waren leider sehr gut darin den Kindern die traurige Wahrheit beizubringen. Alexanders Fall war da bei Weitem nicht der Schlimmste. Natürlich abgesehen davon, dass es sich um unsere eigene Familie handelte. Wir wollten es ihm sagen, doch dann… hatte mein Theodor nicht mehr die Gelegenheit dazu.«

Ich kann nicht anders, als ihr stumm zu lauschen. Mir fehlen die Worte.

»Ich war egoistisch, habe nach dem Tod meines

Mannes nicht mehr an den Jungen gedacht, der nun schon wieder ein Familienmitglied verloren hatte. Und als sein Vater ein paar Jahre später ebenfalls plötzlich verstarb, war es zu spät für die Wahrheit. Was hätte es noch genützt, ihm zu sagen, dass sein Vater ein Versager war, der die ganze Familie in den Ruin gestürzt hatte?«

Elli sieht mich aus großen, traurigen Augen an. Ich hole tief Luft und versuche so den Stein, der sich auf meine Brust gelegt hat, zu vertreiben.

»Ich habe ihn zu mir eingeladen. Wir sind die letzten Griffins dieser Linie. Wir sind eine Familie. Ich wollte, dass er bei mir bleibt. Doch er war außer sich vor Wut. Er ließ mir keine Sekunde, um zu erklären. Natürlich, er war mittlerweile ein erwachsener Mann, der in einer Lüge aufgewachsen ist. Wie konnte ich ihm seine Reaktion verübeln? Er muss mich genauso gehasst haben wie sein Vater.«

»Sein Vater hat dich nicht gehasst.«, unterbreche ich sie, in Erinnerung an das, was ihr Neffe mir gestern erzählt hat.

Als Elli mich fragend ansieht, erzähle ich es ihr.

»Er hat von Alexander verlangt, dass er auf dich aufpasst.«

»So?«, stößt sie ungläubig aus, dann lächelt sie.

»Ach herrje, das nenne ich mal ein gewaltiges Schlamassel!«, witzelt sie.

»Weißt du, Kindchen, ich war mir sicher, ich würde dieses Geheimnis mit ins Grab nehmen. Ich dachte, mein Neffe würde mich hassen, weshalb ich keinen Grund mehr hatte, ihn aufzuklären. Jeder Besuch endete im Streit und als er mir plötzlich mit dieser Maren ankam, die alles an sich reißen wollte, da fürchtete ich mich davor, wie weit dieser Mann wohl gehen würde, um seinen Hass auf mich zu befriedigen. Ich habe bis heute Morgen keine Möglichkeit gesehen, diesen Hass zu vertreiben.«

»Willst du noch einmal mit ihm sprechen?«

Elli lächelt vor sich hin, dann sieht sie durch das Küchenfenster in den Garten.

»Jetzt nicht. Er muss diese Nachricht erst einmal verdauen. Aber er wird sich beruhigen. Und vielleicht werden wir dann doch wieder eine Familie.«

»Meinst du er wird jetzt nicht mehr hinter deinem Geld her sein?«

Er mag mir zwar leidtun, aber er war es auch, der Elli loswerden wollte.

»Wer weiß? Aber vielleicht, wenn er die Wahrheit

zulässt, dann wird er erkennen, dass es nicht das Geld ist, was wichtig ist, sondern was du damit tust.«

*

Nach diesem Gespräch muss ich erst einmal etwas runterkommen. Das Chaos in der Küche, wo sich die Teller und Schüsseln von gestern stapeln, kommt mir da gerade recht.

Während ich die Spülmaschine einräume, schweifen meine Gedanken ab. Zu Alexander Griffin, der mir zu Beginn so unheimlich war und der mir jetzt einfach nur noch schrecklich leidtut.

Was er mit Maren, Ellis vorheriger Haushaltshilfe, für Pläne geschmiedet hat, war nicht in Ordnung. Doch wahrscheinlich hat er mittlerweile erkannt, wie aussichtslos dieser Plan war. Er war blind vor Wut.

Bleibt die Frage, was Maren hier erlebt hat, um dem ganzen Geld fluchtartig den Rücken zu kehren?

Ziehe ich die Möglichkeit in Betracht, dass es sich tatsächlich um den Geist von Theodor Griffin handelt?

Ich schüttele den Kopf. Unheimlich und unwahrscheinlich. Zumindest möchte ich sehr gerne glauben, dass es keine Geister gibt.

»Kindchen, da möchte jemand mit dir sprechen.«, sagt Elli hinter mir.

Mit mir? Wer könnte… Callum?

Mein Herz schlägt schneller, ich bin nervös. Ich habe ihn seit unserer kleinen Aussprache nicht mehr gesehen. Wo war er? Was will er mit mir besprechen? Wird er mir jetzt endlich die Wahrheit über sich erzählen?

Ich schlucke, dann führt Elli mich zur Haustür. Warum kommt er nicht einfach rein? Er hat doch einen Schlüssel.

Doch im Rahmen der Tür, erhellt vom strahlenden Licht der Morgensonne, steht nicht Callum, sondern Andrew.

Mir rutscht das Herz in die Hose. Was will der denn hier?

»Hi.«, begrüßt er mich zurückhaltend und hebt dabei leicht die Hand.

Was soll das werden? Runde zwei unserer Diskussion? Ich hatte mich eigentlich schon damit abgefunden, dass ich ihn nie wieder sehen werde.

»Hi.«, antworte ich ebenso zaghaft.

Stille. Dann wirft Andy einen fragenden Blick auf Elli, die mit verschränkten Fingern tippelnd hinter mir steht.

Ein Ruck geht durch ihren Körper.

»Oh! Ihr möchtet allein sprechen. Zu schade. Dann geh ich mal. Bis später, Kindchen.«

Sie zwinkert mir zu und dackelt davon. Ich habe ihr Zeichen verstanden, aber ich kann noch nicht versprechen, ob ich ihr die Einzelheiten des folgenden Gespräches erzählen möchte. Dennoch lässt mich ihre Sensationslust grinsen.

»Können wir reden?«, fragt Andy verlegen.

Ich nicke, schnappe mir den Schlüssel und leite ihn, ohne zu fragen, zu dem Feldweg, den ich auf meinem ersten Spaziergang zum See entdeckt habe. Im Haus würde ich mich eingeengt und vor allem beobachtet fühlen.

Der Mais steht noch immer, ragt über unsere Köpfe. Als die Straße nur noch ein schmaler Strich hinter uns ist, beginne ich zu reden.

»Also, worüber möchtest du sprechen?«

Andy holt Luft, schweigt aber dann doch.

»Okay, dann fange ich an. Es tut mir leid, dass ich nicht ehrlich zu dir war. Ich habe dir falsche Hoffnungen gemacht und unsere Freundschaft riskiert. Ich fühle mich furchtbar deswegen.«

So, es ist raus. Das lief doch ziemlich glatt.

»Ich habe mir selbst falsche Hoffnungen gemacht.«, entgegnet Andy.

Ich will gerade fragen, wie er das meint, da setzt er seine Erklärung schon fort.

»Ich war so lang allein. Du warst wie eine Erlösung für mich. Ich mochte dich vom ersten Moment an. Du hast mich an sie erinnert. Ich wollte es so sehr. Ich hatte gehofft ich könnte mit dir über Lydia hinwegkommen. Ich habe dich benutzt und am Ende habe ich dich auch noch einfach stehen lassen, weil ich so wütend war. Auf dich, ja, aber vor allem auf mich selbst. Das ist mir in den letzten Tagen klar geworden.«

Ich bin sprachlos. Ich hatte mich darauf eingestellt, dass er mir nach allen Regeln des Dramas eine Ansage macht, weil ich bei unserem Date mit fremden Männern Händchen halte. Mit allem hatte ich gerechnet, aber nicht mit so etwas wie einer Entschuldigung.

Hätte ich mir tatsächlich Hoffnungen gemacht, wäre ich nach diesem Geständnis wohl am Boden zerstört. Doch ich kann mein Glück kaum fassen! Ich bleibe stehen und sehe ihm direkt in seine Schokoladenaugen. Ich kann mir gut vorstellen, dass man sich darin verlieren kann. Ich habe keine Worte für ihn. Nichts kann annähernd ausdrücken, wie erleichtert ich bin. Ich liebe ihn. Auf eine ganz eigene Art und Weise.

Also höre ich auf mein Herz, schlinge die Arme um seinen Hals und ziehe ihn in eine feste Umarmung. Andrew versteift sich, anscheinend habe ich ihn überrascht. Als er erkennt, dass ich ihn nicht erwürgen will, kann ich spüren, wie die Anspannung ihn verlässt und er erwidert meine Umarmung. So stehen wir eine ganze Weile da, niemand sagt etwas, wir sind einfach nur glücklich.

Als wir unseren Weg fortsetzen, erzähle ich ihm von meinem Streit mit Liv.

»Ja, davon habe ich gehört.«, teilt Andy mir mit.

Es wundert mich nicht.

»Sie war sehr wütend, oder?«

»Es ist Liv. Sie fährt sehr schnell aus der Haut. Ich kann gar nicht mehr zählen, wie oft wir uns bis aufs Blut gestritten haben. Doch wir haben uns immer wieder vertragen. Sie ist definitiv nicht der Engel, für den manche sie halten.«

Also für einen Engel habe ich sie von Anfang an nicht gehalten. Eine Sache interessiert mich jedoch noch.

»Hast du Liv dazu gebracht, mich vor unserem Date anzurufen?«

Andy stockt dann schüttelt er langsam den Kopf.

»Sie hat dich angerufen?«

Er hat die Augen weit aufgerissen, als er die Frage stellt. Diese Information scheint ihn wirklich zu überraschen.

»Sie wollte wissen, ob ich in dich verliebt bin.«

»Ich gebe ja zu, dass Liv mir gegenüber Andeutungen in diese Richtung gemacht hat. Aber du musst mir glauben, dass ich sie nie beauftragt habe, dich auszufragen. Ich verstehe nur nicht, warum sie das getan hat.«

Ich habe da so eine Idee.

»Andy kann es sein, dass Liv dich mehr mag, als du glaubst?«, äußere ich meine Vermutung.

Andy sieht aus, als hätte ich ihm in den Magen geboxt.

»Das... glaube ich nicht. In all den Jahren hat sie nie irgendwelche Anstalten gemacht. Wobei...«

Er überlegt kurz, dann scheint ihm etwas einzufallen.

»Nach der Sache mit Lydia war sie immer an meiner Seite. Ich dachte, sie wollte mir in dieser Zeit einfach beistehen. Wir haben uns seitdem kaum noch gestritten.

Sie war nie gut auf Lydia zu sprechen und wollte, dass ich aufhöre, sie zu treffen. Doch ich bin immer davon ausgegangen, dass sie sie einfach nicht leiden kann. Meinst du etwa, sie könnte eifersüchtig gewesen sein?«

»Möglich. Vielleicht wollte sie jetzt einfach wissen, wie ernst es mir mit dir ist, um ihre eigenen Chancen abzuschätzen.«

Ich ende mit meinem Verdacht, da erreichen wir wieder die Hauptstraße. Andy sieht in die Ferne auf die versetzt stehenden Häuser.

»Ich muss mit ihr sprechen.«, beschließt er.

Scheint, als wäre heute ein Tag mit klärungsbedarf.

Vorher begleitet er mich allerdings noch bis zur Haustür. Ganz der Gentleman.

Erleichtert schließe ich die Tür hinter mir. Das lief ja wirklich wie geschmiert!

Ich richte meinen Blick nach vorne, da erregt eine Bewegung in meinem linken Augenwinkel meine Aufmerksamkeit. Schuhspitzen ragen am Türrahmen des Wohnzimmers hervor. Ich muss grinsen.

»Ich kann dich sehen, Elli.«, lasse ich sie wissen, woraufhin die alte Dame schuldbewusst um die Ecke getippelt kommt.

»Und? Wie war es? Habt ihr euch geküsst?«, fragt sie geradeheraus.

Ich erröte.

»Elli! Nein, wir haben uns nicht geküsst. Wir sind nur Freunde. Wirklich nur Freunde und zwar einvernehmlich.«, kläre ich sie auf.

Ihr Gesicht scheint vor Enttäuschung zusammenzufallen.

»Oh. Wirklich schade. Der Gute hätte ehrlich ein nettes Mädchen wie dich verdient. Nach allem, was er durchstehen musste.«, erwidert Elli traurig.

Moment, was?

»Woher kennst du denn Andy?«

»Ach, er hat es dir nicht erzählt? Er war doch mit dem Mädchen zusammen, das den Unfall mit dem Feuer hatte.«, berichtet Elli und mir wird schlecht.

»Warte. Soll das heißen seine Lydia ist das Mädchen, das in dem Haus am Ende der Straße fast im Feuer gestorben ist?«

Der Schock schnürt mir die Kehle zu.

Elli nickt.

»Es war schrecklich. Ich habe die beiden oft zusammen gesehen, sie waren sehr glücklich. Doch wie ich hörte, wollte sie nach dem Unfall nichts mehr mit ihm zu tun haben. Eine Schande ist das.«, erzählt sie weiter.

Mein Mund ist trocken. Deshalb wusste er, ohne nachzufragen, wo ich wohne, als er mich nach Hause gefahren hat. Aber warum hat er mir das verschwiegen?

»Kindchen? Ist alles in Ordnung? Lass dich von dem Geschwätz der Leute nicht verrückt machen.«

Ich verstehe nicht.

»Was meinst du damit?«

»Ein Großteil der Leute vermutet, dass Andrew der Schuldige ist. Sie haben sich an dem Abend wohl gestritten und kurz darauf stand das Haus in Flammen. Ich war an jenem Abend nicht anwesend, doch ich habe sehr wohl mitbekommen, wie hartnäckig der Junge versucht hat, den wahren Täter zu fassen. Wenn du mich fragst, war alles ein dummer Zufall.«, erklärt Elli.

Ein dummer Zufall? Möglich, dass Andy mir nichts erzählt hat, weil er nicht wollte, dass auch ich ihn für den Brandstifter halte. Oder weil er vertuschen möchte, was wirklich passiert ist. Ein Schauer läuft mir über den Rücken.

*

Am nächsten Tag habe ich die Informationen, die ich von Elli habe, noch immer nicht verdaut. All diese kleinen Bruchstücke aus Erzählungen scheinen sich nach und nach zu einem großen Bild zusammenzufügen. Wenn ich ehrlich bin, weiß ich nicht, ob ich noch mehr erfahren möchte.

Einzig die Tatsache, dass ich heute wieder für das Mittagessen zuständig bin, hebt meine Laune.

Elli ist zu Mathilde gefahren, um mit ihr den neuesten Klatsch und Tratsch auszutauschen.

Ich würde es zu gerne genießen, etwas allein zu sein und meditativ meine Kartoffeln zu schälen, doch ich höre ein altbekanntes Poltern von draußen. Callum ist hier. Ich versuche mich unsichtbar zu machen. Der Gedanke, noch einmal mit Callum zu sprechen, verursacht mir Magenschmerzen. Zwar würde ich gerne wissen, wo er sich die letzten Tage versteckt hat, doch allein die Vorstellung, unser Gespräch könnte eine unschöne Wendung nehmen, lässt den Stein auf meinem Herzen schwerer werden.

Also bleibe ich mir treu und gehe der Situation aus dem Weg, bis sie mich unausweichlich einholt. Auch wenn ich nahezu eine Stimme flüstern hören kann, die mir sagt, dass ich gefälligst zu ihm gehen soll. Aber das kann sie vergessen! Ich belasse es dabei, mich hinter der Hauswand zu verstecken. Die Stimme soll sich gefälligst in den Wänden zu Theodor Griffins Geist gesellen!

Moment.

In mir wächst etwas. Nur der Hauch eines Gedankens, doch er setzt sich, schlägt Wurzeln und wächst heran, bis die Erkenntnis wie ein gewaltiger Baum vor mir steht.

Ich lege die halb geschälte Kartoffel auf den Rand des Spülbeckens und begebe mich in Theodors Zimmer. Tatsächlich. Es liegt unter dem Zimmer, aus dessen Wand das Schnarchen kam. Ich trete etwas zurück, um die Größe besser einschätzen zu können und stelle fest, dass das kleine Arbeitszimmer genau unter der dicken Wand liegt. Durch diese Erkenntnis bestätigt, gehe ich hinein.

Der alte Schreibtisch steht verlassen wie eh und je am Fenster. Obwohl ich diesen Raum mittlerweile des Öfteren abgestaubt habe, ergreift mich jedes Mal wieder ein Schauer, wenn sich die Erinnerung an mein Gespräch mit Alexander Griffin vor meinem inneren Auge abspielt. Ich hoffe inständig, er lässt Elli in Frieden, nachdem er verstanden hat, dass sein Plan total bescheuert und vor allem sinnlos ist.

Ich beginne das Zimmer abzusuchen. Das Regal mit Büchern links von mir ist zwar verlockend, doch ich habe das Gefühl, dass dort nicht ist, wonach ich suche. Schon allein, weil Alexander es erst vor Kurzem leergefegt hat.

Mein Blick wandert an die Decke. Ich hoffe so etwas wie eine Luke zu finden, doch einzig die Deckenlampe strahlt mir entgegen.

Es zieht mich an die Wand vor mir. Bilder von Elli und Theodor an den verschiedensten Orten dieser Welt strahlen mir entgegen. Auf einem stehen sie neben einem süßen Babyelefanten, auf einem anderen sind sie in einer Wildwasserbahn, wobei Elli begeistert die Arme hochreißt, während ihr Mann ängstlich nach unten sieht. Ich wünschte, ich hätte ihn kennenlernen dürfen. Man kann die beiden regelrecht durch die Bilder lachen hören.

Ich muss mich konzentrieren!

Den Blick von den Bildern abwendend fokussiere ich die dahinter liegende Wand. Taste sie Stück für Stück ab.

Ich kann nichts entdecken, auch mein gelegentliches Klopfen bleibt unbeantwortet. Habe ich mich doch getäuscht? Gut, es wäre auch ziemlich verrückt zu glauben, dass… einen Augenblick!

Da! Ich folge der Linie, an der zwei Tapetenbahnen sich treffen, nach oben. Doch etwa zwanzig Zentimeter bevor sie oben angelangt, verläuft sie horizontal. Kaum zu erkennen, doch wenn man ganz genau hinsieht, ergeben die Linien ein Rechteck, welches groß genug ist, um eine kleine Tür zu sein. Ich klopfe dagegen, doch nichts geschieht. Meine Hände sind schweißnass vor Aufregung. Habe ich hier tatsächlich ein Geheimnis entdeckt? Ich suche die Wand nach einem Schalter ab, kann jedoch nichts finden. Frustriert wende ich mich schon zum Gehen, da drehe ich mich doch noch einmal um und lausche an der Wand. Ich presse mich dagegen, doch ich kann nichts hören. Enttäuscht stoße ich mich ab, woraufhin die Wand zu meinem großen Schrecken unter meinem Gewicht mit einem leisen Klicken nachgibt. Nicht viel, doch genug, um zu erkennen, dass man die ganze Platte eindrücken kann.

Laut nach Luft schnappend weiche ich ein Stück zurück. Das kann doch nicht wahr sein! Ich habe tatsächlich etwas entdeckt! Mein Puls rast, ich stehe wie versteinert da. Soll ich es wagen? Vielleicht gibt es von dem, was ich dort entdecke, kein Zurück mehr…

Ich sammle meinen ganzen Mut und lege beide

Hände auf die Wand.

Sie lässt sich weiter nach innen drücken, ein zweites Klicken folgt, dann kann ich die Platte schließlich zu Seite schieben. Die Öffnung ist gerade groß genug für einen Menschen. Höher als ich groß bin, aber nur gerade so breit wie eine Tapetenbahn. Perfekt getarnt. Ich atme noch einmal tief durch, dann trete ich in die Dunkelheit.

Du kommst mir gefährlich nahe, mein Engel. Ich kann nicht zulassen, dass du mein Geheimnis lüftest! Zu viele sind beteiligt, dabei sollte dies eine Privatvorstellung allein für mich werden! Wage nicht, mich zu verlassen! Ich muss handeln. Schnell. Bevor es mir erneut verwehrt wird, dich zu besitzen.

Wahrheit

Es fällt nicht viel Licht in die kleine Kammer. Ein muffiger Geruch von altem Holz strömt mir entgegen. Ich strecke meinen rechten Arm und berühre so die kahle Wand neben mir.

Doch wirklich interessant ist, was sich links von mir befindet. Eine Leiter wird von schwachem Licht beleuchtet, welches seinen Ursprung darüber zu haben scheint.

Soll ich nachsehen? Was, wenn noch jemand hier ist?

Ob Elli von diesem Raum weiß? Natürlich tut sie das, immerhin ist es ihr Haus. Ich mache mich vermutlich komplett zum Affen.

Also fasse ich mir ein Herz und beginne die Leiter hochzusteigen.

Jetzt erkenne ich die Quelle des Lichtes. Ich befinde mich in einem winzigen Raum von vielleicht zwei Metern Breite. In der Ecke flimmert eine Lampe, deren Schalter ich allerdings nirgends entdecken kann. Die Wände sind mit Holz verkleidet, was diesen Ort noch düsterer macht.

Doch das Erschreckendste an dieser ganzen Sache ist nicht der geheime Raum, auch nicht das schwache Licht, sondern die Tatsache, dass vor mir auf dem Boden eine alte Matratze, ein Kissen und eine Decke liegen.

Irgendjemand wohnt hier.

Panik steigt in mir auf. Also habe ich mir diese Gestalt nicht eingebildet! Wir werden beobachtet und wer weiß, was diese Person mit uns vorhat? Oder weiß Elli etwa davon? Sie war so unbekümmert, als ich ihr von den Geräuschen erzählt habe. Steckt sie hier etwa mit drinnen? Bin ich in Gefahr? Was hat die Stimme aus Theodors Arbeitszimmer durch die Wände geflüstert? Was ließ Maren von hier fliehen?

Ich muss hier raus, muss das alles erst verarbeiten. Da fällt mein Blick auf ein Buch neben der Lampe. Ich kann meine Neugier nicht zügeln und gehe zu ihm hinüber, um einen Blick hinein zu werfen. Roter Stoff ist um die Buchdeckel gespannt.

»Geheimnisse der Natur – Band 6« ist in goldenen Lettern vorne aufgedruckt. Ich kenne diese Art von Buch. Die restlichen Ausgaben stehen unten in Theodors Bücherregal. Mit meinem Daumen lasse ich die Seiten schnell durchblättern, als etwas aus dem Buch fällt.

Ich halte es zunächst für ein Stück Papier, doch als ich es aufhebe und im schwachen Licht betrachte, stockt mir der Atem. In meiner Hand halte ich, gepresst und getrocknet, eine einzelne gelbe Nelke.

Ich verstehe nichts von Blumen, doch diese eine kenne ich, als wäre sie ein Teil von mir. Genauso wie er ein Teil von mir ist. Was hat das alles zu bedeuten?

»Deliah!«, ruft Callum erschrocken meinen Namen, als er mich hier oben stehen sieht.

Mitten in seinem Versteck.

Ich lasse die Blume fallen, sie segelt genüsslich zu Boden, sie hat keinen Grund, sich zu beeilen. Auch ich habe das Gefühl, die Zeit würde stillstehen. Was soll ich tun? Ich weiß nicht, wie ich reagieren soll. Callum hat sich hier ein Versteck gebaut. Doch wozu? Ist er etwa gar nicht der Engel, für den ich ihn gehalten habe? Ist er letztendlich… der Teufel?

Er macht einen Schritt auf mich zu, ich weiche so weit zurück, wie es der winzige Raum zulässt. Die Wände scheinen näher zu kommen.

Callum hebt beschwichtigend die Hände.

»Ich werde dir nicht wehtun, Deliah.«, beschwört er

mich.

Das würde jetzt ja wohl jeder sagen! Mein Herz fühlt sich an, als würde es zerrissen werden.

Das ist Callum! Der Mann, in den ich verliebt bin! Das ist sein Geheimnis. Wie viel von diesem Geheimnis ist mir noch verborgen und wie schlimm ist dieser Teil?

Tränen rinnen über meine Wangen. Der Schmerz ist unerträglich. Ich erschaudere vor dem, was ich entdeckt habe und welche Geschichte dahintersteckt.

»Lass es mich erklären, Deliah.«, redet er auf mich ein und kommt näher.

»Bleib da stehen! Keinen Schritt weiter!«, schreie ich ihm entgegen, doch er schüttelt kaum merklich den Kopf.

»Callum hör auf!«, flehe ich ihn an.

Ich fürchte mich vor ihm und es bricht mir das Herz. Meine Augen brennen, Verzweiflung droht mich zu übermannen. Nicht, weil ich hilflos bin, sondern weil ich nicht glauben möchte, dass Callum der Böse hierbei ist.

Als er noch immer nicht stehen bleibt, habe ich keine andere Wahl. Meine Tränen haben ihm den Eindruck vermittelt, dass ich schwach wäre, weshalb ich ihn überrumpele, als ich ihm mit voller Wucht das dicke Sachbuch ins Gesicht werfe.

Ein schmerzerfüllter Schrei ist mein Zeitfenster, in dem ich an ihm vorbei husche.

Die Leiter wirkt länger als vorher. Ich muss aufpassen, dass ich in der Hast nicht eine Sprosse übersehe. Genau genommen kann ich überhaupt nichts sehen.

Die Tür! Callum muss sie geschlossen haben!

Panisch taste ich die Wand ab, drücke, schiebe, doch es regt sich nichts. Verzweifelt hämmere ich dagegen in der Hoffnung, dass Elli zurück ist und mich hier rausholt.

Da greifen starke Hände um meine Handgelenke. Ein fester Griff hält mich gefangen.

»Lass mich los!«, kreische ich, während ich versuche mich zu befreien, wobei ich mir nur selbst wehzutun scheine.

»Deliah, bitte beruhige dich! Ich tue dir nichts!«, redet Callum ruhig auf mich ein.

Ich kann nicht mehr. Er ist zu stark, ich kann mich nicht befreien.

»Was hast du jetzt vor?«, schluchze ich.

Wenn Elli nichts von diesem Raum weiß, wird nie jemand meine Leiche finden. Meine Eltern werden daran zerbrechen. Warum konnte ich nicht einfach den Rest meines Lebens im »A Tavola« bleiben?

»Bitte hör auf zu weinen. Ich will wirklich nur mit dir sprechen. Sieh her.«, beschwört Callum mich mit sanfter Stimme, dann greift er über mich, zieht an einer Art Griff, den ich vorher nicht bemerkt habe und öffnet die Tür.

»Du kannst gehen. Lass es mich erklären oder lass mich zurück, es ist deine Entscheidung. Aber bitte hab keine Angst vor mir.«

Mit diesen Worten lässt er meine andere Hand auch noch los und ich bin frei. Und jetzt? Ich muss raus. Raus aus diesem unwirklichen Raum.

Callum folgt mir. Jedoch mit Abstand.

»Bitte Deliah.«, versucht er mich zurück zu locken.

An der Haustür lehne ich mich an das Geländer. Hier sind doch alle verrückt! Ich will nach Hause! Jetzt!

Ich zerre meine Turnschuhe aus dem hölzernen Schuhschrank.

»Deliah, bitte lauf nicht weg.«

Doch ich kann ihm nicht antworten. Ich bin durcheinander. Ich will das alles nicht mehr. Ein Griff an das Brett neben mir und ich halte meinen Autoschlüssel in der Hand.

»Bitte verlass mich nicht.«, flüstert Callum hinter mir und ich erstarre.

Es ist, als hätte der Blitz in mein Herz eingeschlagen.

Meine Hand schwebt über dem Türgriff, meine Gedanken stehen still.

»Sieh mich an Deliah.«, beginnt er erneut.

Seine Stimme ist zittrig, als würde es ihm die Kehle zuschnüren.

Ich drehe mich um und erblicke einen gebrochenen Mann. Kein Zeichen mehr von seiner stolzen, aufrechten Haltung. Die Haare hängen wild ins Gesicht, sein Atem geht kurz und flach.

So stehen wir da und schweigen uns an, während tausend Worte zwischen uns stehen. Ich ertrage das nicht mehr. Ich will weg.

Da fällt sein Blick hinter mich, wo kurz darauf ein Schlüssel im Schloss zu hören ist.

Elli betritt das Haus.

»Ich bin wieder zurück, Kindch… oh!«, unterbricht sie ihre Begrüßung, als sie uns erblickt.

»Was ist denn hier los?«, fragt sie verwirrt.

Callum schweigt, sieht mir einfach in die Augen. Sein Blick fleht nicht, fordert nicht, sondern wartet einfach auf meine Antwort. Wie damals beim Stadtfest. Er ergibt sich. Ich habe es in der Hand. Lasse ich ihn auffliegen, ohne seine Geschichte zu kennen? Oder halte ich meine Entdeckung geheim und riskiere doch in eine Falle gelockt zu werden? Ich suche in seinem Gesicht nach der Wahrheit, doch ich kann kein Zeichen erkennen. Keine Regung von ihm verrät mir, was ich tun soll. Er steht einfach vor mir und wartet ab, ob ich ihm den Todesstoß gebe.

Dann antworte ich.

»Nichts. Hier ist alles in Ordnung.«

Keine Ahnung, ob Elli mir glaubt, zumindest fragt sie nicht weiter nach und geht in die Küche.

Callum starrt auf den Boden vor meinen Füßen. Es scheint, als hätte er eine andere Antwort erwartet. Stille breitet sich zwischen uns aus, legt sich um meinen Hals. Ich weiß nicht, was ich sagen oder tun soll. Ich habe Fragen, doch bin mir nicht sicher, ob ich die Antwort wissen möchte.

Callum bricht die Anspannung, indem er sich umdreht und geht.

Ich kann die Hintertür hören, er ist in den Garten gegangen.

Und jetzt? Dieses Thema ist noch nicht vom Tisch, doch ich bin Callum dankbar für seine Reaktion. Ich muss mich erst beruhigen, bevor ich mit ihm darüber sprechen kann und hoffe, ich habe keinen Fehler begangen, indem ich ihn vor Elli gedeckt habe.

Ich stürze mich in Arbeit, um nicht weiter darüber nachdenken zu müssen, doch mein Plan scheitert.

Natürlich hat sich der Vorfall in der versteckten Kammer in meinen Kopf eingenistet und dreht sich dort wie ein Karussell. Ich habe das Gefühl, mein Leben findet nur noch in meinen Grübeleien statt.

Dieses Geheimnis erklärt so viel. Die koketten Formulierungen auf der einen und diese plötzliche Kälte auf der anderen Seite. Ich war ihm zu nah. Hätte sein Geheimnis aufgedeckt. Zumindest diesen Teil davon. Wollte er es mir offenbaren, als er plötzlich auf dem Stadtfest aufgetaucht ist? Hatte er damals beschlossen, mir zu vertrauen?

Da erinnere ich mich plötzlich an das Mädchen und die unheilvolle Warnung, die sie ausgesprochen hatte. Mit einem Mal wird mir klar, wer dieses Mädchen war. Lydia. Das Mädchen, das das Feuer nur knapp überlebt hatte. Das Feuer, dessen Ursache noch immer ein Mysterium ist. Ist es das? Ist das dein Geheimnis, Callum? Aber was hätte das mit seinem Versteck hier zu tun?

Wie dem auch sei, es gibt nur eine Möglichkeit, die Wahrheit zu erfahren.

Den ganzen Nachmittag hatte mein Herz so laut geklopft, dass ich fürchtete, es würde aus meiner Brust springen. Ich habe Angst vor diesem Moment und dem, was er offenbart. Doch ich muss stark sein. Meinen Weg gehen, wie Elli es gesagt hat. Dazu gehört eben auch Mut und Mut bedeutet Dinge zu tun, obwohl man Angst vor ihnen hat.

Es ist still im Haus. Alle Lichter sind gelöscht. Da ich jetzt weiß, worauf ich achten muss, habe ich mich auf die Lauer gelegt und den Moment mitbekommen, in dem Callum sein nicht mehr ganz so geheimes Versteck betreten hat. Ob er ahnt, dass ich ihn beobachte? Kurz hatte ich befürchtet, er würde seine Sachen packen und verschwinden, doch das ist jetzt eine Stunde her.

Ich lege meine Hände auf die unsichtbare Tür und drücke dagegen. Diesmal fällt es mir leichter, sie zu bedienen, da ich weiß, worauf ich achten muss. Ich trete ein, erkenne sofort die Leiter im warmweißen Schein der Lampe.

»Callum?«, frage ich flüsternd.

Ich weiß nicht einmal, warum ich flüstere. Elli wird sicher nicht aufwachen. Etwas in mir scheint einfach zu hoffen, dass das alles nicht wahr ist.

»Deliah?«, dringt es verblüfft zu mir herunter, gefolgt von einem Lockenkopf über mir.

»Was machst du... wieso bist du...?«, stammelt er mir entgegen, doch ich lasse ihn nicht zu Wort kommen.

»Du schuldest mir eine Erklärung. Ich bin hier, um sie zu hören.«

Callum sitzt auf seinem improvisierten Bett. Er ist wie versteinert, als ich die Leiter nach oben steige. Fürchtet er sich, die Wahrheit auszusprechen? Dabei bin ich es doch, der die Knie schlottern, als ich die Stufen zu diesem Mann erklimme, der mir vielleicht doch noch etwas antun möchte. Ich habe mir den ganzen Tag über die wildesten Geschichten ausgemalt, die all das hier erklären würden, doch letztendlich kann mich nur die Wahrheit von meiner Grübelei erlösen.

Die Hände in die Hüften gestemmt, stehe ich vor ihm.

»Also. Rede!«, fordere ich ihn auf.

Ich höre mich stärker an, als ich bin.

»Sind wir hier bei einem Verhör? Setz dich doch bitte

hin, du machst mich ganz nervös.«, bittet Callum, doch ich schüttele nur langsam den Kopf und nicke ihm dann auffordernd zu, damit er zu erzählen beginnt.

Noch vor ein paar Stunden hätte ich mich am liebsten auf seinen Schoß gesetzt.

Schweigen.

Warum zögert er? Was hat er noch zu verheimlichen? Nachdrücklich hebe ich die Augenbrauen, woraufhin er tief Luft holt.

»Wo soll ich anfangen?«, richtet er sich an mich.

»Warum versteckst du dich hier?«, frage ich härter, als ich wollte.

Diese winzige Furcht, dass er sich auf mich stürzen und verletzen könnte, sitzt wie ein Dämon neben mir. Wobei eine kleine Verletzung meine geringste Sorge ist, sollte mein Verdacht mit Lydia und dem Feuer sich bestätigen.

»Von Anfang an also.«, erwidert Callum, dann atmet er tief durch und beginnt mit seiner Geschichte.

»Meine Mutter war krank, mein Vater ein Säufer. Klingt sehr nach Klischee, ich weiß, aber so war es nun einmal. Sie starb, als ich sechzehn war. Der einzige Halt in meinem Leben, von heute auf morgen, einfach weg.

Zurückgelassen mit einem Menschen, der mich am liebsten tot gesehen hätte, waren die nächsten zwei Jahre die Hölle für mich.

Am Tag meines Abschlusses hat er mich in mein Zimmer eingesperrt. Ich würde ihn nur unnötig Geld kosten, außerdem sei ich viel zu verkommen, um je einen vernünftigen Job zu bekommen. Ich glaube, er hatte einfach Angst, dass ich ihn verlassen würde, da der Alkohol bereits seine Spuren an ihm hinterlassen hatte. Dieser Typ brauchte nur jemanden, der sich um ihn kümmerte, wenn er im Suff nicht einmal mehr nach Hause fand.

Ich konnte mich an jenem Tag aus dem Haus schleichen, was mir eine Tracht Prügel einbrachte. Doch anstatt es wie sonst einfach über mich ergehen zu lassen, habe ich mich gewehrt. Habe ihm seine scheiß Bierflasche gegen den Schädel geschlagen. Danach bin ich abgehauen. Ziellos in der Gegend umhergeirrt. Zwei Nächte habe ich im Freien geschlafen. Ich wollte auf keinen Fall zu ihm zurück.

Ich weiß nicht, warum ich nie die Polizei gerufen habe. Vielleicht aus Angst, was aus mir werden würde. Oder aus dem abstrusen Gefühl heraus, meine Familie nicht verraten zu dürfen.

Wie dem auch sei, ohne Geld und ohne richtige Unterkunft war es doch sehr schwer, zurecht zu kommen. Also bin ich doch zurückgegangen. Ich hatte vor, ihn einfach rauszuschmeißen.

Was ich dort allerdings vorfand, war das absolute Chaos. Alles war verwüstet. Scherben auf dem Boden, Flecken an der Wand. Lampen von der Decke gerissen, es roch nach Urin und Erbrochenem.

Mein Erzeuger? Keine Spur von ihm. Ich weiß bis heute nicht, wo er ist. Vielleicht ist er auch schon tot. Ich war verzweifelt. Da fiel mir eine Person ein, die immer nett zu mir gewesen war. Ich kannte sie aus der Schule, da sie mit ihrem Mann immer wieder wohltätige Organisationen unterstützt hatte. Eleonore Griffin.

Ich beschloss, zu ihr zu gehen, um Hilfe zu bitten und vielleicht würde ich sogar etwas zu essen bekommen.

Doch als ich ankam, war das Haus leer. Eleonore und Theodor waren wieder einmal auf Reisen. Es sollte ihre letzte Gemeinsame sein, wie ich später schmerzlich erfahren habe. Ich war schon im Begriff zu gehen, da hörte ich ein Geräusch. Es klang wie das Knarzen einer Tür. Ich schlich um das Haus herum und tatsächlich war ein Fenster nicht richtig geschlossen worden.

Mein Glückstag!

Ich überlegte nicht lange und stieg ein. Ich würde verschwinden, sobald die Griffins zurückkämen. Erst einmal einen klaren Kopf bekommen.

Die Tage vergingen und ich begann mich umzusehen.

Die Bücher im Arbeitszimmer von Theodor zogen mich nahezu magisch an. Ich sog alles in mich auf, meine Leidenschaft für die Natur war geweckt.

Auf dieses Geheimzimmer stieß ich, wie du, nur zufällig. Ich hatte nie die Absicht, mich hier zu verstecken. Schon gar nicht über Jahre hinweg.

Doch als Elli zurückkam, war alles anders. Sie und ihr Mann hatten einen Autounfall gehabt. Er war sofort tot.

Ich konnte doch nicht zu einer Frau gehen, deren Leben gerade zutiefst erschüttert wurde und sie um Asyl bitten. Also beschloss ich, mich hier zu verstecken und als Gegenleistung machte ich ihr kleine Freuden. Ich habe alle Menschen gemieden, die mich kannten. Zu meinem Glück hatte ich nie wirklich Freunde. Keiner hat mich vermisst.

Eines Nachts begann ich Zimtkekse für Elli zu backen und am nächsten Morgen habe ich mich rausgeschlichen, an der Haustür geklingelt und sie ihr übergeben. Irgendwann fing ich an, den Garten herzurichten. Theodor hatte das früher immer gemacht, weshalb er mittlerweile recht verwildert war. Elli schien es zu gefallen und so ging es einfach weiter. Irgendwann ist die Zeit einfach verflogen. Ich hatte nicht mehr das Bedürfnis, ihr die Wahrheit zu sagen, denn zum ersten Mal in meinem Leben spürte ich Frieden.«

Als er mit seiner Geschichte endet, bemerke ich die Tränen, die mir die Wangen hinunterrinnen. Das soll ich ihm glauben?

»Du bist hier überhaupt nicht angestellt? Und wie verdienst du dann dein Geld?«, frage ich skeptisch.

»Gar nicht. Ich habe hier alles, was ich brauche. Essen, Trinken, ein Bad, einen Schlafplatz und eine Beschäftigung. Elli steckt mir ab und an einmal etwas zu, wovon ich mir Kleidung kaufe. Ich habe mir nur ein einziges Mal Geld von ihr genommen.«

Da fällt es mir wieder ein.

»Du! Du hast das Geld vom Tisch gestohlen!«

»Es war wichtig.«, verteidigt er sich.

»Oh bitte, was kann so wichtig sein, dass man eine alte Frau bestiehlt?«

»Ich brauchte es für einen besonderen Anlass. Zu meinem Bedauern kam es nie dazu. Doch letztendlich hat es einen ähnlichen Zweck erfüllt. Mit diesem Geld konnte ich an jenem Abend in die Stadt kommen. Um bei dir zu sein.«

Die Erkenntnis trifft mich wie ein Faustschlag in den Magen. Das Sommerfest! Er sagte damals, er würde in der Stadt wohnen. Er wollte bei mir sein?

Meine Furcht verflüchtigt sich und ich beginne über seine Geschichte nachzudenken. Ich kann mir nicht vorstellen, wie er gelitten haben muss. Dass er den Mut hatte, in seiner Verzweiflung in ein fremdes Haus einzubrechen. Hätte ich es genauso gemacht? Keine Ahnung. Ich bin völlig anders aufgewachsen, ich kann es nicht einmal ansatzweise nachvollziehen.

»Bitte sag doch etwas.«, flüstert Callum.

Doch ich schweige. Keine Worte können beschreiben, was in mir vorgeht. Es könnte eine Falle sein.

Ein Teil von mir zweifelt, glaubt ihm kein Wort und flüstert, ich solle davonlaufen. Ein anderer Teil jedoch sieht die Wahrheit und die Verzweiflung in seinen Augen. Dieser ist stärker.

Langsam nähere ich mich ihm wie ein scheues Reh.

»Du hast Maren verjagt, indem du sie glauben ließest, sie würde Geister hören, habe ich recht?«

Er nickt.

»Ich konnte nicht zulassen, dass sie ihren Plan durchzieht. Das hier ist mein Zuhause. Elli ist meine Familie.«

Ich komme näher zu ihm.

»Du lässt Elli seit Jahren glauben und hoffen, dass sie ihren toten Mann hört.«

Näher.

»Du hast mich beim Schlafen beobachtet.«

Ich bin direkt vor ihm und knie mich ihm gegenüber auf den Boden.

»Und du hast mich belogen. Immer wieder. Warum sollte ich dir noch trauen?«

Ich sehe ihm direkt in die Augen.

Er erwidert meinen Blick.

»Weil ich dir nie etwas angetan habe. Und weil du Licht in meine dunkle Welt gebracht hast. Weil ich dich brauche.«, antwortet er mit einer solchen Wahrhaftigkeit, die mich dahinschmelzen lässt.

Ich will etwas erwidern, doch er kommt mir zuvor, beugt sich zu mir und küsst mich.

Ich bin wie versteinert, doch nach und nach gebe ich mich ihm hin, bis ich den Kuss schließlich erwidere.

»Ich wollte dich nie verletzen!«, flüstert er an meine Stirn gelehnt, »Und ich wollte dich nie belügen.«

»Was ist das zwischen uns?«, flüstere ich meine Frage.

Wir kennen uns kaum, sind uns eigentlich fremd und doch scheinen wir uns immer wieder anzuziehen. So, wie er es an meinem ersten Tag hier zu mir gesagt hat.

»Ich weiß es nicht.«, antwortet Callum, »Doch was immer es ist, es ist das Schönste und Wahrhaftigste, was ich je gefühlt habe. Ich wusste nicht, dass mir etwas fehlt, bis ich dich im Garten stehen sah. Ich wusste nicht, dass ich jemanden so begehren könnte, bis du mit deinem tonnenschweren Koffer durch die Tür kamst.

Ja, ich war einmal bei dir. Nachts. Du warst so eiskalt zu mir. Ich musste einfach in deiner Nähe sein. In dieser Nacht wollte ich mit dir sprechen, wollte es dir erzählen, deshalb stand ich an deinem Bett, als du aufgewacht bist. Doch dann hat mich der Mut verlassen.«, erklärt er, während er seine Finger eng mit meinen umschlingt.

Atemlos sehe ich ihm tief in die Augen. Ich bin so erleichtert, dass sein Geheimnis nun nicht mehr zwischen uns steht. Jetzt ist es an mir, ehrlich zu sein.

»Ich war zu feige, um dir zu zeigen, wie sehr ich dich mag. Ich war auch nicht ehrlich zu dir. Ich war nicht besser als du. Ich war vielleicht sogar schlechter. Du hast zwar das Date zerstört, aber wenn ich ehrlich bin, hatte Andy auch keine Chance. Ich war das Monster in dieser Szene.«, gestehe ich mir ein.

»Nein. Nein, das warst du nicht. Du warst einfach nur hilflos während du versucht hast das Richtige zu tun.«, tröstet er mich.

»Du scheinst mich wirklich beobachtet zu haben.«, witzele ich.

Ein vorsichtiges Lächeln stiehlt sich auf sein Gesicht.

»Nur ein wenig. Aber eines muss ich klarstellen. Ich habe dein Date neulich nicht zerstört. Ich habe an jenem Abend lediglich eine offene Tür eingerannt.«

Und wie er das hat!

Wir umarmen uns, küssen uns erneut, werden eins.

Diese Geschichte scheint doch noch ein Happy End zu haben.

Du treibst mich in die Enge, mein teuflischer Engel. Unangenehme Fragen über mich, das dulde ich nicht mehr! Niemand darf sich mehr einmischen! Die Zeit ist reif! Ich muss meinen Plan vollenden, bevor du mir entgleitest! Die Zeit ist gekommen!

Flammen

Es ist zu schön, um wahr zu sein! Ich fühle mich noch immer, als wäre ich auf Wolke sieben.

Callum und ich haben beschlossen, mit Elli zu sprechen. Er kann sein Leben nicht zwischen den Wänden verbringen. Außerdem ist er jetzt nicht mehr allein. Gemeinsam werden wir unseren Weg gehen.

Ich wünschte, ich könnte jetzt bei ihm sein, doch die letzte Nacht hat uns schmerzlich gezeigt, wie klein dieser Raum wirklich ist. Also liege ich heute allein in meinem Bett, mit dem Wissen, dass der Mann meines Herzens wenige Meter entfernt ist. Allein das ist Grund genug, um mit Elli zu reden und ihn endlich aus dieser Kammer zu befreien. Jetzt kann es nur noch besser werden! Nach all der Zeit scheine ich endlich eine Art inneren Frieden gefunden zu haben. Mit den Gedanken bei Callum gleite ich schließlich in einen traumlosen Schlaf.

Ich erwache durch ein Poltern. Etwas scheint auf den Boden gefallen zu sein. Ich öffne die Augen und sehe... nichts.

Völlige Schwärze.

Was ist mit meinen Augen? Warum kann ich nichts sehen? Als der Schlaf sich schlagartig verflüchtigt, erkenne ich, dass ich eine Augenbinde trage.

Ich höre jemanden atmen. Callum? Was ist hier los?

Ich will aufstehen, doch meine Füße sind gefesselt. Ebenso meine Hände hinter meinem Rücken. Hat er mich etwa belogen? Bin ich ihm in die Falle gegangen?

Mir ist, als hätte jemand einen Dolch in mein Herz gestoßen.

»Callum? Callum bitte!«, flehe ich, doch ich bekomme keine Antwort.

Nur ein scheinbar amüsiertes Schnauben.

Lacht er etwa über mich? Was soll ich nur tun? Um Hilfe rufen? Was sollte Elli schon gegen ihn ausrichten? Wenn es ihr denn gut geht. Oh Gott!

»Bitte! Mach mich los! Bist du so feige, dass du mir nicht einmal in die Augen sehen kannst?«, schreie ich ihn an.

Was darauf folgt, ist ein stechender Schmerz in meiner

Wange, der meinen Kopf zur Seite wirft. Er hat mich geschlagen!

»Du elender Scheißkerl!«, wimmere ich.

Mein Herz zerspringt in tausend Teile. Wie konnte ich auch so dämlich sein und dem Mann vertrauen, der sich seit Jahren in einem fremden Haus versteckt?

Bestimmt ist seine ganze Geschichte gelogen! Was hat er jetzt mit mir vor?

Ich höre, wie die Tür aufgestoßen wird.

»Was ist hier los? Du?«, kann ich Callums entsetzte Stimme hören.

Moment, wenn er es ist, der gerade hereingekommen ist, wer ist dann noch hier? Wer hat mich gefesselt?

Lautes Klopfen und Poltern lässt mich darauf schließen, dass ein Kampf begonnen hat. Ich versuche irgendwie meine Fesseln zu lösen, doch keine Chance, sie sind zu fest.

Ich höre ein Summen, spüre die Vibration neben mir. Mein Handy!

Ich robbe an den Rand meines Bettes. Wer auch immer mich gefesselt hat, er war nicht schlau genug, mir mein Handy wegzunehmen, welches auf dem Schränkchen neben meinem Bett steht. Blind taste ich nach der Kante, wobei ich mir fast die Schulter auskugele. Immer wieder greife ich ins Leere, doch dann kann ich es endlich fühlen. Panisch versuche ich auf dem Display herum zu wischen, um den Anruf anzunehmen.

Ich werde immer zittriger, da meldet sich endlich eine Stimme.

Leise, ich muss mich konzentrieren, um das Gesagte zu verstehen. Das Poltern des Kampfes hat sich entfernt, trotzdem muss ich genau hinhören. Ich wage nicht blind die Lautsprecher Taste zu suchen und vielleicht meine einzige Chance auf Hilfe zu vermasseln.

»Deliah? Ich weiß, es ist spät, aber ich muss unbedingt mit dir sprechen. Ich glaube, du hattest recht. Es geht um Liv. Sie ist nach unserem Gespräch völlig ausgeflippt.«, berichtet Andy.

»Hilf mir! Hilf mir!«, schreie ich und hoffe, er hat mich aus der Entfernung gehört.

Ein Ton verrät mir, dass jemand aufgelegt hat. Da ich nicht befreit werde, kann es nicht Callum sein. Sofort schießen mir Tränen in die Augen.

»Was hast du mit ihm gemacht?«, will ich wissen.

Es muss etwas passiert sein. Er würde mich nie hier zurücklassen.

Ein Stechen fährt an meinem nackten Bein entlang, als würde jemand die Flamme eines Feuerzeuges darüberstreichen lassen. Ich rieche brennende Kerzen. Es müssen einige sein, denn der Geruch ist sehr penetrant.

»Was willst du von mir?«, frage ich mit zitternder Stimme.

Ein unterdrücktes Lachen folgt meiner Frage.

»Ich wünschte wirklich, wir könnten das alles mehr genießen. Doch die Zeit drängt.«, sagt mein Peiniger mit einer mir sehr gut bekannten Stimme.

»Liv?«, stoße ich schockiert aus.

Da wird mir die Augenbinde heruntergerissen und ich sehe sie komplett nackt vor mir stehen.

»Was zum Teufel, Liv?«

»Pscht.«, sagt sie, während sie den Finger vor ihre Lippen hält.

»Kein Grund aggressiv zu werden, mein Engel. Du solltest dich freuen! Ich habe dich auserwählt. Du wirst erblühen in der Flamme meiner Liebe und wenn du gänzlich zerflossen bist, werde ich dich in mir aufnehmen. So werden wir für immer vereint sein.«

»Du willst *was* mit mir machen?«, frage ich schockiert.

»Dich in Flammen aufgehen lassen, meine Schöne.«, erklärt Liv, als wäre es das Normalste der Welt.

Eiskalte Furcht ergreift mich. Sie wird mich töten!

»Warum?«

Panisch suche ich den Raum nach einer Möglichkeit ab, mich zu befreien.

Liv lacht.

»Na, weil du mein Engel bist, Dummerchen. Ich dachte vor einigen Jahren, es wäre Lydia. Doch, oh, wie ich mich getäuscht habe! Sie hatte nicht annähernd deine Perfektion! Sie ist so schwach! Erst hat sie aus Angst vor mir die Beziehung zu Andy beendet und dann hat sie mich nicht einmal an die Polizei verraten, obwohl ich sie fast getötet hätte! Damals hielt ich es noch für eine fürchterliche Schande, dass dein blonder Vollidiot so lange Steine an ihr Fenster geworfen hatte, bis sie aufgewacht ist. Danach hatte ich keine Zeit, mein Werk richtig zu vollenden, doch ich dachte, es würde reichen. Dieser Scheißkerl war es auch, der die Feuerwehr gerufen hat. Dass ich ihm hier wieder begegne und mich endlich rächen kann, ist eine wunderbare Genugtuung für mich. Er hat mich damals nicht erkannt, doch ich habe mir sein dämliches Gesicht genau eingeprägt. Nach all der Zeit, in der ich nach ihm suchte und er mir doch verborgen blieb, ist es wahrlich Schicksal, dass wir uns hier treffen.«, erzählt Liv, während sie wie in Trance weitere Kerzen anzündet.

Ich kann es nicht fassen. Natürlich! Der Brand, in dem Lydia fast gestorben wäre, ist passiert, als Elli und Theodore auf ihrer letzten Reise waren. Callum hat damals schon hier gelebt und konnte alles mitansehen. Er hat Lydia das Leben gerettet. Und Lydia wollte mich auf dem Sommerfest vor Liv warnen. Liv, die an jenem Abend so plötzlich aufgetaucht ist. Sie war der Grund für Lydias Flucht. Sie muss wahnsinnige Angst haben, dass Liv ihr Vorhaben von damals beenden könnte.

»Wie bist du hier reingekommen?«, will ich wissen.

Ich brauche einen Plan!

»Wenn man das Haus gut kennt, ist es ein Leichtes sich ein Hintertürchen offenzulassen.«, antwortet sie mit überheblichem Grinsen.

»Wieso kennst du das Haus?«, frage ich verblüfft.

Liv beugt sich zu mir, ein breites, schon fast wahnsinniges Lächeln auf den Lippen.

»Na, weil wir Nachbarn sind.«

Ich bin sprachlos. Wie bitte? Aber, dann hätte ich sie

doch bemerkt. Wobei, ich habe nie wirklich darauf geachtet, wer in den anderen Häusern lebt, auch wenn ich einige Leute gesehen habe.

»Einmal hättest du mich fast erwischt. Als du das abgebrannte Haus inspiziert hast. Ich wäre dir fast über den Weg gelaufen, doch ich konnte mich noch verstecken. Fast hättest du mir mein Vorhaben um einiges erschwert. Ein Glück, dass du dich so zu diesem Garten hingezogen fühlst. Hinter den Büschen war es so viel einfacher, dich zu beobachten, als durch dein Fenster zu klettern.«, erzählt Liv und mir dreht sich der Magen um bei dem Gedanken daran, dass ich die ganze Zeit über von ihr beobachtet wurde.

Wie leicht sie es hatte. Wie unbekümmert ich war, während sich hinter meinem Rücken ein Sturm zusammenbraute.

Die Luft wird immer schlechter, ich muss husten.

»Was stimmt nicht mit dir?«, röchele ich.

Sie dreht sich langsam zu mir.

»Was mit mir nicht stimmt? Oh, nein, nein, nein. Du stellst die falschen Fragen, mein Engel! Was stimmt nicht mit der Welt? Du wirst allein in diese Welt geworfen und sollst bestehen. Eine Welt, in der Mord, Gewalt und Tod an der Tagesordnung stehen. Ich bin in Furcht vor dieser Welt aufgewachsen! Ich habe gebetet, zu einem Engel habe ich gebetet, dass er mich beschützen möge. Doch jeder, der kam, hat mich eines Tages wieder verlassen. Das hier!«, sie macht eine umfassende Bewegung, »Das hier ist der einzige Weg dich, mein Engel, der du mir erschienen bist, in mir aufzunehmen und für immer zu behalten! Ich werde nie wieder allein sein!«

Die Augen weit aufgerissen, starrt sie mich an.

»Gewalt, Mord, Tod. Genau das ist es doch, was du mir antust! Wie kannst du dich dagegen aussprechen und doch selbst dazu beitragen?«, konfrontiere ich sie.

Sie stockt. Kurz hoffe ich, sie zur Besinnung gebracht zu haben, doch weit gefehlt. Ich habe sie gereizt. Mit einer schwungvollen Bewegung holt sie aus und schlägt mir erneut ins Gesicht.

»Das ist nicht das Gleiche!«, schreit sie mich an.

»Ich erlöse dich, mein Engel! Es dient dem Guten! Genau wie das Vieh, das zur Schlachtung geführt wird, um die Hungrigen zu nähren!«

Sie erhebt ihre Stimme, als würde sie vor Hunderten predigen. Wie kann diese selbstsichere Frau, die ein eigenes Café führt, nur so eine Schattenseite haben? Ich habe keinen Fluchtplan, ich weiß nicht, wo Callum ist, ob er noch lebt und ich habe keine Ahnung, ob Andy meinen Hilferuf überhaupt wahrgenommen hat. Ich bin am Ende.

»Nun denn, lass uns beginnen.«, sagt Liv, dann kommt sie mit einer Kerze zu mir und steckt mein Bett in Brand.

Die Flamme nährt sich von dem Stoff, verzehrt sich nach mehr. Die Hitze lässt die Stelle brennen, an der Liv mich mit dem Feuerzeug verbrannt hat. Tränen der Verzweiflung steigen in mir auf.

Doch ich darf nicht aufgeben, ich muss kämpfen!

Da bemerke ich eine Bewegung hinter Liv. Callum?

»Warte!«, rufe ich.

Liv stoppt.

»Letzte Worte, mein Engel?«, fragt sie mit einem so zuckersüßen Grinsen, dass mir schlecht wird.

Was soll ich nur tun?

»Bitte, ich habe noch einen letzten Wunsch!«, flehe ich sie an.

Ich muss überlegen. Was kann ich verlangen, um diese Wahnsinnige abzulenken? Um ein Glas Wasser bitten? Denk nach Deliah oder du wirst hier sterben!

»Sprich!«, fordert Liv mich auf.

Ich atme flach und hektisch. Ein Wunsch, etwas, das

sie mir gern erfüllen wird und zwar bevor diese Flamme mich erreicht hat.

»Ein Kuss. Küss mich!«, spreche ich meine Bitte aus.

Das muss als Ablenkung doch wohl reichen, auch wenn mir allein bei dem Gedanken schlecht wird. Der Hass, der sich in mir aufgebaut hat brennt heißer, als das Feuer neben mir, das mittlerweile gefährlich nahe ist.

Liv schweigt. Dann kommt sie näher. Ich fürchte, sie würde mich wieder schlagen, doch dann…

»Nun gut, mein Engel. Soll dies das Letzte sein, an das du denken wirst, während meine Wärme dich erfüllt.«, verkündet sie.

Widerlich.

Ich lächle so liebevoll, wie es mir nur gelingt, hebe den Kopf und erwarte sie.

Liv kommt näher, öffnet leicht die Lippen und schließt die Augen. Als sie so nah ist, dass ich ihren Atem auf der Haut spüren kann, nehme ich all meinen Mut und meine Kraft zusammen und schlage so stark ich kann mit meinem Kopf gegen ihren.

Erschrocken und vor Schmerz gekrümmt, taumelt Liv rückwärts von mir weg.

»Du kleine Schlampe!«, presst sie, sich den Kopf

haltend, hervor.

Ich sehe kleine Sternchen durch das Zimmer tanzen und muss mehrmals blinzeln. Das hat gesessen. Leider auch bei mir. Ich huste, der Qualm wird immer schlimmer.

Was als Nächstes geschieht, bekomme ich nur unscharf mit. Jemand nähert sich Liv und schlägt ihr mit voller Wucht einen Gegenstand auf den Hinterkopf, woraufhin diese taumelt, Kerzen umstößt und schließlich zusammenbricht. Die Vorhänge fangen augenblicklich Feuer, ebenso die Jacken, die an der Tür des Kleiderschrankes hängen. Ich huste und keuche und als ich die Augen wieder öffne, steht mein Retter vor mir.

»Was zum Donnerwetter ist denn hier los? Geht es dir gut, Kindchen?«, fragt Elli, als sie meine Fesseln löst und ich mich im letzten Moment vor den Flammen retten kann.

»Elli!«, rufe ich freudig aus und umarme sie vor Erleichterung.

»Jaja, ist ja gut Kindchen, keine Zeit für Liebkosungen, wir müssen verschwinden!«, krächzt Elli gefasst.

Sie ist wirklich die mutigste alte Dame, die ich je

kennengelernt habe. Sie schubst mich hastig Richtung Tür, doch etwas hält mich zurück.

»Wir können sie doch nicht hier liegen lassen!«, protestiere ich mit einem Blick auf Liv.

»Gnade, wem Gnade gebührt, doch dieses Mädchen hat seine Chance verwirkt!«, protestiert Elli und drängt mich aus dem Zimmer.

Schnell entfernen wir uns aus dem brennenden Raum. Als wir im Flur ankommen, schnürt es mir die Kehle zu.

Dort auf dem Boden, völlig reglos, liegt Callum.

»Nein!«, schreie ich meinen Schmerz aus mir heraus, dann stürze ich zu ihm. Mein Magen dreht sich, ich fürchte, ich muss mich übergeben. Mit einem Mal ist es mir völlig egal, was mit Liv passiert. Soll sie doch in ihrer eigenen Hölle verbrennen!

Elli kniet sich zu uns und begutachtet Callum. Ihr faltiges Gesicht ist von tiefen Furchen geprägt.

»Er ist ohnmächtig. Schau!«, sie weist auf seinen Brustkorb, der sich sachte hebt und senkt.

In meiner Panik hatte ich das gar nicht bemerkt. Er lebt!

»Wir müssen ihn hier rausbringen!«, beschwöre ich Elli.

»Wie stellst du dir das vor, Kindchen? Glaubst du, ich werfe mir den Zwei-Meter Riesen über die Schulter?«, fragt sie mich.

»Nimm seine Arme, wir tragen ihn gemeinsam!«, schlage ich vor.

»Nimm seine Beine und halte sie hoch!«, befiehlt sie.

Ich gehorche so schnell ich kann und warte darauf, dass sie seine Arme ergreift, doch sie beugt sich zu ihm und tätschelt ihm sacht die Wangen.

»Komm schon, Jungchen, wir brauchen deine Hilfe.«, sagt sie zu ihm.

Quälend langsam vergehen die Sekunden, bis Callum blinzelnd die Augen öffnet.

»Halt die Beine weiter oben!«, befiehlt Elli.

Das Knistern des sich ausbreitenden Feuers ist nun deutlich lauter zu hören.

Callum nimmt einen tiefen Atemzug, gefolgt von einem starken Husten. Vor Erleichterung hätte ich fast losgelassen.

»Deliah?«, fragt Callum mit gebrochener Stimme.

Elli, die noch immer über ihn gebeugt ist, lächelt zufrieden.

»Ich nehme das als Kompliment, Jungchen, du alter

Charmeur!«, krächzt sie ihm entgegen.

Wir helfen ihm aufzustehen, doch der Schwindel lässt ihn am Boden kleben. Rauch umhüllt uns.

»Callum, bitte! Wir müssen hier raus! Du kannst dich draußen hinlegen!«, flehe ich ihn an.

Auf Elli und mich gestützt, schaffen wir es schließlich ihn mehr oder weniger stabil aufzurichten. So taumeln wir Schritt für Schritt zur Treppe, der dichte Qualm stets hinter uns.

Wir haben es fast geschafft, haben gerade das Geländer erreicht, da reißt uns plötzlich etwas nach hinten. Callum bricht zusammen und zieht mich mit sich auf den Boden.

Liv.

Schnell springe ich wieder auf die Beine.

Wie eine Göttin der Hölle steht sie vor uns, die Haut gerötet, die Haare teilweise abgebrannt.

Sie hat Elli gepackt und von uns weggezerrt. Elli, die völlig überrumpelt wurde, stolpert und schlägt hart auf dem Boden auf. Dann rührt sie sich nicht mehr.

»Elli!«, rufe ich erschrocken aus.

Das Gesicht zu einer hässlichen Fratze verzogen nähert Liv sich Callum und mir. Doch nicht etwa mit der

Eleganz, die ihr stets innewohnte, sondern wie eine blutverschmierte Löwin auf der Jagd stürzt sie sich auf uns.

Ich weiß nicht, wohin.

Links Callum, der sich kaum auf den Beinen halten kann, rechts die glatte Wand und hinter mir die Treppe, die sich bedrohlich nach unten schlängelt.

Mit aller Kraft versuche ich mich stabil zu positionieren, um Livs Angriff abzuwehren. Diese sprüht vor blinder Wut.

In diesem Moment, diesem Bruchteil einer Sekunde, wird mir klar, dass ich sie nicht aufhalten kann.

Mit einem lauten Schrei stürzt Liv sich auf uns.

Dann geht alles ganz schnell. Callum steht auf, packt mich um die Taille, zieht mich zur Seite und Liv stürzt ungebremst die Treppe hinunter. Poltern, Schreie, ein lautes Knacken, dann bewegt sie sich nicht mehr.

Gegen die Brüstung gestützt gibt Callum mich frei.

Ich eile so schnell wie ich kann zu Elli, die noch immer am Boden liegt. Sie hat die Augen leicht geöffnet.

»Kindchen.«

Es ist lediglich ein Flüstern.

»Elli, komm! Steh auf, wir müssen hier raus!«,

beschwöre ich sie.

Mittlerweile vernebelt der Qualm den Flur.

»Nein, Kindchen. Mein Theodor ruft mich zu sich.«, sagt sie mit einem leichten Lächeln auf den Lippen, dann schließt sie die Augen.

»Nein! Elli! Wach auf!«, rufe ich und versuche sie zu tragen.

Der schlaffe Körper macht mir Probleme, ich hebe sie an, kann mich jedoch nicht aufrichten.

Dann eben so!

Mit all meiner Kraft schleife ich Elli Richtung Treppe. Plötzlich steht Callum vor mir und nimmt sie mir ab. Sein Gesicht ist starr vor Konzentration, er sammelt seine ganze Kraft, um uns zu helfen. Er hebt Elli hoch, als wöge sie nichts und läuft vorsichtig Schritt für Schritt nach unten. Dabei bemerke ich das Blut, das sein Haar am Hinterkopf verklebt.

Wir husten und unsere Augen tränen. Hin und wieder muss ich Callum stützen, damit er nicht das Gleichgewicht verliert. Die sonst so vertrauten Stufen scheinen einen Kampf gegen uns zu führen.

Plötzlich erklingen Sirenen von draußen.

Wir sind gerade unten angekommen, da kann ich

bereits Stimmen hören. Klare Anweisungen werden gerufen. Ich öffne die Tür und werde von blauem Licht geblendet. Männer und Frauen in Uniform eilen zu uns. Einige widmen sich Liv, die reglos neben uns am Boden liegt. Zwei weiß gekleidete Personen nehmen Callum Elli ab.

Menschen reden auf mich ein, als ich aus dem Haus taumele. Ich kann sie nicht verstehen, sehe verschwommen die blauen Lichter und eine Menge, die sich um das Haus versammelt hat.

Das Letzte, was ich wahrnehme, ist ein geschockter Andy, der zu mir eilt. Dann breche ich im Hof zusammen.

Epilog

Durch die Glastüren, die links und rechts den Weg frei machen, dringt kühle Luft.

Die Sonne steht hoch am Himmel, die Blätter der Bäume beginnen sich zu verfärben. Es ist, als hätte ich eine Zeitreise gemacht. Vor dem Eingang des Krankenhauses warten Andy und Lydia bereits auf uns.

Ich habe Andy die Wahrheit erzählt. Über den Brand in jener Nacht, als seine Freundin so schwer verletzt wurde. Sie haben sich daraufhin ausgesprochen und scheinen sich nun wieder näher zu kommen. Ein verhaltenes Lächeln umspielt ihre Lippen, als ich zu ihnen nach draußen gehe.

»Da kommt ja unsere Heldin.«, begrüßt Andy mich und zieht mich in eine feste Umarmung.

»Und?«, fragt er mich erwartungsvoll.

»Er ist gleich so weit.«, antworte ich ihm.

Da erscheint, wie auf Kommando, Callum in der Tür.

Ich ergreife seine Hand, als er bei uns steht. Diese

furchtbare Nacht hat ein schier unzerstörbares Band zwischen uns gewebt, auch wenn der Schock noch tief in uns sitzt.

»Ende gut, alles gut.«, ergreift Lydia das Wort.

»Nicht ganz.«, widerspricht Callum ihr.

Betretenes Schweigen breitet sich aus.

»Hast du sie dabei?«, richtet Callum seine Frage an mich und ich nicke stumm.

»Wollen wir?«, fordert Andy uns auf.

Einstimmiges Nicken, dann machen wir uns auf den Weg.

Ich hätte nicht gedacht, dass mir das Herz auch nach der Beerdigung noch so sehr schmerzen würde, wenn ich vor dem Grab stehe.

Eleonore und Theodor Griffin.

Endlich wieder vereint, doch hinterlassen sie ein riesiges Loch in unseren Herzen.

Erneut überwältigen mich meine Tränen. Ich bin traurig, dass diese wundervolle Frau nie wieder an meiner Seite sein wird. Gleichzeitig bin ich so unendlich dankbar für jeden Tag, den ich erleben durfte.

Der Schlag auf Ellis Kopf war schlimmer, als es

zunächst aussah, doch sie musste nicht leiden.

»Deliah?«, ruft es hinter uns.

Meine Eltern sind hergekommen, um mich abzuholen. Um uns abzuholen.

Ich nicke meiner Mutter als stilles Signal zu.

Andy, Lydia und Callum legen je eine Blume auf das frische Grab. Callum versucht stark zu sein, er lässt sich nichts anmerken. Und doch weiß ich, dass er gerade zum zweiten Mal seine Mutter verloren hat. Als alle sich zum Gehen wenden, knie ich nieder, lege meine Rose neben die anderen und füge noch eine Kleinigkeit hinzu, um die Callum mich gebeten hat.

Neben vier Rosen funkelt der Zucker eines Zimtplätzchens in der Sonne.

Wir verabschieden uns von Andy und Lydia.

Andy zieht mich erneut in eine feste Umarmung.

»Kommt so schnell wie möglich wieder!«, sagt er an mich gepresst.

»Und du!«, wendet er sich an Callum, »Pass mir ja gut auf sie auf!«, warnt er ihn.

»Keine Sorge, ich werde nicht von ihrer Seite weichen.«, verspricht er.

Nachdem ich mich von Lydia verabschiedet habe,

steige ich auf die Rückbank des Autos meiner Eltern. Callum nimmt neben mir Platz.

»Na, nervös, was uns in Zukunft erwarten wird?«, frage ich ihn.

Er schüttelt den Kopf.

»Ich bin mir sicher, was auch kommen mag, wir werden es gemeinsam bewältigen.«

Ich greife nach seiner Hand, verschränke meine Finger mit seinen.

Und so fahren wir los. Hinter uns mein Vater, der mein Auto fährt und vor uns eine leuchtende Zukunft voller Möglichkeiten und Liebe.

Ich werde meinen Weg gehen!

All die Zeit, in der ich versucht habe herauszufinden, was meine Rolle in diesem Spiel ist. Und schließlich war es Callum, der mir von Anfang an sagte, was meine Aufgabe bei Eleonore Griffin war.

Ich war ihre Beschützerin.

Doch am Ende war sie es, die mich gerettet hat.

Printed in Great Britain
by Amazon